Oxford Handbook of
Sport and
Exercise
Medicine

Edited by

Domhnall MacAuley
School of Life and Health Science,
University of Ulster;
Department of Epidemiology,
The Queen's University of Belfast,
Northern Ireland

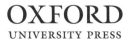

OXFORD
UNIVERSITY PRESS

617.1027
OXF

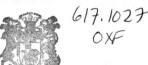

OXFORD
UNIVERSITY PRESS

Great Clarendon Street, Oxford OX2 6DP

Oxford University Press is a department of the University of Oxford.
It furthers the University's objective of excellence in research, scholarship,
and education by publishing worldwide in

Oxford New York

Auckland Cape Town Dar es Salaam Hong Kong Karachi
Kuala Lumpur Madrid Melbourne Mexico City Nairobi
New Delhi Shanghai Taipei Toronto

With offices in

Argentina Austria Brazil Chile Czech Republic France Greece
Guatemala Hungary Italy Japan Poland Portugal Singapore
South Korea Switzerland Thailand Turkey Ukraine Vietnam

Oxford is a registered trade mark of Oxford University Press
in the UK and in certain other countries

Published in the United States
by Oxford University Press Inc., New York

British Library Cataloguing in Publication Data
Data available

Library of Congress Cataloging in Publication Data
Data available

Typeset by Newgen Imaging Systems (P) Ltd., Chennai, India
Printed in Italy
on acid-free paper by
Legoprint S.p.A.

ISBN 0–19–856839–8 (flexicover: alk.paper)   978–0–19–856839–1 (flexicover: alk.paper)

10 9 8 7 6 5 4 3 2 1

Foreword

The excellent authoritative *Oxford Handbook of Sport and Exercise Medicine* is published at a singularly appropriate time. The Government has just, belatedly many think, recognized an NHS Faculty of Sport and Exercise Medicine. The new Faculty was launched at the Royal College of Physicians by HRH Princess Royal, herself an Olympic equestrian medallist now having a daughter with equal equestrian achievements.

It is fortunate that Professor Domhnall MacAuley has agreed to edit this remarkable volume. To his credit he has been one of the leaders of the campaign for the Faculty as well as advancing sports medicine practice and teaching (and is now a Senior Editor with the *BMJ*). He is to be congratulated on this book which, though rather modestly described as a handbook, is in fact a comprehensive encyclopaedia of sport and exercise medicine. Its layout and indexing make it a quickly accessible practical guide to all sports injuries both common and rare. It will be welcomed by all sports medicine practitioners, both doctors and all the others in allied professions like physiotherapy. It is a worthy successor to the *Oxford Textbook of Sports Medicine,* first published by Oxford University Press in 1994 under the editorship of Mark Harries, then physician to the British Olympic Medical Centre, with his colleagues Clyde Williams, William Stanish, and Lyle Michaeli

You may ask why official recognition of sport and exercise medicine is so important. The reason is that by its very nature sports medicine is a polymorphous animal comprising an unusually large number of disparate and loosely linked subspecialties: respiratory and cardiac physiology and medicine, physical medicine, physiotherapy, and orthopaedics to name but a few. For the past 50 years it has not been possible to create an overall umbrella body within which all can cooperate and work together. The faculty will now do just this. Though the success of joining the pantheon of 70 recognized specialties is a triumph in itself, it is only the beginning: more NHS posts are needed, more skilled A&E sports medicine trained staff. Also recognized is the inclusion of sports medicine in qualifying and advanced examinations. A significant victory has been advanced but many more battles lie ahead before sport and exercise medicine finds a proper place in British medicine.

The government may have been persuaded that this was the right moment for recognition with the realisation that in 2012 some 10,000 athletes from around the globe will converge on London for the Olympic Games. Britain can be a showcase for sports medicine as the sports men and women will need and rightly expect the highest quality of care for injuries they sustain, which inevitably occur when bodies are strained to the limit and beyond. It should never be overlooked too that prompt and effective treatment of sports injuries brings benefits to the health service as a whole by encouraging better management of comparable traumatic injuries in civilian life.

A further factor the government has recognized is that with average television viewing of nine hours a week for our children, coupled with bad diets, we face an obesity epidemic more serious than almost any country. The habit of exercise must be gained in childhood. Exercise for exercise's sake alone rarely appeals to the young. But, almost all will respond with enthusiasm to some kind of sport well taught and supervised. This is badly neglected in many schools, with playing fields sold off and sports teaching a minor part of teacher training and curriculum time. Such a programme including competitive sport needs alongside it a better sports injury service.

So, the future is bright for the *Oxford Handbook of Sport and Exercise Medicine* and for sports medicine in Britain. The success of both is fully deserved and I wish both well.

Sir Roger Bannister
October 2006

Preface

Sport medicine is fast and reactive. You need an immediate answer to most problems but you may not need the breadth of a major textbook or the detail of the specialist work. What is needed is a quick and accessible overview—and one you can easily carry around. This book is designed as your companion in everyday sport and exercise medicine. All you need in one source.

From ankles to altitude, blood doping to bursitis—everything you ever wanted to know about sport and exercise medicine—in your pocket. Arranged by systems, focused on the patient, it offers an immediate guide to all aspects of diagnosis and treatment, exercise benefits, and epidemiology.

Sports medicine is an evolving discipline. The science and research base is expanding and there are changing views on the value of many treatment modalities, the utility of preventive strategies, and the optimal exercise prescription. Clinicians are looking for evidence and patients are increasingly aware of the need for a scientific approach. This book brings together the common problems and diagnoses in sport and exercise medicine with a focused summary of the latest strategies, management plans, and evidence-based protocols.

The aim is to provide a rapid access overview of sport and exercise medicine. The objective is to produce a comprehensive text that is filled with essential information presented in a user-friendly, easily accessible format. It has all the essential information, with blank pages for the readers' own updates, local procedures, or personal notes. We set out to provide a comprehensive basic text. It is directed at the increasing numbers of students of physiotherapy, sport therapy, sports science, and exercise and rehabilitation who are searching for a suitable textbook. It is particularly relevant to post-graduate students on masters courses in sport medicine, and undergraduate medical students, many of whom undertake electives, special study modules, and intercalated degrees in sport and exercise medicine. It should also be the first line reference handbook for general practitioners with a special interest, and the foundation text for career professionals in the emerging specialty of sport and exercise medicine. It has been compiled by expert educators in the field, all of whom have been involved in teaching at undergraduate, masters, and specialist level and it has an international flavour, in keeping with worldwide development of the discipline.

Contents

Acknowledgements

Like sport, if it looks easy, it probably means thorough preparation, hard work, talent, and teamwork. If you enjoy this book, then the credit must go to the great team of people involved in putting it together. Each contributor wrote a number of sections that were moved around and finally placed together to build the chapter structure. It is essentially a huge jigsaw where some chapters have up to four authors. We had a team of reviewers who worked hard to ensure that chapters were up-to-date and comprehensive. They were excellent. We must also give credit to those pioneers of academic sport and exercise medicine who defined the boundaries of this new discipline, sought specialist recognition, formed colleges, and created the examination structure. We are only following in their wake. And thank you to the friends, partners, and families who keep the show on the road, while we follow our love of sport and exercise medicine.

Acknowledgements

Contributors

Chris Bleakley
University of Ulster,
Northern Ireland

Carolyn Broderick
University of New South Wales,
Australia

Michael Cullen
Musgrave Park Hospital, Belfast,
Northern Ireland

Bernard Donne
Trinity College, Dublin,
Ireland

Jonathan Dugas
University of Cape Town,
South Africa

Phil Glasgow
Sports Institute Northern Ireland

Peter Gregory
University of Nottingham, UK

Scott Grindel
Ferris State University,
Michigan, USA

W. Stewart Hillis
University of Glasgow, UK

Zoe Hudson
University of London, UK

Tim Jenkinson
University of Bath, UK

Paul McCrory
University of Melbourne,
Australia

John A. MacLean
The National Stadium Sports
Medicine Centre,
Glasgow, UK

Nicola Maffulli
Keele University, UK

Nick Mahony
Trinity College, Dublin,
Ireland

Niall Moyna
Dublin City University,
Ireland

Moira O Brien
Trinity College, Dublin,
Ireland

Tim Noakes
University of Cape Town,
South Africa

Mark Ridgewell
University of Wales Institute,
Cardiff, UK

Ian Shrier
McGill University,
Canada

Murali Krishna Sayana
Royal College of Surgeons in
Ireland, Ireland

Cathy Speed
Addenbrooke's Hospital,
Cambridge, UK

Simon Till
University of Sheffield, UK

Nick Webborn
University of Brighton, UK

Catherine Woods
Dublin City University, Ireland

Reviewers

Anjali Chandra

Dr Amy Jones

Dr Carys Williams

Dr Richard Walter

Dr Cathy Speed

Dr Jane Dunbar

Dr Judy Ross

Dr Chris Blakely

Symbols and abbreviations

↑	increased
↓	decreased
≈	approximately
ACE	angiotensin converting enzyme
ACL	anterior cruciate ligament
ACSM	American College of Sports Medicine
ACTH	adrenocorticotrophic hormone
ADH	antidiuretic hormone
ADP	adenosine diphosphate
AED	automated external defibrillator
AITFL	antero-inferior tibio-fibular ligament
ANCOVA	analysis of covariance
ANOVA	analysis of variance
AP	antero-posterior
APL	abductor pollicis longus
ASIS	anterior superior iliac crest
ATFL	anterior talofibular ligament
ATLS	advanced trauma life support
ATP	adenosine triphosphate
AVN	avascular necrosis
a-vO$_2$ diff	arterio venous difference in oxygen concentration
BLa	blood lactate
BMD	bone mineral density
BMI	body mass index
BMR	basal metabolic rate
CABG	coronary artery bypass graft
CDC	Center for Disease Control
CFL	calcaneofibular ligament
CHF	cardiac failure
CHO	carbohydrate
CISS	Comite International Sports des Sourds
CMC	carpo-metacarpal
CNS	central nervous system
CON	concentric
COPD	chronic obstructive pulmonary disease
CP	cerebral palsy
CP	creatine phosphate
CP-IRSA	Cerebral Palsy International Sport and Recreation Association
CPK	creatine phosphokinase
CPR	cardio-pulmonary resuscitation

CRP	C-reactive protein
CSF	cerebro-spinal fluid
CT	computer tomography
CTD	connective tissue disease
CVD	cardiovascular disease
DCO	doping control officer
DCS	diffuse cerebral swelling
DEXA	dual energy X-ray absorptiometry
DIP	distal interphalangeal
DM	diabetes mellitus
ECC	eccentric
ECG	electrocardiogram
ECRB	extensor carpi radialis brevis
ECRL	extensor carpi radialis longus
ECU	extensor carpi ulnaris
EEA	energy expenditure for activity
EIA	exercise-induced asthma
EIB	exercise-induced bronchospasm
EMG	electromyography
ENMG	electoneuromyography
EPB	extensor polaris brevis
EPO	erythropoetin
ER	external rotation
ESR	erythrocyte sedimentation rate
ET	endurance trained
EVH	eucapnic voluntary hyperpnoea
FABER	flexion abduction external rotation
FBC	full blood count
Fe CO_2	expired air carbon dioxide concentration
Fe O_2	expired air oxygen concentration
FCR	flexor carpi radialis
FCU	flexor carpi ulnaris
FDS	flexor digitorum superficialis
FH	family history
FPL	flexor policis longus
FSH	follicle stimulating hormone
GCS	Glasgow Coma Scale
GFR	glomerular filtration rate
GH	growth hormone
GnRH	gonadotrophin releasing hormone
Hb	haemoglobin
HDL	high density lipoprotein
HMB	beta-hydroxy-beta-methylbutyrate
HR	heart rate
Hct	haematocrit
HT	highly trained
IBD	inflammatory bowel disease

ICP	intracranial pressure
IGF-1	insulin-like growth factor 1
IHD	ischaemic heart disease
HIS	International Headache Society
IOC	International Olympic Committee
IR	internal rotation
ITB	ilio-tibial band
ITBFS	inio-tibial band friction syndrome
IVP	intravenous pyelogram
IZ	injury zone
LDL	low density lipoprotein
LH	luetinizing horming
LMA	laryngeal mask airway
LOC	loss of consciousness
LV	left ventricle
LVH	left ventricular hypertrophy
MANOVA	multivariate analysis of the variance
MCL	medial collateral ligament
MCS	microscopy and culture
MDI	measured dose inhaler
MPHR	maximum predicted heart rate
MRI	magnetic resonance imaging
MRSA	methicillin-resistant *Staphylococcus aureus*
MSU	mid-stream urine sample
MTPJ	metatarsophalangeal Joint
NGB	National Governing Body
NSAIDs	Non-steroidal anti-inflammatory drugs
OA	Osteoarthritis
OCD	osteochondritis dissicans
OCP	oral contraceptive pill
ORIF	Open reduction internal fixation
OTC	over-the-counter
PCL	posterior cruciate ligament
PCR	phospho-creatine (energy system)
PCS	post-concussion syndrome
PEA	pulseless electrical activity
PFJ	patello-femoral joint
Pi	inrganic phosphate
PIN	posterior interosseous nerve
PIP	proximal interpharongeal
PMH	past medical history
PNF	proprioneurofacilitation
POMS	profile of mood states
POP	plaster of Paris
PRICE	protect, rest, ice, compression, elevation
PSIS	posterior superior iliac crest
PSYM	parasympathetic

PTFL	posterior talofibular ligament
Q	cardiac output
QID	4 times a day (quarter in die)
QSART	quantitative sudomotor axon reflex tests
RCC	red cell count
RM	repetition maximum
ROM	range of movement
RR	respiratory rate
RSO	resting sweat output
RTA	road traffic accident
RV	residual volume
SAH	subarachnoid haemorrhage
SAID	specific adaptations to imposed demand
SARA	sexually acquired reactive arthritis
SCAT	Standardised Concussion Assessment Tool
SEM	sports and exercise medicine
SIJ	sacro-iliac joint
SLAP	superior labrum anterior to posterior
SLE	systemic lupus erythematosus
SLR	straight leg raise
SPECT	single photon emission computer tomography
SYM	sympathetic
SV	stroke volume
TBI	traumatic brain injury
TFCC	triangular fibrocartilage complex
TLac	lactate threshold (aerobic/anaerobic threshold)
TUE	therapeutic use exemption
UCL	ulnar collateral ligament
URTI	upper respiratory tract infection
US	ultrasound
UT	untrained
ULTT	upper limb tension test
VA	alveolar ventilation
VF	ventricular fibrillation
VE	minute ventilation
VI	visually impaired
VMO	vastus medialis obliquus
VO_2	oxygen uptake
VT	ventricular tachycardia
WADA	World Anti-Doping Agency
WCC	white cell count

Detailed contents

Immediate care

Sports first aid

- Assess the Airway, Breathing, and Circulation (ABC).
- Assess and monitor level of consciousness.
- Direct the casualty on to the appropriate agency.
- Keep within recognized first aid guidelines.
- We all have a Duty of Care (Good Samaritan) but will have a different Standard of Care, whether doctor, nurse, physio, etc.
- In children there is an additional responsibility. Contact parents immediately—you are *'locum parentis'*—responsible for their care and management. Must have written consent to 'administer' medication.

Roles and responsibilities of first aider

- *Assess*—what has occurred.
- *Protect*—self and others.
- *Identify*—nature of illness/injury.
- *Treat*—by severity and safety.
- *Transport*—remove to care.
- *Accompany*—remain with casualty.
- *Report*—to doctor or paramedic.
- *Isolate*—to prevent cross infection.
- *Secure*—valuables and clothing.
- *Inform*—family.

Recording incidents

Health & Safety Executives (HSE) have a form to record.

- Name and address of casualty
- Date and time of incident
- Details
- Witnesses
- Injury
- Treatment
- Disposal.

Include your name and contact details.

First aid facilities at venues

It is important to know the venue and the key staff including the location of the first aid room, medical help, and the particular emergency procedures for the venue. Remember when telephoning for help to give the exact location and try to meet the ambulance where possible. This is especially important at a large venue.

The Taylor Report has set criteria for safety at sports grounds with specific advice regarding doctors, ambulances etc. Depending on the expected crowd size.

Make sure that the first aid room is open and has the following:
- Telephone—with emergency contact numbers.
- Large, clean room with good lighting.
- Stretcher.
- Couch, pillows, and blankets.
- Hot & cold running water with soap and towels.
- Ice and bags.
- First aid kit.

Crisis management: the primary survey

DRS ABC

D = Danger
R = Response
S = Shout or Send for help
ABC = Assess and treat as required

Danger could include hazards such as electricity, water, and height. Remember that in a sporting situation the most common danger is the game and its participants so always:

STOP THE GAME!

For ABC see Basic Life Support.

Basic life support

Introduction

Following an initial assessment of the possible DANGER to those carrying out the resuscitation and the RESPONSE of the casualty, basic life support (BLS) comprises:

1. Airway maintenance.
2. Rescue breathing.
3. Chest compression.

BLS guidelines are for out-of-hospital, single rescuer, adult basic life support, and imply no equipment is employed—a simple airway or facemask should be used if available.

Purpose of BLS

- Maintain adequate ventilation and circulation until means can be obtained to reverse the underlying cause of the arrest.
- BLS is a 'holding operation'—on occasions, particularly when the primary pathology is respiratory failure, it may itself reverse the cause and allow full recovery.
- Failure of the circulation for three to four minutes (less if the victim is initially hypoxic) will lead to irreversible cerebral damage.
- Current 'thoracic pump' theory proposes that chest compression, by increasing intrathoracic pressure, propels blood out of the thorax, forward flow occurs because veins at the thoracic inlet collapse while the arteries remain patent.
- Even when performed optimally, chest compressions do not achieve more than 30% of the normal cerebral perfusion.
- Assessment of the carotid pulse is time-consuming and leads to an incorrect conclusion (present or absent) in up to 50% of cases. For this reason, training in detection of the carotid pulse as a sign of cardiac arrest is no longer recommended for non-healthcare persons.
- The risk to the rescuer during CPR is minimal.
- As blood oxygen remains high initially, ventilation is less important than compressions. Thus the priority is to start with compressions.
- Jaw thrust is not recommended for lay rescuers but for more experienced personnel in cases of suspected neck injury.

Guideline changes

The Resuscitation Council recently updated the BLS Guidelines to reflect the fact that an interruption in chest compressions is associated with a reduced chance of survival for the victim. The update stresses the need to maximize the chest compressions while minimizing interruptions and simplifies the skills to aid layperson resuscitation.

Two other changes are included:

1. Chest compression only resuscitation is now recommended for those unable or unwilling to perform rescue breathing.
2. The removal of the check for 'signs of circulation' in an unresponsive victim—the absence of breathing is now the main sign of cardiac arrest.

Sequence of events for BLS

- Check for danger (rescuer and victim).
- Check for response—squeeze and shout.
- If response, place casualty in the recovery position, send for help if required, and reassess regularly.
- IF NO RESPONSE:
  - Shout for help.
  - Turn casualty on his back.
  - **Open the airway**—head tilt, chin lift, and remove any visible loose objects from mouth. Leave well-fitting dentures and gum-shields.
  - If cervical spine injury suspected then use jaw lift instead of head tilt.
- **Look, listen, and feel for normal breathing** for no more than 10 seconds. If in doubt, act as if the casualty is not breathing.
  - Look for chest movement.
  - Listen at the casualty's mouth for breath sounds.
  - Feel for air on your cheek.
- If breathing, place casualty in the Recovery Position, send for help if required, and reassess regularly.
- **If not breathing**:
  - Send for help. If on your own go for help at this stage and return to continue BLS. In some circumstances it is recommended that 1 min of CPR is given before a lone rescuer goes for help. see below.
- **If the casualty is not breathing do not check for signs of circulation but proceed immediatly to commence chest compressions**.
  - Kneel by the side of the casualty.
  - Place the heel of one hand in the centre of the casualty's chest and place the heel of the other hand on top of the first. Less emphasis on exact hand placement is encouraged in the revised guidelines to prevent further time being lost prior to commencing compressions.
  - Interlock fingers of both hands, extend arms vertically above the sternum, and depress the sternum 4–5cm x 100 times each minute. Pressure should be on the centre of the sternum, not the lower sternum, ribs, or upper abdomen. Compression and release should take an equal amount of time.
- After 30 compressions open the airway again (head tilt/chin lift), pinch the soft part of the nose with thumb and index finger, take a normal breath, place your lips around the casualty's mouth ensuring a good seal, and blow steadily into the mouth watching for the casualty's chest to rise—the breath should take 1 second—this is an effective **Rescue breath**. Repeat for a second rescue breath.
- Return hands to the correct position on the sternum and give a further 30 compressions.
- Continue with chest compressions and rescue breaths in a ratio of 30:2.
- Continue until:
  - More qualified help arrives and takes over.
  - The victim shows signs of life—unlikely.
  - Exhaustion.

When to go for help

When there is more than one rescuer, then one should go for help immediately. With a single rescuer and if the casualty is an adult, then assume the cause is cardiac and go for help before commencing cardiac compressions.

It may be worthwhile performing resuscitation for one minute before going for help if:
- The cause is respiratory.
- Trauma.
- Choking.
- Drug or alcohol intoxication or poison.
- Drowning or extreme cold.
- The casualty is a child.

Two-person resuscitation

- Send one person for help as the second commences resuscitation.
- Work on opposite sides of the casualty.
- Maintain airway at all times.
- Ensure a smooth and quick transition between ventilation and compressions.

Resuscitation of children

The fear of causing harm to a child as a result of resuscitation is unfounded. For ease of teaching and retention, laypeople should be taught that the adult sequence should be used for children who are not responsive and not breathing.

The following minor modifications to the adult sequence will make it more suitable for use in children:
- Give five initial rescue breaths before starting chest compressions.
- Lone rescuers should perform CPR for one minute before going for help.
- Compress the chest by approximately 1/3 of its depth.

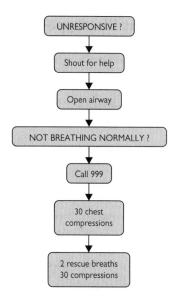

Fig. 1.1 BLS algorithm. Reproduced with permission from the Resuscitation Council (UK). *Resuscitation Council Guidelines.*

Advanced adult life support

Introduction

Heart rhythms associated with **cardiac arrest** can be divided into two groups:

- Ventricular fibrillation/pulseless ventricular tachycardia (VFVT).
- Other rhythms include asystole and pulseless electrical activity (PEA), which is also known as electromechanical dissociation (EMD).

The main difference between the two is the need for defibrillation in those with VFVT.

All other actions including chest compressions, airway management and ventilation, venous access, administration of adrenaline, and correction of contributing factors are common to both.

Where any of these contributing factors are present, resuscitation will require specific intervention to treat/reverse the cause.

Ventricular fibrillation/pulseless ventricular tachycardia

- In adults, VF is the commonest rhythm at time of arrest.
- May be preceded by a period of VT or supraventricular tachycardia (SVT).
- Best survival rates in this group—especially when shock delivered promptly.
- Survival rates decline by 7–10% for each minute that the arrhythmia persists—BLS can slow but not halt this decline.
- It is vital that patient rhythm is determined early via monitoring electrodes or defibrillator paddles.
- Start BLS if any delay in defibrillation but this should not delay shock delivery.
- **Single praecordial thump** of use only in monitored/witnessed arrest when defibrillator not immediately to hand.

Defibrillation

- Up to 3 shocks—200J (joules), 200J, and 360J—aim to deliver in less than one minute.
- Leave paddles on the chest with manual defibrillators during recharging, while observing monitor for changes in rhythm.
- Successful defibrillation is normally followed by a few seconds of true asystole—'electrical stunning'.
- Palpate carotid pulse after every shock/sequence of 3 shocks if monitor indicates a rhythm capable of providing a cardiac output.
- When a rhythm compatible with a cardiac output is restored, there may be a period of temporary impairment in myocardial contractility—known as 'myocardial stunning'—resulting in a weak impalpable pulse. Allow one minute of CPR before reassessing rhythm and further pulse check.
- Initial 200J will cause minimal myocardial damage while adequate to defibrillate most recoverable situations.
- Having restored a spontaneous circulation, if VF/pulseless VT recurs, the algorithm is applied again from the beginning, i.e. the first shock is 200J.

Chest compressions, airway, and ventilation

If ventricular fibrillation persists after the initial 3 shocks, the best chance of restoring a perfusing rhythm still lies with defibrillation, but myocardial and cerebral viability must be maintained with chest compressions and ventilation of the lungs (CPR).

- Commence 1 minute of CPR at ratio of 30 compressions to 2 ventilations.
- Consider reversible causes—see below.
- Check electrode/paddle positions, gel pads etc.
- The patient's airway should be secured:
  - Tracheal intubation is most reliable if adequate training/experience.
  - Alternatives include laryngeal mask airway (LMA).
  - Aim is to ventilate the patient's lungs and deliver the highest possible concentration of oxygen, preferably 100%.
  - Once the patient's trachea has been intubated, chest compressions, at a rate of 100/min, should continue uninterrupted (except for defibrillation or pulse checks when indicated), and ventilation should continue at approximately 12 breaths/min.
  - Chest compressions uninterrupted for ventilation result in a substantially higher mean coronary perfusion pressure.
  - LMA use should enable interrupted compressions and ventilation. If leakage is excessive revert to 30:2 ratio.

Intravenous access and drugs

- Intravenous access should be established if this has not been achieved already.
- The central veins provide the optimal route as they allow drugs to be delivered rapidly into the central circulation.
- Peripheral venous cannulation is quicker, easier to perform, and safer in inexperienced hands.
- Drugs administered by the peripheral route must be followed by a flush of at least 20ml of 0.9% saline to assist their delivery into the central circulation.
- Adrenaline (epinephrine) is administered, 1mg by the intravenous route or 2–3mg via the tracheal tube (diluted to at least 10ml with sterile water) and followed by five ventilations to disperse the drug into the peripheral bronchial tree and aid absorption.
- The role of adrenaline is to improve the efficacy of CPR—alpha-adrenergic actions cause vasoconstriction, which increases myocardial and cerebral perfusion pressure.
- The evidence supporting the use of any antiarrhythmic drugs in VF/VT is weak and no pharmacological interventions for cardiac arrest have yet been found to improve survival to hospital discharge.
- Consider amiodarone (300mg made up to 20ml with dextrose, or from a prefilled syringe) to treat shock-refractory cardiac arrest due to VF or pulseless VT.
- Lignocaine should not be given if the patient has received amiodarone but may be used as an alternative if amiodarone is not available.

- If the patient remains in VF after one minute of CPR then 3 further shocks, each at 360J (or biphasic equivalent) are administered, and the monitor is checked between each.
- Adrenaline 1mg is given every 3 minutes.
- The use of bicarbonate (50mmol) may be considered if the arterial pH is less than 7.1 and/or if the cardiac arrest is associated with a tricyclic overdose or hyperkalaemia. Where blood gas analysis is not possible, it is reasonable to consider sodium bicarbonate after 20–25 minutes, particularly if resuscitation may have been sub-optimal or delayed.

When do you stop resuscitation?

The number of times the loop is repeated during any individual resuscitation attempt is a matter of clinical judgement, having regard to the circumstances and the perceived prospect of a successful outcome. If it was considered appropriate to start resuscitation, it is usually considered worthwhile continuing as long as the patient remains in identifiable VF/VT.

Non-VF/VT rhythms

- Outcome relatively poor unless a reversible cause can be found and treated effectively.
- If apparent asystole or PEA occurs directly after delivery of a shock, the rhythm and pulse should be rechecked after just one minute of CPR and before any further drugs are given.
- If asystole or PEA is confirmed, appropriate drugs are given and a further two minutes of CPR is given to complete the loop.

Asystole

It is essential that the correct diagnosis is made and, most importantly, that VF is not missed.

Asystole must be confirmed by:
- Checking that the leads are attached correctly.
- Checking the gain.
- Viewing the rhythm through leads I and II.

If there is any doubt, treatment for VF should be started, as the risks of not treating VF, with its greater potential for a successful outcome, are greater than for three unnecessary shocks administered to an asystolic heart.

- Chest compressions and ventilation should be undertaken for three minutes within each loop (or for one minute if directly after a shock), during which the airway can be secured, intravenous access obtained, and the first dose of adrenaline given.
- Give atropine, 3mg intravenously or 6mg via the tracheal tube (in a volume of 10–20ml).
- Whenever a diagnosis of asystole is made, the ECG should be checked carefully for the presence of P waves or slow ventricular activity, because this may respond to cardiac pacing.
- CPR is continued and adrenaline is administered every three minutes.
- Any reversible or aggravating factors should be identified and treated promptly.

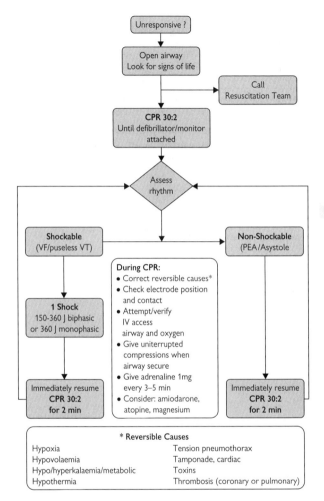

Fig. 1.2 ALS Algorithm. Reproduced with permission from the Resuscitation Council (UK). *Resuscitation Council Guidelines.*

Pulseless electrical activity

Definition: clinical signs of a cardiac arrest with an ECG rhythm compatible with a cardiac output. The patient's best chance of survival will be by prompt identification and treatment of any underlying cause.

- CPR is started immediately; the airway and ventilation managed as appropriate, and intravenous access obtained.
- Adrenaline 1mg intravenously is administered every 3 minutes.
- If PEA is associated with a bradycardia (< 60/min) atropine 3mg intravenously or 6mg via the tracheal tube should be given.

Potential causes or contributory factors

During any cardiac arrest, potential causes or aggravating factors for which specific treatment exists should be considered. For ease of memory, these are divided into two groups of four based upon their initial letter—either H or T:

The four 'Hs'
- Hypoxia.
- Hypovolaemia.
- Hyperkalaemia, hypocalcaemia, acidaemia.
- Hypothermia.

The four 'Ts'
- Tension pneumothorax.
- Cardiac tamponade.
- Toxic substances or therapeutic substances in overdose.
- Thromboembolic or mechanical obstruction (e.g., pulmonary embolus).

Automated external defibrillators

- Electrical defibrillation is well established as the only effective therapy for cardiac arrest due to VF or pulseless VT.
- The scientific evidence to support early defibrillation is overwhelming, the single most important determinant of survival being the delay from collapse to delivery of the first shock.
- The chances of successful defibrillation decline at a rate of 7–10% with each minute.
- Basic life support will help to sustain a shockable rhythm but is not a definitive treatment.

The 'chain of survival'

The chances of survival following cardiac arrest are considerably improved if appropriate steps are taken to deal with the emergency. These steps are:

- Recognition of cardiac arrest.
- Early activation of appropriate emergency services.
- Early basic life support.
- Early defibrillation.
- Early advanced life support.

Manual defibrillation has been widely available for many years, but the requirement for training in arrhythmia recognition limits the application of this technique to medical practitioners, nurses working in critical care areas, and ambulance paramedics.

Recent developments in automated external defibrillators (AEDs) have enabled increasing numbers of individuals to perform defibrillation safely and effectively.

Increased provision of early defibrillation through the widespread deployment of AEDs is now considered a realistic strategy for reducing mortality from cardiac arrest due to ischaemic heart disease.

Equipment

- AEDs must be totally reliable, simple to operate, of low weight, require little routine maintenance, and be competitively priced.
- It is recommended that AEDs are provided with a sturdy carrying pouch, which should contain spare electrodes, strong scissors, and a disposable safety razor, as well as spare electrodes.

Training

- Any individual with responsibility for the management of cardiac arrest in the hospital or community should be trained in, and authorised to perform defibrillation using an AED.

- The Resuscitation Council (UK) also recommends the provision of AEDs and training in early defibrillation for other individuals who may be called upon to provide emergency cardiac arrest management. These might include police officers, fire fighters, security personnel, airline cabin crew, and others.
- AEDs should be deployed within a medically controlled system under the direction of a medical adviser who should ensure adequate training of AED users, with periodic refresher training.
- General practitioners should be proficient in basic life support and, certainly when responding to a patient with symptoms of chest pain, should bring an AED with them. There is substantial research to show that general practitioners are capable of performing successful early defibrillation.
- There may be occasions when it is appropriate for staff other than nurses and doctors to defibrillate. These may include physiotherapists supervising cardiac rehabilitation exercise classes, and physiological measurement technicians supervising exercise tests. In the community it may be appropriate to train dental surgeons and pharmacists. These individuals should be trained in defibrillation using an AED.
- AEDs have been used successfully in the community by lay first responders, including police officers, fire fighters, security staff, airline cabin crew, and members of first aid and rescue organizations. The Resuscitation Council (UK) recommends that AEDs be made available wherever large crowds gather, for example at sports stadiums, pop concerts, theatres, cinemas, and shopping complexes.
- AED use by lay bystanders, operating outside a medically controlled system, is an attractive concept, but evidence of the safety and efficacy of this strategy is insufficient to recommend widespread lay use at this time.

Sequence of actions for AED

Basic life support skills must also be taught, assessed, and refreshed in accordance with current guidelines.
- Assess casualty.
- Check response: gently shake his shoulders and shout.
- Open airway; check for breathing: tilt head and lift chin. Give 2 effective breaths.
- Check for signs of circulation.
  For lay rescuers this means look, listen, and feel for normal breathing, coughing, or movement by the victim. Take no more than 10 seconds to do this. For health care providers this will also include checking the carotid pulse.
- If signs of circulation **are** present:
  - If breathing is present put victim into recovery position.
  - If not breathing start rescue breathing and re-check for a circulation every minute.
- If **no** signs of a circulation:
  - Start BLS if defibrillator is not immediately available.
  - Switch on defibrillator and attach the electrode pads.
  - Follow spoken/visual directions.

- Ensure that nobody touches the victim whilst the AED is analysing the rhythm.
- If a shock **is** indicated:
  - Ensure that everybody is clear of the victim.
  - Push shock button as directed.
  - Repeat 'analyse' or 'shock' as directed.
  - Do not perform pulse checks between the first 3 shocks.
- After three shocks check for signs of a circulation:
  - (a) If **no** circulation present:
  - Perform CPR for one minute.
  - After one minute stop CPR and 'analyse' rhythm (most AEDs will automatically initiate this analysis).
  - Continue the AED algorithm as directed by voice and visual prompts.
  - (b) If signs of circulation **are** present:
  - Check for breathing.
  - If breathing is present, put casualty into recovery position.
  - If no breathing, start rescue breathing and re-check circulation every minute.
- If **no** shock indicated:
  - Look for signs of circulation.
  - If no circulation present, perform CPR for one minute.
  - After one minute stop CPR and 'analyse' rhythm (most AEDs will automatically initiate this analysis).
  - Continue the AED algorithm as directed by voice and visual prompts.
  - Continue to follow AED instructions until ALS is available.

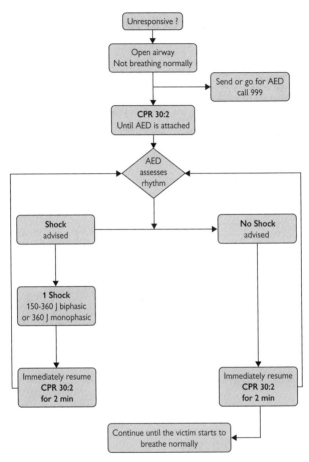

Fig. 1.3 AED algorithm. Reproduced with permission from the Resuscitation Council (UK). *Resuscitation Council Guidelines.*

Major emergencies in sport

- Bleeding and shock.
- Head injuries.
- Cervical spine injuries.
- Choking.
- The unconscious casualty.
- Severe facial injuries.
- Hypothermia, heat stroke, and altitude sickness.
- Abdominal trauma.
- Cardiac and pulmonary emergencies.
- Major limb injuries:
  - Fractures and dislocations.
  - Major ligament injuries.
- Medical emergencies:
  - Diabetes.
  - Seizures.
  - Acute asthma attack.
  - Severe allergic reaction.
  - Poisoning.

The unconscious athlete

Lack of *oxygen* or *nutrient* to the *brain*

Causes of unconsciousness:
- *Lungs*: respiratory problem, injury, or poison.
- *Heart*: lack of adequate circulation to brain.
- *Metabolism*: diabetes, drugs, alcohol, infection, too hot, too cold.
- *Brain*: lack of oxygen, head injury, epilepsy.

Management
- DRS ABC + recovery position if no C-Spine suspected.
- Look for clues as to cause.
- Treat if possible.
- Monitor casualty continuously.
- Call for help.

Monitoring the unconscious casualty

Glasgow Coma Scale most widely used worldwide but difficult for first-aider to understand and use. Simpler versions are available including AVPU:

AVPU scale

A = Alertness	Avpu = Alert
V = Verbal	aVpu = responsive to speech
P = Pain	avPu = responsive to pain
U = Unresponsive	avpU = Unresponsive

Choking

Choking is serious. It may lead to the casualty becoming unconscious, and is potentially fatal if the obstruction is not removed.

- If blockage is partial and the casualty is conscious and breathing, support the casualty and **encourage to cough**.
- If coughing does not remove the object then try carefully to remove any obvious objects from the mouth. Take care not to push anything further down the airway.
- Call 999.
- If casualty shows signs of exhaustion but is conscious, then ensure someone has called 999.
- Carry out back blows x up to 5. These are done with the heel of the hand between the scapulae.
- If the back blows fail, carry out abdominal thrusts (casualty bending forwards, both hands in clenched fist placed just below lower edge of sternum, and pull inwards and upwards).
- If the casualty becomes **unconscious** proceed to BLS.

Choking child

- Only clear superficial debris—danger of moving objects further down airway and increasing obstruction.
- Alternate abdominal thrusts with chest thrusts.

Management of shock and bleeding

Introduction

Bleeding most commonly arises as a result of trauma:

- Externally due to direct trauma—wounds, facial, and nasal injuries etc.
- Internally including head, chest, or abdominal injury, or from major fractures—particularly to the pelvis and long bones.

The major hazard of significant bleeding in sport is the development of shock.

Management of shock

Shock is defined as an inadequate perfusion of the body's vital organs.

Clinical shock is very different and much more serious that the layper-sons description of 'shock' which refers to fright or surprise.

The body will put into place compensatory mechanisms to maintain perfusion and blood pressure initially, so hypotension is **not** an early sign of shock, especially in children and healthy young adults.

Causes of shock

- Cardiogenic = pump failure.
  - Myocardial infarction/myocarditis.
  - Thoracic aortic dissection/acute valvular regurgitation.
  - Cardiac arrhythmias.
  - Cardiac depressant drug overdose.
- Hypovolaemia.
  - Blood loss—external or internal haemorrhage.
  - Other fluid loss such as diarrhoea, vomiting, burns etc.
- Anaphylaxis.
  - Food allergy especially peanuts.
  - Insect stings especially bees and wasps.
- Spinal—neurogenic shock may occur in a cervical spine injury.
- Systemic.
  - Sepsis.
  - Liver or adrenal failure.
  - Drug overdose e.g. vasodilators, paracetamol.

Management of bleeding

Initial 'First Aid' history and assessment may give clues as to the cause, e.g. bleeding wound, chest pain, bee sting etc.

If blood pressure is so low that it is unrecordable then treat as a medical emergency and call for an ambulance and any available medical assistance immediately.

- Assess danger and response.
- Assess/open airway—look for obstruction, vomit, or blood and clear if possible.
- Check breathing—classically rapid and laboured.
- Check cardiac rhythm—pulse weak and thready ? arrhythmia.

- Check skin—cold and clammy in pump failure and hypovolaemia. May be fevered in sepsis but beware peripheral shutdown in severe sepsis with cold skin.
- Check for signs of blood loss—open wound, evidence of fracture, abdominal trauma, etc.
- Check for any evidence of allergic reaction—wheeze, stridor, soft tissue swelling, etc.
- Assess conscious level.

First aid

- Danger, response, ABC and send for help.
- Give oxygen if available.
- Try to stabilize cause if possible e.g. stop bleeding.
- Lie casualty flat with head down and feet up—those with asthma or cardiac aetiology may feel uncomfortable in this position.
- Maintain temperature.
- Reassure.
- Monitor ABC and conscious level.
- Do not give anything to eat or drink.

In-hospital management includes aggressive intravenous fluid support, insertion of a central line, catheterization, assessment and treatment of the underlying condition, and investigations such as CXR, ECG, bloods (U&E, FBC, LFTs, cross match, septic screen, cardiac screen, etc).

Sports injury

Injury management

The initial management of an acute sporting injury is vital as optimal treatment will shorten the recovery time, protect the athlete from further injury, and enable the athlete to return to training and competition as soon as possible. Delayed or inappropriate treatment has the opposite effect and may adversely affect an athlete's career.

Good initial management requires on-site recognition of the injury and prompt initiation of treatment. It requires a team approach with experienced medical and physiotherapy staff working with coaches, referees, and administrators.

Sports injuries may be as a result of trauma or overuse and can involve any of the tissues of the body. The most commonly involved are muscles, ligaments, and tendons (soft tissue injury) or the bony skeleton. Some serious joint injuries may involve a combination of bone and soft tissue.

Injuries to the head and cervical spine or the thoracic and abdominal organs are potentially life threatening.

Acute injury
- Bleeding occurs with tissue damage.
- Immediate swelling and the resultant pressure on surrounding structures causes secondary effects.
- Response follows the classical inflammatory pattern—see chapter on NSAIDs for an explanation.
- Local oedema increases tissue pressure, further delays healing, and lengthens rehabilitation.
- In immediate treatment of acute injury, the objective is to interrupt this cycle, limit bleeding and swelling, reduce inflammation, and reduce the size and extent of the injury.

Overuse injuries
This type of injury leads to the same cycle of response, without local bleeding. Continued activity causes repetitive micro-trauma, tissue inflammation, and damage. The treatment of overuse injury follows the same plan.

Soft tissue inflammation
This follows the classic pattern of:
- Swelling.
- Heat.
- Erythema.
- Pain and loss of function.

The treatment plan is based on this process and cycle as described above.

General management plan for acute sports injuries

Preparation and planning
The management of sports injury requires preparation and planning. Factors include:
- Equipment and facilities.
- First aid kit and doctors bag.
- Liaison with officials, administrators, and coaches.
- Membership of 'The Medical Team' which includes a variety of health professionals.

On-site availability
On-site availability allows:
- Initiation of the appropriate management immediately.
- Direct observation of the mechanism of injury—this aids accurate diagnosis.

This, ideally, includes presence at both training and matches or competition. This helps to build trust with the coaching staff and the athletes. It also allows further input into the athlete's preparation in areas such as:
- Pre-season screening and assessment.
- Fitness assessment.
- Planning of training schedules.
- Monitoring rehabilitation, arranging surgical opinions/operations etc.

Event management
Medical input may be needed in planning of events, and may include advice on playing surface, equipment, adequate time for warm-up and rest, training facilities, and first aid equipment. Good event management will not only limit injury risk (e.g. by not playing on dangerous surfaces) but will also ensure prompt and appropriate management at the time of the injury.

Observation
This includes:
- Observation of training and warm-up etc to ensure good technique.
- Observation of exact injury mechanism will result in prompt and appropriate treatment.
- Observation of the sport so that the doctor is familiar with the rules and likely injuries which will result.

History
An appropriate history is vital to ensure correct diagnosis and treatment. In acute sports injury the athlete may be distressed by the pain or the implications of serious injury.

The exact nature and location of the pain will give a guide as to the structures injured. In achilles tendon or anterior cruciate ligament rupture, for example, the athlete may describe an audible 'pop'.

Clinical examination

Early examination, before swelling and the inflammatory response ensues, may give clues as to the diagnosis, which are more difficult to elicit at a later time. Initial pitchside assessment is usually helpful but at times it may be more appropriate to carry out a clinical examination at a better location e.g. first aid room. Protective equipment should be removed to allow full examination, unless this will worsen the injury e.g. fractured tibia.

The initial examination should:

- Establish a preliminary diagnosis.
- Determine whether the athlete can continue.
- Determine whether further treatment is required e.g. at hospital.

Treatment

- Emergency care—injuries to the head, cervical spine, and chest, and those to major joints or bones should be considered as an emergency and managed appropriately.
- Triage—this includes transport from the field and, if required, onwards to hospital for X-ray, further examination etc. Good communication with the hospital and the athlete/coach to ensure appropriate after care. Arrangements for review as soon as practical.
- Immediate injury care—if standard care is appropriate it should follow the PRICES regimen—see management of acute soft tissue injury.

Return to play

Return to training and competition is determined by:

- Return will not worsen the injury.
- Return will not increase the risk of further injury.
- The athlete will be able to perform at pre-injury level.
- The athlete's return will not place other competitors at risk.

This decision should take into account factors such as the importance of the event, time left in the event, future schedule, and playing conditions.

The medical team should observe the athlete closely on their return to ensure rehabilitation is complete and no further damage is taking place.

Judgement on return to play should be based solely on the health of the athlete and should take precedence over the wishes of the coach, relatives, club, supporters and, sometimes, the wishes of the athlete him/herself.

Management of acute soft tissue injury

The 'PRICES' mnemonic incorporates the various treatment modalities for acute soft tissue injuries:

P = Protect
R = Rest
I = Ice
C = Compression
E = Elevation
S = Support

Protect

This refers to a number of types of protection such as:
- Protect the athlete so they do not make the injury worse.
- Protect and support surrounding structures.
- Protect other competitors.
- Protection of the injured part may include crutches, splints, slings, braces, taping, strapping etc.

Rest

True rest is difficult to enforce—and in practice usually unnecessary.

Absolute rest

Severe soft tissue injuries may require a short period of bed rest or immobilisation in plaster or brace to limit movement to a minimum. Absolute rest will also be required initially after an operation.

Relative or active rest

An athlete can often maintain some activity. This will usually be part of the treatment programme and is important psychologically. Relative activity ensures:
- Maintenance of muscle strength.
- Maintenance of general cardiovascular conditioning and aerobic fitness e.g. hydrotherapy.

Exercise is a recognized part of the treatment programme for soft tissue injury. Damaged ligaments benefit from the 'stress' of weight bearing and movement. Excessive rest will prolong the inflammatory phase and lengthen the time to return to play.

Ice

The application of cold (cryotherapy) has been advocated since the classical description of inflammation by Celsus in the 1st century AD (redness, swelling, heat, and pain) to which Virchow, in 1858, added loss of function. Theoretical benefits of cryotherapy:
- Limitation of bleeding via vasoconstriction. The theory of reflex vasodilatation remains controversial.
- Limitation of swelling.
- Limitation of inflammation and further tissue damage. This may be due to the effect of histamine on vascular membranes and on neutrophils and leucocytes.
- Reduction in metabolism in local tissues. This reduces enzyme function, inhibits pain and decreases swelling and oxygen consumption.

- Assists with pain control—however, beware the athlete who becomes 'pain free' with ice and wishes to resume playing. Ice inhibits pain in 2 ways:
  - Relief of surrounding muscle spasm.
  - Slowing of sensory pain impulses.

How to apply ice

Ice comes in a variety of forms including crushed ice (better than ice cubes as the contact is better), chemical ice packs, reusable gel cold packs, and those combined with compression e.g. cryocuff.

Coolant sprays work by evaporation thus reducing skin temperature. They do not achieve sufficient depth of cooling to be effective in reducing muscle temperature.

Debate continues as to the optimum frequency and time of application. An intermittent protocol is more effective than continued application. Repeated applications of 10 minutes × 3 each day for the first 48–72 hours is usually effective.

Ice works via conduction. As adipose tissue is an excellent insulator, ice application may have to be extended in those areas with greater body fat.

Contraindications to using ice

- Broken or damaged skin.
- Where nerve damage is suspected and sensation altered.
- Altered circulation is suspected.
- When ice application increases pain.

Compression

The early use of compression will:
- Support the injured area.
- Decrease swelling.
- Ice can be combined with compression. Later, compression can be replaced by a supportive bandage or strapping. Taping is best done by an experienced sports physiotherapist to achieve maximum benefit.

Elevation

- Contributes to the reduction in blood flow and as a result, swelling.
- Must be at a significant angle i.e. greater than 45 degrees for a lower limb.
- Should be combined with support of the elevated part e.g. pillows.
- Should be maintained over the first 24 hours.

Support

Support aims to help to stabilize the injured tissue and prevent further injury. Under controlled conditions it may allow the athlete to return to competition earlier.

Support also allows an early commencement of controlled and monitored activity such as weight bearing, which will shorten the rehabilitation period and facilitate an earlier return to sport.

Care of wounds, cuts and grazes

A *wound* is defined as a 'disruption of the tissues produced by an external mechanical force'. Wounds include:
- Contusions.
- Abrasions.
- Lacerations.
- Incised and puncture wounds.

Open wounds are very common in contact sports such as football, rugby, hockey and ice hockey, American football etc. They are also common in sports where falls often occur such as cycling and riding. Wounds account for 25–30% of the workload in emergency departments.

Prognosis is dependent on the type of trauma and the extent of the damage.
- Severe bleeding and clinical shock.
- Infection.
- Complications secondary to the extent of the damage e.g. blood vessel, nerve, and tissue damage.

Abrasions

An abrasion (Latin abradere–to scrape) is a superficial injury. Damage is only to the epidermis so it should not actively bleed (though in practice abrasions may extend into the dermis). A scratch is linear, while a graze suggests a broader impact.

The cause is normally a glancing contact with a rough surface. Tangential impact produces a moving abrasion, which indicates direction by the pattern of damage to the epidermis and may leave trace material such as grit. This type is most common in sport on artificial surfaces such as astroturf.

Direct impact produces an imprint abrasion with the pattern of the causative object.

All abrasions reflect the site of impact (contrast contusions).

Contusions (bruises)

A *contusion* involves bleeding into the soft tissue due to the rupture of a small blood vessel resulting from a direct, blunt force e.g. a punch. A haematoma is a contusion where a larger amount of bleeding results in a pool of blood.

Contusions and strains comprise 60–70% of all sports injuries and are of variable severity from simple skin damage to contusions of internal organs. Most go unreported and untreated. Typically caused by blunt trauma such as a blow or a fall. Uncomplicated contusions do not breach skin surface and there is no external bleeding.

It is important to exclude other causes of bleeding including abnormalities of the clotting system in diseases such as leukaemia, thrombocytopenia, liver disease, and vitamin deficiencies (Vitamin C).

Pathology

Trauma causes rupture of capillaries and possible venules (arterial damage rare). After impact, bleeding may continue for some time due to circulatory pressure. If the volume of bleeding is sufficient, swelling occurs. If extravastrated blood collects in a pool it is known as a haematoma. Local inflammatory reaction occurs at a site with necrotic tissue, caused by macrophage infiltration.

Site of bruising does not always indicate exact site of injury, as blood will track through tissues under influence of gravity and body movement. E.g. bruising along lower border of foot in ankle ligament and thigh bruising in fractured hip.

Deeper bruising will result in a slower appearance of surface skin discolouration. Changes in colour will give an inaccurate estimate of the time of the initial impact.

Signs and symptoms
- Soreness and pain with active movement.
- Visible trauma and swelling.
- Residual function is unaffected compared to injuries such as a muscle rupture.
- Will require formal assessment before return to play.

Differential diagnosis
Soft tissue injury including muscle rupture, ligament sprain etc.

Wound healing
- Most wounds are treated by primary closure with a close approximation of the wound edges—primary intention. This may involve suturing or items such as steristrips or wound glue.
- Secondary wound healing occurs when the wound is initially left open. This may occur when there is infection or in the case of a crush injury with extensive tissue damage.
- Wound healing may also be affected by:
  - *Anatomical site*—poor over tibia.
  - *Vascular supply*—poor in peripheral vascular disease.
  - *Movement* e.g. over a joint.
  - *Wound configuration* e.g. jagged edges.
  - *Mechanism of injury*—incised wounds heal quickly.
  - *General health and nutrition of the casualty*—older patients, those on steroids etc.

Assessment of wounds

It is important to obtain an accurate history (with accurate note taking) including:
- Time of injury.
- Mechanism of injury.
- First aid treatment—if any.
- Tetanus immunization status—if any.
- Allergies or hypersensitivities (esp. tapes, dressings, etc.).
- Medication—if any.

A formal examination and assessment of the wound is then made which should include:

- Anatomical site.
- Size—width and length.
- Depth.
- Configuration—straight, jagged edge, etc.
- Tissue loss.
- Deformity.
- Loss of function including motor and/or sensory loss.
- Pain.
- Bleeding—actual and estimated.

Management

First aid

- Elevation with support.
- Direct pressure—with sterile dressing if available.
- Pressure dressing—not tourniquet.
- Apply closure strips if appropriate triage measure until hospital transfer is possible.

Cleaning

- Essential to prevent infection and remove foreign body fragments.
- Protective barrier effect of skin is broken in wounds allowing microorganisms to enter deeper tissues.
- Wounds that 'look' clean are not necessarily sterile—consider all traumatic wounds as contaminated.
- May require pain relief (including entonox) and/or anaesthetic to ensure adequate cleansing.

Which cleansing agent?

- Irrigate to remove contaminants with water—sterile if available. No evidence of increased infection with drinking-quality tap water.
- There are a variety of antiseptic solutions, which will assist wound cleansing. For an anti-bacterial action is has been suggested that 20 min contact time is required.

Wound closure

- Variety of methods are available depending on nature of wound, time since injury etc. Some wounds may be best treated by delayed closure.
  - Sutures.
  - Steristrips.
  - Staples.
  - Adhesive.

Dressings

Many now commercially available. Choice depends on factors such as:

- Nature and location of wound.
- Presence and risk of infection.
- Amount of exudates.

Tetanus

All casualties should have current tetanus status established and be immunized as per current Department of Health guidelines.

Return to sport

This will depend on a number of factors including:
- Nature of wound—size, method of closure, edges etc.
- Site of wound especially if over a joint.
- Nature of sport.

Non-steroidal anti-inflammatory drugs (NSAIDs)

As the level of competition increases and greater competitive perform-ance is required, there is a point where the 'strain' on the skeletal framework exceeds that which body can withstand, resulting in damage to connective tissues and joints.

The inflammatory response

- Enables the body's defensive and regenerative resources to be channelled into tissues which have suffered damage or are contaminated with abnormal material (eg invading microorganisms).
- The term inflammation is derived from the Latin inflammare—to set on fire. It is used to describe the pathological process that occurs at the site of tissue damage. Classical description by Celsus 1st century AD.
- Signs of inflammation are four—redness, swelling, heat, and pain. Virchow (1858) added loss of function.
- Prior to the 20th century *phagocytosis* was considered the primary movement of inflammatory reaction with specialized cells able to move 'amoeba-like' to the site of the noxious agent, to ingest and destroy foreign material such as bacteria. The importance of a vascular system was later recognized—without this there would be no redness or heat associated with the inflammatory response.
- Inflammation is a dynamic process which may, at times, cause more harm to the organism than the initiating noxious stimulus itself. Hayfever, for example, can be incapacitating but occurs as a consequence of our defence system to harmless airborne pollen.
- Not all inflammatory reactions are useful—there are no benefits from the inflammatory reactions that occur in diseases such as rheumatic fever or rheumatoid arthritis.

Vascular changes

- The immediate reaction of skin is redness due to increased bloodflow through the inflamed area. Its duration depends on the severity of the stimulus.
- Skin temperature rises and approaches that of the deep body temperature.
- The whole capillary bed at the damaged site becomes suffused with blood at an increased pressure as capillaries dilate and closed ones open up. Venules open up with increased venous flow.
- Thus two of the cardinal signs of inflammation *heat* and *redness* are caused by this increase in blood flow to the affected area.

Swelling

- Results from changes in the permeability of the blood vessel wall to protein. Normally the tissue fluid is composed of water with some low-molecular-weight solutes. The very low protein content compared to the blood is because of the impermeability of the blood vessel wall which inhibits protein movement from blood vessel to the surrounding tissues.

- Normally the vascular pressure generated from the heart forces water out of the blood at the arteriolar end, while the colloid osmotic pressure exerted by the protein in the blood draws water back at the venous end. Without the presence of the plasma protein, blood volume would rapidly diminish due to net movement of water from the blood to the tissues.

Pain

- May also be due to release of pain-inducing chemicals at the site of the reaction.
- Due in part to the increased pressure on sensory nerves caused by the accumulation of the oedematous fluid.

Mediators

- Lewis first proposed the *mediator* concept in 1927—he called this the H-substance. The first class discovered were **prostaglandins**—formed by the action of cyclo-oxygenase on arachidonic acid.
- Abundant in body—stored in granules in mast cells—found in high levels in lungs, GI system, and skin.
- Produce vasodilatation—redness and temperature and increased blood vessel permeability to protein—swelling.
- At high concentration can also produce pain.

Leucocytes in inflammation

- More persistent inflammatory reactions involve the influx of leucocytes, of which the most important in inflammation is the polymorph/neutrophil. Normal extra vascular tissue contains few polymorphs but, in inflammation, these cells pass from the blood into damaged tissue.
- Polymorphs are the first inflammatory cells to accumulate at the site of injury—they are *phagocytic* and ingest and digest invading microorganisms and tissue debris.

Acute inflammation will gradually resolve in time with no damage or, if more severe, synthesis of connective tissue to form a scar.

The inflammatory response

1. An influx of blood giving rise to the characteristic *heat* and *redness*.
2. A movement of plasma protein and associated water into the tissue, causing *swelling*.
3. An influx of phagocytic cells that have the potential to cause tissue destruction.
4. *pain*, perhaps due to pressure on the nerve endings caused by the swelling or to the effect of chemical mediators of pain being released.
5. Finally, and perhaps most importantly to the sportsman, *loss of function*—Virchow's fifth sign.

The use of anti-inflammatory drugs to treat inflammatory conditions

- Hippocrates mentions chewing of willow bark. MacLagan (1876) used an extract of willow bark called *salacin* to treat rheumatic fever. In 1899, a synthetic analogue of salacin, produced by Bayer, called *acetylsalicilic acid* was given the trade name *aspirine*.
- Now 20 or so aspirin-like drugs are available—aspirin and ibuprofen are on general sale.
- No clear evidence of any single agent being more effective than others—or indeed more effective than aspirin!

Mechanism of action
- In 1971, John Vane and his colleagues published 3 papers in *Nature* which outlined their ability to suppress the synthesis of prostaglandins. Their activity is to:
  - Reduce the symptoms of heat and redness as prostaglandin normally promotes an increased blood flow.
  - Reduce pain as there will be no hyperalgesia without prostaglandin.
  - Reduce oedema and swelling as the permeability increasing effect of chemical agents on blood vessel walls would not be subject to the normal exaggerating action of prostglandin.
- The use of NSAIDs in inflammatory conditions is well-established and they are a simple and relatively safe means of reducing the inflammatory response to injury and assist return to competitive fitness more rapidly.
- There is no unequivocal evidence that newer agents have more efficacy but less gastric side-effects.
- Advantages in the early treatment of inflammatory responses to injury, in early post-injury stage.
- Effectiveness of treatment over longer periods is less apparent. In self-limiting injuries the differences between treatment and placebo groups diminish with time.
- Early NSAIDs were all based on aspirin but now there are more than 20 individual drugs. Ibuprofen is most widely used and available for purchase over the counter.
- Newer drugs were developed to lessen the gastric side effects, and in particular GI bleeding, which is especially important in the elderly. The most recent drugs which selectively inhibited cyclo-oxygenase 2 (COX 2), appeared to have an excellent initial side-effect profile. Recent reports suggest an increased risk of cardiovascular events.

Topical NSAID agents

- Their concept is to maximize level of drug at site of injury while minimizing systemic, especially gastrointestinal, adverse effects.
- There is evidence that they achieve high levels of the active drug in the underlying tissues.
- Clinical trials demonstrate the active drug to be more effective than placebo but the differences slight.
- *British National Formulary* concludes that they '…may provide some slight relief of pain…'

Strain and sprain

A strain is a partial or complete tear of a muscle or tendon. The most commonly strained muscles are those that cross two joints during an eccentric, rather than concentric, contraction. Lower limb muscles like rectus femoris, biceps femoris, semitendinosus, adductors, hamstrings, and medial head of the gastrocnemius are more frequently injured. Muscle strain more commonly occurs at the myotendinous junction, the weakest link in the muscle. Ligament injury is very common in sports medicine. Knee, ankle, elbow, shoulder, and fingers most common joints affected.

• *Grade 1 injury:* small number of fibres damaged, resulting in some pain and swelling, with minimal loss of strength, function, or stability.
• *Grade 2 injury:* more fibres damaged, with moderate pain, swelling, and loss of function, strength, or stability.
• *Grade 3 injury:* complete tear of the tissue. May result in instability of a joint or a gap in the muscle fibres.

Diagnosis is by clinical examination. An ultrasound scan or an MR scan may be helpful.

Ligaments

Anatomy and physiology
- Ligaments are of variable shapes and sizes with fibres running parallel between two bony points of insertion. Some appear as less distinct sheets of connective tissue.
- Most are extra-articular (though cruciates are intra-articular).
- Variable blood supply—e.g. poor for cruciates, good for medial collateral of knee.
- Most research on the cruciate ligaments because of their vital role in knee stability.
- Ligament tensile strength is lost with immobility—plaster cast immobilization for 8 weeks required 9-month rehabilitation to recover tensile strength.
- Conversely there may be an increased ligament strength with a formal training programme.

Histology
- Parallel collagen fibres running in a wave pattern to allow a spring-like stretch and lengthening. This allows an adjustment of tension and reduces the risk of injury.
- At the ligament insertion into the bone there is a transition from fibrous tissue to fibro-cartilage, which becomes mineralized as it attaches to bone.

Composition
- Mainly type I collagen (some type III), elastin and proteoglycans. 65% by weight is water.
- The stiffness of the ligament increases with loading, which allows limited movement but resists excessive load.

Function of ligaments
- Maintenance of joint alignment and the gliding motion of joint surfaces. Ligament disruption will result in malalignment and subsequent early joint degeneration.
- Proprioception around the joint.
- Support the skeleton e.g. spinal ligaments.
- Maintain pressure on articular cartilage.

Classification of ligament injuries
- *Grade I*—mild sprain with no instability and a firm end-point on stressing.
- *Grade II*—moderate sprain with mild instability and softer end-point on stressing.
- *Grade III*—severe sprain with significant instability.

Mechanism of injury

Injury may occur as a result of direct trauma, or indirectly when there is a sudden mechanical stress to the joint. One of the most common ligament injuries is to the medial collateral ligament of the knee when there is a forced valgus injury. This may occur, even when the point of contact is distal, due to the long levers of the lower leg. If, for example, the sportsman is struck on the lateral side of the lower leg when the foot is fixed, the knee joint is forced medially. This tends to open up the medial side of the joint and, unfortunately, may also damage the meniscus and cruciate ligament(s).

Ligament healing

Classically ligament healing is divided into 3 phases:

Inflammatory or substrate phase

This begins immediately after the acute injury with the classical inflammatory response of bleeding, swelling, cellular infiltrate of inflammatory cells, and white blood cells with later fibroblast aggregation.

Cellular proliferation phase

From 4 days until 2–3 weeks after injury. Fibroblasts proliferate and collagen is produced. Macrophages and mast calls are abundant. A new capillary network is established.

Remodelling phase

Ongoing and probably continuous. Fibroblast infiltration and collagen production peak and diminish. Collagen scar forms which gradually remodels from the healing type III to type I collagen fibres.

Factors affecting ligament healing

The degree of injury

The injury itself is the initial stimulus for repair. Traumatically torn tissue usually disrupts the length of the ligament and incomplete tears repair more easily.

Wound stress

A topic of much debate and research. Initial protection of the site (for about 2 weeks) allows some strength to be regained. Later, however, mobilization and a degree of stress is essential if maximal repair is to be achieved.

Adequate blood supply and nutrition

Adequate blood supply is important for:
- Transport of inflammatory cells that initiate wound healing.
- Ensure optimum wound healing.
- Decrease the risk of infection.
- Improve wound healing if infection ensues.

It has also been suggested that vitamin C, protein, and cystine will facilitate tissue healing.

Prevention of ligament injury

Factors which may help to prevent or limit damage and consequently time lost from sport include:

- Understanding the risk—high-risk sports are those played at high velocity where direct trauma is more likely. These result in a higher risk of ligament injury.
- Rules of the sport—modification of the rules in contact sports may reduce the injury risk.
- Sporting environment—certain climatic conditions, such as heavy rain or ice, will alter the surface on which sport is played and thus the injury risk.
- Use of protective equipment and devices—these include both protection to prevent injury, such as protective padding, and also the use of protective braces and supports to minimize repeated injury to an already damaged, incompletely healed ligament.
- 'Prehabilitation'—while the immediate goal of training programmes is to optimize performance, it will also have the additional benefit of reducing the incidence of injury. This can be achieved by:
  - High standard of coaching and training.
  - Warm-up and stretching programmes.
  - Endurance and strength training.
  - Proprioceptive, flexibility, and agility training.
- Medical screening of the athletes—assessment of:
  - Previous injury and degree of rehabilitation achieved.
  - Excessive ligamentous laxity may be picked up on screening examination.
  - Incompetence of other supporting ligaments.
  - Poor muscle strength.
  - Other factors such as the use of alcohol or drugs may increase injury risk.
- As with all febrile illness, athletes should not return to sport until fever subsides.

Bone

The human body comprises a variety of different materials, which can be divided into 2 groups based on function.
- Active structures which produce force—muscles.
- Passive structures, which do not produce force—bones, cartilage, ligaments, and tendons.

Functions of bone

The adult human skeleton consists of 206 individual bones. These:
- Provide support.
- Act with muscles as levers to transfer force.
- Protect the internal organs.
- Metabolic—calcium storage and metabolism.

Types of bone

1. *Cortical:* (Latin meaning bark) also known as compact bone.
- Predominant in limbs—appendicular skeleton.
- Surrounds trabecular bone as a protective covering.
- Main role is to provide skeletal strength.
- 3 layers—outer periostium, middle intracortical layer and inner endostium, next to the marrow cavity.
- Contain neurovascular 'haversian canals' with capillaries and nerve fibres.
2. *Trabecular:* (Latin 'trabs' means timber). Also known as cancellous or spongy bone.
- Forms bones of axial skeleton e.g. skull, rib cage, and spine.
- Minimal part of skeletal strength.
- Major metabolic role.
- Made up of strands or trabeculae of bone whose pattern is determined by the forces applied to the bone.

Classes of bones

1. *Long bones*—hollow shaft and two extremities e.g. humerus and tibia. Found in limbs and act as levers to transmit force generated by muscles.
2. *Short bones*—cubical in shape, cortical cover, and spongy core. Include carpal and tarsal bones.
3. *Flat bones*—layers of cortical bones with spongy centre. Include sternum, skull bones, ribs, and scapula. Provide large area for tendon attachment and protective function.
4. *Irregular bones*—adapted shape for particular function. Include pubis, maxilla, and vertebrae.

Bone metabolism

Bone composition

- Bone cells—osteoclasts and osteoblasts.
- Bone matrix:
  - 40% organic—type 1 collagen, proteoglycans, and growth factors.
  - 60% inorganic—calcium hydroxyapatite.

Calcium metabolism
- Regulated by parathormone (PTH) and vitamin D.
- Recommended daily intake = 1000mg.
- Excreted by kidneys.

Bone turnover
- Balance of osteoblast and osteoclast activity.
- Affected by hormones such as oestrogen, glucocorticoids and thyroxine.
- Bone 'stress' is important.

Normal bone metabolism
- Peak bone mass in early adulthood.
- Plateau until 35–40 years.
- Rapid annual decline (1–2%/year) in women after the menopause.
- Male loss begins later (45 yrs) and at a slower rate.
- Osteoporosis is the decrease in bone mass (per unit volume). Primary osteoporosis is normally post-menopausal and is determined by reduced oestrogen. Other risk factors include:
  - Race.
  - Heredity.
  - Early menopause/hysterectomy.
  - Smoking/alcohol/drug abuse.
  - Calcium intake.

Standard investigations include measurement of bone density (DEXA scan) and calcium metabolism. Treatments include dietary measures, calcium and vit D, hormone replacement therapy and bisphosphonates. Screen for osteoporosis in those with a fracture or 2 or more risk factors.

Secondary osteoporosis can result from a variety of causes such as:
- Poor diet.
- Endocrine causes.
- Drug induced e.g. steroids.
- Chronic disease e.g. rheumatoid arthritis and chronic renal disease.
- Malignancy.

Bone biomechanics

Wolff's law (1892) stated that 'The shape of bone is determined only by the static stressing…'. While in general terms this is largely true, the effect of stress on bone is not as simple. Stress can have a variety of effects; as seen in a healing fracture or in bone atrophy. Wolff did not take into account the effect of heredity, where stress will not influence an inherited bone deformity.

When loaded, bone becomes increasingly 'stiff', thus less likely to fracture under load (spine). Fracture will occur, however, when the load exceeds the ultimate strength of the bone.

Stress fractures are clinical manifestations of bone fatigue. This occurs due to increased load repetitions which, individually, are within the normal acceptable load. Animal studies, for example, show a 5-fold increase in stress fractures from walking to jogging. The bones of the lower limb are more highly loaded and react with less strain at a given level of stress.

Fracture, which is the pathological result of load, may result from:
- Excessive force.
- Weakened bone.
- Small bone diameter.
- Excess frequency of load.
- Reduced recovery time between repeated loading.

Bone remodelling is a slow process. A gradual progression in training intensity allows bone response which prevents stress fractures.

Bone shape is optimal for a normal load pattern so that bone deformity or an excessive load both contribute to the risk of skeletal injury.

Bones in children and adolescents deform at a lower load than in adults. The bone is weaker than the attached ligaments or tendons and is thus more likely to suffer avulsion fractures.

Bone and physical activity

1. *Effect of gravity*: bone mass has a positive correlation to body mass. Astronauts suffer an increased excretion of calcium and decreased bone mineralization that is not reversed by exercise in non-weight bearing conditions.
2. *Effect of inactivity*: bed rest induces a weekly loss of bone mass with a mineral loss of up to 30%. The effects of prolonged bed rest may not be reversible.
3. *Effects of muscular activity*: muscular activity has a positive loading effect on the skeleton. Less activity and deteriorating muscle mass in the elderly increases fracture risk.
4. *Effects of physical activity*: multiple studies show a positive correlation bet bone mass and physical activity benefits at any age.
5. *The female athletic triad*: is a combination of excessive athletic activity, negative effects on bone metabolism, amenorrhoea, and eating disorder.

Sports injury in children

- Acute sports injuries occur 1.8–2.5 times more often in boys than girls.
- The highest incidence of sports injuries is in children between the ages of 5 and 15 years (twice that of the general population).
- Peak rate of injury is aged 12 years in girls and 14 years in boys.
- In contact sports, injuries occur more commonly in post-pubertal than pre-pubertal children.
- Peak fracture incidence coincides with time of peak height velocity.
- Winter sports appear more injurious than summer sports for children.

Mechanisms of injury

How children differ from adults

- Immature skeleton requires special consideration.
- Identical mechanisms of injury produce different pathologies in children when compared with adults.
- Existence of growth plates and apophyses (insertion of muscle-tendon units into immature bone) largely account for the different injury profile observed in children.
- Ligaments and tendons are stronger than bone in children.
- In children growth plate injuries and avulsion fractures are more common than ligament and tendon tears.

Osteochondroses

Pathology

- Group of conditions affecting the growing skeleton and articular cartilage.
- May be intra-articular (e.g. osteochondritis dissecans), physeal (e.g. Scheuermann's disease) or extra-articular (e.g. traction apophysitis).

Cause and prognosis

- Vary in aetiology and frequency of occurrence.
- More common in boys than girls.
- Causative factors are not fully understood.
- Stress, ischaemia, and genetics are all implicated to varying degrees.
- Differ in treatment and prognosis—some resolve spontaneously, others require surgical intervention.

Conn JM et al. (2003). Sports and recreation related injury episodes in the US population. *Inj Prev* **9**:117–123.

Traction apophysitis

Cause
Combination of growth and excessive loading of the vulnerable tendon-growth plate interface.

Treatment
- Local anti-inflammatory measures.
- Unloading the inflamed tendon-bone interface by avoiding or reducing provocative activities (usually running and jumping).
- Improving flexibility of the involved muscle-tendon unit.
- Graduated strengthening program.
- Gradual reintroduction of activity.

The specifics of these conditions will be discussed later under the region they affect.

Benefits of exercise

Benefits of exercise

The benefits of exercise can be divided into those that reduce mortality and those that reduce morbidity. Most studies are observational but there are randomized controlled trials in selected high-risk populations.

Epidemiological outcomes

- Reduces mortality in healthy, post-MI, and diabetic patients. This is also true for healthy 'weekend-warriors'.
- It is estimated that an inactive lifestyle is associated with the same risk of dying as smoking 1pk/day.
- Reduces obesity, incidence of diabetes, cancer, hypertension, osteoporosis (impact exercise), stroke, falls in the elderly, and depression.
- Improved cognition in the elderly.
- Improved self-esteem.
- Improved outcomes in pregnancy.
- Reduces absenteeism from work.

Physiological outcomes

Cardiovascular profile

- Increases collateral circulation.
- Increases response to nitric oxide.
- Improves lipid-risk profile.
- Improves lipid and carbohydrate metabolism.
- Decreases myocardial oxygen requirements in response to an absolute increase in workload (heart rate and blood pressure response is less).

Musculoskeletal profile

- Improves endurance, strength, power, and range of motion.
- Improves balance.
- Minimizes bone and muscle mass loss associated with ageing.

Miscellaneous

- Decreases lymphoedema following breast surgery.

Avoiding injuries in beginners

- Start at an obviously easy level.
- Increase gradually at about 10–20% per week. Factors included when increasing based on FITT principle:
  - Frequency (number of sessions per week).
  - Intensity (effort, e.g. speed, resistance, hills).
  - Timing (duration of exercise session).
  - Type (less of an increase if cross-training added vs more of the same exercise).
- These same principles can be used for rehabilitation following any injury.
- Begin at a level that does not cause pain and slowly increase.

Exercise in prevention

In addition to the prevention of mortality, exercise is an important primary and secondary prevention tool for injury. In many cases, specific exercise programs are targeted for specific injuries associated with a given sport.

Primary prevention

Primary prevention refers to the prevention of disease among healthy individuals.

- Tai Chi prevents falls in the healthy elderly.
- Proprioceptive training reduces anterior cruciate ligament tears in women.
- Eccentric hamstring strengthening reduces hamstring strains.
- Suggestion for cohort studies that it may help prevent cancer.
- Moderate exercise may prevent common cold (J-shaped curve effect on immunity).

Secondary prevention

Secondary prevention refers to the prevention of disease among people who already have a disease. In general, this is considered to apply to a second occurrence of the illness or injury.

Falls in the frail elderly are decreased with:

- Tai Chi.
- Weight training.
- Balance training.

Ankle sprains

- Strengthening reduces re-injury.
- Balance training reduces re-injury.

Medical

- Type II diabetes mellitus in subjects with impaired glucose tolereance.
- Obesity-related consequences.
- Reduces mortality in post-MI patients.
- Impact (e.g. jogging) or high resistance exercise prevent worsening of osteoporosis.

Tertiary prevention

Tertiary prevention refers to minimizing the worsening of the illness or injury. In the case of sport medicine, this is generally the field of rehabilitation and is beyond the scope of this chapter.

Cardiovascular disease

Cardiovascular disease is a broad term that describes a number of pathological conditions that can affect the heart and blood vessels. These conditions include angina, myocardial infarction, cerebrovascular disease, hypertension, and chronic heart failure.

Cardiovascular disease:
- Is the leading cause of death in Europe and the US.
- Kills 4 million people in Europe and 1.5 million in the EU per year.
- Causes 41% of all deaths in the EU and 48% of all deaths in Europe.
- Kills more people every year than the next five leading causes of death combined (cancer, chronic lower respiratory tract disease, accidents, diabetes mellitus, and influenza and pneumonia).
- Negatively affects individuals and their quality of life as well as being a major economic burden.

Benefits of physical activity
- Incremental levels of regular physical activity are inversely proportional to long-term cardiovascular mortality when controlled for the presence of other risk factors in both men and women.
- The relative risk for cardiovascular mortality is 6 times higher in the least fit or active compared with the most fit or active.
- Risk of death from CVD becomes progressively lower as physical activity levels increase from an expenditure of 500 to 3500kcal/wk.
- There is approximately a 25% reduction in cardiovascular mortality in men and women who expend >2000kcal/wk.
- Walking at 3.5 mph for 1 hr/week is associated with substantial reductions in the incidence of coronary events among women.
- Inactive individuals who become active have a significant reduction in cardiovascular risk compared with those who remain inactive.
- There is 24% reduction in all-cause mortality and a 25% reduction in cardiovascular mortality in patients with known CVD who undertake an exercise rehabilitation compared with control subjects.
- High levels of physical fitness, when measured with an exercise tolerance test, are associated with a significantly lower subsequent cardiovascular mortality rate among men and women.
- Benefits associated with regular physical activity are similar in magnitude to the benefits associated with maintaining blood pressure, normal glucose, normal cholesterol levels, not smoking, and maintaining an ideal body weight.

Possible biological mechanisms for the observed benefits
- Reduction of resting and exercise heart rate.
- Reduction of resting and exercise blood pressure.
- Reduction of myocardial oxygen demand at submaximal levels of physical activity.
- Increase in myocardial contractility.
- Increase in peripheral venous tone.
- Favourable changes in fibrinolytic system.
- Increased endothelium-dependent vasodilatation.

- Enhanced parasympathetic tone.
- Possible increases in coronary blood flow, coronary collateral vessels, and myocardial capillary density.
- Reduction of obesity.
- Enhanced glucose tolerance.
- Improved lipid profile.

Cancer

Cancer is a group of more than one hundred diseases characterized by uncontrolled growth and spread of abnormal cells. This can occur in the epithelial cells, blood cells, immune cells, and connective tissue.

- Cancer accounts for 25% of all deaths in the United States.
- The death rate among women suffering from lung cancer in Britain is almost double the EU average.
- Lung, breast, and colorectal are the most commonly diagnosed cancers.
- The most common causes of cancer death are lung , stomach, and liver cancer.
- Breast cancer is the most prevalent cancer worldwide.

Benefits of physical activity

- Physical activity and diet are the most important modifiable determinants of cancer risk in non-smokers.
- Protects against overall cancer risk, with a graded dose-response association in men and women.
- The amount of physical activity required to reduce various forms of cancer is approximately 4h/week of at least moderate intensity (>4–5 MET).
- Moderate intensity physical activity (>4.5 MET) is associated with a 10–70% decrease in colon/colorectal cancer and a 30% reduction in pre- and postmenopausal breast cancer.
- Reduction in risk for endometrial cancer of 20–80%.
- Prostate cancer can be reduced by up to 70% in men who expend between 1000 and 3000kcal/week.
- Moderate activity (>4–5 MET), but not light activity (<4–5 MET) reduces the risk of lung cancer independently of smoking and other possible risk factors.

Possible biological mechanisms for the observed benefits

- Improved circulation.
- Improved ventilation and perfusion.
- Shortened bowel transit time.
- Improved energy balance.
- Enhanced immune function.
- Modulates the production, metabolism, and excretion of sex hormones.

Obesity

Overweight is defined as a BMI of 25–29.9kg/m^2 and obesity is defined as a BMI above 30kg/m^2. Obesity is a risk factor for a number of chronic diseases including heart disease, type 2 diabetes, hypertension, stroke, and certain site-specific cancers.

Prevalence

- Global levels of obesity and overweight have increased dramatically in recent years.
- 39.8 million (1 in 6) US adults are affected.
- Approximately 4 in every 10 US adults are overweight.
- Up to 27% of men and 38% of women in the EU are obese.
- There has been an alarming rise in the number of children who are overweight or obese.
- Ireland has the fourth highest prevalence of obese and overweight men in the EU, and ranks seventh highest for the prevalence of obesity and overweight in women.
- Obesity rates in Ireland are growing by 1% annually.
- Obesity-related illnesses are estimated to account for as much as 7% of total healthcare costs in the EU.

Benefits of physical activity

- It is a key strategy along with diet in the primary and secondary prevention of obesity.
- Physically active men and women generally maintain a desirable body composition.
- Can result in significant decreases in visceral, subcutaneous, and total abdominal fat in obese children and adults without changes in caloric intake.
- Average weight is reduced by 1.0kg/month in response to short tem physical activity programs (≤16 weeks) that involve relatively high energy expenditures (~2200kcal/wk).
- Total body fat is reduced in a dose-response manner in response to physical activity programs of ≤16 weeks that involve an energy expenditures of ~2200kcal/wk.
- Long-term physical activity programs (≥16 weeks) that result in an energy expenditure of ~1100kcal result in an average weight loss of 0.25kg/month.
- Mortality levels are lower in obese individuals who have moderate fitness compared to obese individuals who are sedentary.
- Important role in weight loss maintenance.
- Increasing amounts of physical activity may be necessary to effectively maintain a constant body weight in individuals who were previously obese.

Possible biological mechanisms for the observed benefits

- Negative energy balance.
- Favourable alterations in body composition.
- Increased resting metabolic rate.
- Alteration in substrate utilization.
- Improved insulin sensitivity.

Overweight and obesity in children

The incidence of childhood overweight and obesity has increased greatly over the past 20 years in the Western world. The current western culture nurtures obesity.

Epidemiology

- Incidence of overweight and obesity in Australia and the UK doubled between 1985 & 1997.
- 23% Australian children and adolescents are overweight or obese[1].
- Childhood obesity (>3 years of age) is highly correlated with adult obesity[2].
- Parental obesity more than doubles the risk of adult obesity among both obese and non-obese children <10 years of age[2].
- Marked increase in incidence of type 2 diabetes in adolescents.
- Progressive decrease in physical activity after age 11[3].
- Decrease in activity in girls before boys.
- Boys are more active than girls in every age-group[3].

Possible causes

- Unstructured play time has been replaced with inactive pursuits such as watching television, playing video games, and surfing the internet.
- Dominance of the car has meant that walking and cycling are less often used as a mode of transport.
- Safety concerns regarding places where children can exercise ie. local parks and streets.
- Desire for instant meals and the subsequent prevalence of fast food outlets (providing high fat food options).
- Advertising of unhealthy food choices directed at children.

Diagnosis

- International standards now exist for the definition of overweight and obesity in childhood[4].
- BMIs at various ages for boys and girls which will pass through a BMI of 25kg/m^3 (overweight) or 30kg/m^3 (obese) have been determined. See Fig. 3.1.

Complications

- Dyslipidaemia and insulin resistance.
- Two-fold increase in risk of death from IHD over 57 years if overweight in childhood[5].
- NIDDM.
- Sleep apnoea.
- Musculoskeletal concerns eg. slipped upper capital femoral epiphysis.
- Psychological disturbances including low self esteem.

Strategies to increase exercise

- Involve the family in exercise interventions. Having both parents' support for physical activity increased participation rates of girls from 30% to 70%[6].
- Carry exercise equipment in car for impromptu stops.

Age (years)	Body mass index 25 kg/m²		Body mass index 35 kg/m²	
	Males	Females	Males	Females
2	18.41	18.02	20.09	19.81
2.5	18.13	17.76	19.80	19.55
3	17.89	17.56	19.57	19.36
3.5	17.69	17.40	19.39	19.23
4	17.55	17.28	19.29	19.15
4.5	17.47	17.19	19.26	19.12
5	17.42	17.15	19.30	19.17
5.5	17.45	17.20	19.47	19.34
6	17.55	17.34	19.78	19.65
6.5	17.71	17.53	20.23	20.08
7	17.92	17.75	20.63	20.51
7.5	18.16	18.03	21.09	21.01
8	18.44	18.35	21.60	21.57
8.5	18.76	18.69	22.17	22.18
9	19.10	19.07	22.77	22.81
9.5	19.46	19.45	23.39	23.46
10	19.84	1986	24.00	24.11
10.5	20.20	20.29	24.57	24.77
11	20.55	20.74	25.10	25.42
11.5	20.89	21.20	25.58	26.05
12	21.22	21.68	26.02	26.67
12.5	21.56	22.14	26.43	27.24
13	21.91	22.58	26.84	27.76
13.5	22.27	22.98	27.25	28.20
14	22.62	23.34	27.63	28.57
14.5	22.96	23.66	27.98	28.87
15	23.29	23.94	28.30	29.11
15.5	23.60	24.17	28.60	29.29
16	23.90	24.37	28.88	29.43
16.5	24.19	24.54	29.14	29.56
17	24.46	24.70	29.41	29.69
17.5	24.73	24.85	29.70	29.84
18	25	25	30	30

Fig 3.1 International cut off points for overweight and obesity[4]. Reproduced with permission from BMJ Publishing Group.

- Encourage habitual, daily exercise where possible. Walking to and from school or the bus-stop/train station is desirable.
- Introduce a reward system for achieving short and long term activity goals.
- Link TV viewing (or other favoured sedentary activities) to exercise in reluctant exercisers.
- Include home-based, less structured activities.

Prevention and treatment

- Long-term results of current weight loss strategies have been disappointing.
- Treatments used have included: family therapy, cognitive behavioural therapy to promote dietary change and aerobic exercise, school-based interventions, pharmacological and surgical interventions.
- Prognosis is poor if one or both parents are obese.

References

1. Booth ML *et al.* (2001). *Australian & New Zealand Journal of Public Health.* **25**(2):162–9.

2. Whitaker RC *et al.* (1997). *N Engl J Med* **337**(13): 869–873.

3. ABS Australian Bureau of Statistics.

4. Cole TJ *et al* (2000). *BMJ* **320**: 1240–3.

5. Gunnell DJ *et al.* (1998). *Am J Clin Nutr* **67**: 1111–18.

6. Davison KK *et al.* (2003). *Med. Sci. Sports Exgerc* **35**(9): 1589–95.

Hypertension

Hypertension is defined as a systolic blood pressure ≥140mmHg or a diastolic blood pressure ≥90mmHg. Individuals with a systolic BP of 120–139mmHg or a diastolic BP of 80–89mmHg are considered as being prehypertensive. Hypertension is an increasingly important medical and public health issue.

Prevalence

- Worldwide prevalence estimates for hypertension may be as high as 1 billion individuals.
- It is predicted that up to a third of the world's population will be hypertensive by the year 2025.
- Approximately 7.1 million deaths per year are attributed to hypertension.
- WHO reports that sub-optimal BP (>115mmHg SBP) is responsible for 62% of cerebrovascular disease and 49% of ischaemic heart disease among men and women.
- The prevalence of hypertension increases with advancing age—more than 50% of people aged 60 to 69 years, and approximately 75% of those aged 70 years and older are hypertensive.

Benefits of physical activity

- Inverse relation between dynamic physical training and blood pressure.
- Fitness status is inversely associated with ambulatory BP in men and women.
- Individuals with lowest fitness levels have significantly higher 24-h, daytime, and nighttime blood pressure than those in the moderate and high fitness levels.
- Average changes in blood pressure in response to at least 4weeks of dynamic aerobic training is −3.4/−2.4mmHg (SBP/DBP) in normotensives, and −7.0/6.0mmHg in hypertensive individuals.
- Changes in systolic blood pressure are related to duration of training program.
- Dynamic aerobic training between 40% and 70% VO_2max appears to result in similar reductions in systolic and diastolic blood pressure.
- The blood pressure response to dynamic aerobic training is similar for frequencies between 3–5d/wk and for session times between 30–60min.
- Net changes in SBP and DBP are similar to net weekly energy expenditure ranging from 353 to 1899 kcal/week.
- A single bout of moderate intensity exercise can lower BP in prehypertensive men and women into the normotensive range for 18–24 hours.

Possible biological mechanisms for the observed benefits
- Decrease in plasma norepinephrine (noradrenaline) levels.
- Alterations in renal function.
- Improved endothelial vasodilator function.
- Improved left ventricular diastolic filling.
- Reduced arterial stiffness .
- Decreased total and abdominal fat.
- Improved insulin sensitivity.

Diabetes

Diabetes mellitus is characterized by abnormal glucose metabolism resulting from defects in insulin release, action, or both. Type 1 diabetes is insulin-dependent and is an immune-mediated disease that selectively destroys the pancreatic cells, leading to an eventual absence of endogenous insulin production. Type 2 diabetes (type 2 DM) is non-insulin-dependent and accounts for 90% of diabetes cases. It is characterized by a reduction in insulin sensitivity in major organ systems such as muscle, liver, and adipose tissue. Complications of diabetes include heart disease and stroke, hypertension, blindness, kidney disease, nervous system disease, and complications of pregnancy.

Prevalence
- It is estimated that worldwide there are now 150 million people with diabetes, and that this number will rise to 215 million by 2012 and 300 million by 2025.
- Alarming rise in the number of children and adolescents being diagnosed with type 2 DM.
- Associated with substantial morbidity and mortality.
- The number of deaths attributed to diabetes in 2000 was estimated at 3.2 million.
- Globally, at least 1 in 10 deaths in adults aged 36–44 years is attributed to diabetes. This figure rises to 1 in 4 in some parts of the world.

Benefits of physical activity
- Associated with a substantially reduced risk for type 2 DM particularly in individuals at increased risk .
- Linear dose response relation between exercise intensity and the degree of risk reduction.
- Modest improvements in glucose control—0.5–1.0% decrease in HbA1c. There is currently not enough available data to discern whether a dose-response relation exists between exercise volume or intensity, and improvements in glucose control.
- Improvements in glucose control reduce the risk of CVD among persons with diabetes by 33–50%, and the risk of microvascular complications by approximately 33%.
- Acute exercise results in transient improvements in insulin sensitivity.
- Reduced cardiovascular complications. It is likely that many of the beneficial effects of physical activity on cardiovascular risk are related to improvements in insulin sensitivity.

Possible biological mechanisms for the observed benefits
- Improved glucose control.
- Improved insulin sensitivity.
- Decreased intra-abdominal fat.
- Improved cardiovascular function.
- Favourable changes in fibrinolytic system.
- Increased endothelium-dependent vasodilatation.
- Improved lipid profile.

Falls

Accidental injury resulting from falls is a major cause of death and immobilization.

Prevalence

- The number of falls increases progressively with age in both sexes and all racial and ethnic groups.
- Falls are the primary cause of injury, morbidity, and mortality in the elderly.
- Falls are the leading cause of injury-related visits to emergency departments in the US.
- A large number individuals over the age of 65 years die from unintentional injuries, with one out of two of these due to falls.
- Compared with children, elderly persons who fall are 10 times more likely to be hospitalized and eight times more likely to die as the result of a fall.
- More than 90% of hip fractures occur as a result of falls, with most of these fractures occurring in persons over 70 years of age.
- In older people, falls can also lead to further complications such as pneumonia and prolonged bed rest, which can have a negative impact on overall health and quality of life.
- Postmenopausal women are particularly susceptible to fractures resulting from falls.
- Gender differences exist in fall arrest—men are more likely to fall to the side or trip, and women are more likely to fall forward or slip.

Benefits of physical activity

- Maintains neuromuscular function by slowing the age related decline in cognitive performance associated with speed and information processing.
- Improves flexibility, balance, and proprioception.
- Induces beneficial effects on measures of disability, pain, and physical performance.
- Along with increasing calcium intake can assist in the prevention of bone loss and in some cases can induce an increase in bone mass.
- Enables older people to maintain high levels of functional capacity.
- Moderate progressive resistance training can significantly increase muscle strength into the ninth decade of life. Improvements in strength range from 2–132% in men and women over the age of 60 years.
- A linear dose response relation exists between the intensity of exercise and the improvements in strength.

Possible biological mechanisms for the observed benefits

- Increased dynamic and static strength.
- Improved proprioception.
- Enhanced motor unit recruitment and activation patterns.
- Increased gait velocity.
- Improved power in several joints.
- Slows the biological ageing of select neuromuscular functions.

Chronic obstructive pulmonary disease

Chronic obstructive pulmonary disease (COPD) is a category of diseases of the pulmonary system which are characterized by progressive limitation in predominantly expiratory airflow that is partially reversible by bronchodilator or anti-inflammatory therapy. The disease is normally associated with a decrease in exercise tolerance.

Prevalence
- COPD is the fourth leading cause of death worldwide, and is predicted to further increase in the coming decade.
- Smoking is the main determinant of COPD.

Benefits of physical activity
- Improve health status.
- Improve functional capacity by increasing muscle mass, muscle strength, cardiovascular endurance, and the exercise intensity corresponding to the ventilatory or lactate threshold.
- Breathing techniques and aerobic exercise training can improve the strength and endurance of the respiratory muscles. This can reduce the frequency and severity of respiratory symptoms during exercise and allow individuals to perform everyday activities.
- Improve ventilatory function by maximizing arterial O_2 saturation and CO_2 elimination.
- Reduce frequency of hospitalization.
- Attenuate the rate of disease progression.

Physical activity or exercise?

- Physical activity is an umbrella term and it refers to any musculo-skeletal movement that results in energy expenditure. This energy expenditure is more than that normally expended at rest.
- There are five main types of physical activity that are currently measured in self-report physical activity recall questionnaires. These include:
  - Occupational activity.
  - House and gardening activity.
  - Sport and free time (leisure or recreational) activity.
  - Family activity (looking after a sick relative, actively playing with children).
  - Commuting activity (walking or cycling to/from somewhere e.g. school or work).
- Exercise is planned, structured, and repetitive bodily movement done to improve or maintain one or more components of health-related physical fitness.
- The components of health related fitness are muscular endurance, flexibility, aerobic capacity, muscular strength, and body composition.
- So, what's in a word? Most people perceive the term 'exercise' negatively, the word 'workout' with work and drudgery, while the phase 'physical activity' is perceived positively.
- A sedentary individual, for example, is someone who participates in little or no physical activity.
- We all need encouragement to get active and to remain active. To help us in this we need to view physical activity as pleasurable. We need to value the 'entire' process of participation in physical activity, as well as the final 'product' or benefits we may accrue.
- Whatever your age, ability, or condition, you can benefit from being more physically active.

Health and physical activity

Health includes physical, social, and psychological components, each one of equal value. If an individual exercises purely for physical health reasons, for example to lose weight, and they pursue this to the detriment of their psychological or social health, then exercise is detrimental to health.

The shift has been from an 'exercise training—physical fitness' paradigm to include the 'physical activity health' paradigm developed recently. This shift was due to research showing reduced morbidity with an increase in moderate volume and intensity of physical activity. This evidence became known as the dose-response curve, and from this the concept of lifestyle physical activity interventions began to develop.

However, debate over the minimum volume, intensities, and frequencies of physical activity required to confer health benefits is still ongoing. Additionally, although recommendations may be appropriate for prevention of disease and health promotion, as viewed from a biomedical model of health, participation in regular physical activity can provide much more than this.

A more humanistic or biopsychosocial understanding of physical activity is one that sees physical activity as a mixture of physical, psychological, and social factors. Regular physical activity can:
- Provide a way to relax after work.
- Be a way of having fun.
- Help you to meet people.
- Be an opportunity to play.

The positive elements of physical activity such as enjoyment, learning new skills, gaining in confidence, getting to know your body better, developing your mind and body, or just having fun should not be forgotten.

An understanding of personal preferences in relation to participation in physical activity is vital if we are to encourage more people to be more active more often.

Is physical inactivity a problem?

People appear to know that regular physical activity is good for them, but they choose to remain sedentary. Two thirds of the european population have insufficient activity to meet current recommendations. However, over 90% of the population in every european country believe that physical activity has numerous health benefits. There is little variation in these beliefs by age or socio-economic status. The gap between beliefs and behaviour represents a challenge.

The top 10 Health Indicators set by the US Department of Health and Human Services in their Healthy People 2010 document are listed below. The criteria they applied for rank ordering (1 = most important) their selection included:

- Their ability to motivate action.
- Availability of data to measure progress.
- Their relevance as broad public health issues.
    - (i) Physical inactivity.
    - (ii) Overweight & obesity.
    - (iii) Tobacco use.
    - (iv) Substance abuse.
    - (v) Responsible sexual behaviour.
    - (vi) Mental health.
    - (vii) Injury and violence.
    - (viii) Environmental quality.
    - (ix) Immunization.
    - (x) Access to health care.

Inactivity is a problem, but the difficulty is in how exercise scientists, health promoters, and government or national agencies can most effectively provide interventions to increase the percentage of the population who are physically active. Unless this is achieved, all the potential health benefits from regular physical activity available to individuals, communities, and populations may remain unrealized.

Determinants of physical activity

Determinants are reasons for being active, and potential barriers to an active lifestyle.

Reasons to be active include:
- Good health.
- Reduction in stress.
- To meet people.
- Weight management.
- Fun and enjoyment.

Barriers include:
- Perceived lack of time.
- Lack of motivation.
- No perceived need.
- Fear of injury.
- Not the fit or sporty type.

It is important to understand the determinants that may increase or decrease one's likelihood of adhering to, or avoiding physical activity.

Factors, influences, or determinants, all interchangeable words, refer to variables for which there are established reproducible associations or predictive relationships, rather than cause-and-effect connections.

It is important to know the determinants of physical activity so that we can:
- Revise and improve our theoretical basis for understanding physical activity involvement or avoidance.
- Identify inactive individuals easily and allocate scarce resources accordingly e.g. rural women on low incomes.
- Design interventions that work better because they target key determinants e.g. social support, enjoyment.
- Tailor-make interventions for specific populations—what works for city boys aged 15–17 might not work for country boys aged 15–17 (population subgroups).

The determinants can be divided into three key categories. Theses are:
1. Environmental determinants.
2. Personal determinants.
3. Behavioural determinants.

1 Environmental determinants
Environmental determinants are made up of social (cultural, peers, family) and physical (man-made/natural) factors.

Social environment
The social environment includes social support provided as formal and informal encouragement, assistance, and/or information from individuals or groups. It can vary in frequency, durability, and intensity. It is provided by peers, family, friends, or relatives, essentially significant others in your life.

Physical environment

The physical environment can actively and passively influence physical activity patterns. It represents an effective vehicle for increasing physical activity, as it has the potential to influence large groups, even entire populations.

Supportive physical environments possess features such as parks, cycling trails, and footpaths and are conducive to physical activity. Restrictive physical environments lack such relevant features and actively discourage physical activity.

2 Personal determinants

Personal determinants are made up of cognitive/personality, demographic, and biological factors.

Cognitive/personality

- People who don't enjoy exercise don't do it: 'I hate the gym, and therefore don't go'. Enjoyment is a positive determinant of physical activity.
- People who don't identify with exercise don't do it: 'I'm not the sporty type'.
- Behavioural intention, attitudes, beliefs, knowledge, values, perceived competence, and self-efficacy—are all highly associated with physical activity.
- High levels of self motivation are also highly correlated with adherence to physical activity. For example, when self-motivation was combined with %body fat, over 80% of subjects were correctly predicted as either an adherer or a drop-out.
- Individuals who are highly self motivated are thought to be very effective at goal setting, monitoring and rewarding progress, and adjusting their exercise programme to their needs and abilities. These skills are learned through experience, but can also be taught to an individual.

Demographic

- Higher income, and more education implies you are more likely to be physically active.
- 65% of individuals earning less than 15K annually are inactive, as compared to 48% of those earning 50K or more.
- 72% of individuals who have not completed secondary school education are inactive, as compared to 50% of those who have been university educated.

Biological

- Gender: boys are more active than girls.
- Age: activity levels decline with age.
- BMI: adolescent girls with higher BMI are much less likely to exercise.

3 Behavioural determinants

- Previous sport participation (recent participation is more predictive than childhood involvement).
- Past involvement in structured exericse programme is the best predictor of current participation: 'once I was in the programme I knew what it it took to stay active'.
- High-intensity exercise is more stressful on the system than moderate-or low-intensity exercise. It is predictive of drop out for sedentary or unfit individuals and is linked to negative mood states.
- An exercise leader who is knowledgeable, likeable, and provides positive feedback regularly is more likely to encourage exercise adherence.
- Group exercise sessions can lead to increased social support and enjoyment, they provide an opportunity to compare progress, and tend to enhance commitment to the exercise programme as the individual becomes affiliated to the group. They are more likely to increase adherence than individual sessions.

Caution

The relationship between the determinant and physical activity is not always clear.

- Higher exercise self-efficacy is more likely to lead to exercise involvement.

But

- Increased fitness due to exercise involvement can increase exercise self-efficacy.

Determinants of physical activity are not isolated variables. They influence, and are influenced by each other in terms of exercise.

Understanding behaviour change

Change is a dynamic process that occurs over time. As an individual changes their behaviour they progress through a series of five stages of change. Each stage of change has two components—one is behaviour, the second is intention or readiness to change.

Very few individuals are physically unable to take part in moderate or light physical activity. Many, however, are not psychologically ready to take on the challenges of changing their lifestyle to accommodate physical activity.

There are five stages of exercise behaviour change. These are:
• Pre-contemplation (sedentary individuals who have no intention of changing).
• Contemplation (sedentary individuals and 6-month intention to change).
• Preparation (irregularly active and 30-day intention to become more regularly active).
• Action (regular physical activity for the last 6 months).
• Maintenance (regularly physically active for longer than 6 months).

In order to 'stage' an individual you must know their exercise behaviour and their behavioural intention.

Ensure you define regular physical activity using the American College of Sports and Medicine (ACSM) (1998) guidelines of the minimum requirements for disease prevention and health promotion. This incorporates both the moderate accumulative message and the continuous fitness message, and is worded to include frequency, intensity, time, and type of activity.
• *Frequency*: most, preferably all days of the week.
• *Intensity*: moderate or above (e.g. brisk walking).
• *Time*: accumulating 30 minutes or more per day.
• *Type*: any aerobic activity that is preferred by the individual.

To develop and maintain aerobic fitness the continuous message recommends continuous aerobic activity 3–5 days per week, for a minimum of 20 minutes per session, of at least a moderate intensity (60–90% of maximum heart rate).

An individual can be staged into one of the following five categories:
I currently…
• Do not exercise, and do not intend to start exercising in the next 6 months.
• Do not exercise, but am thinking about starting to exercise in the next 6 months.
• Exercise sometimes, but not regularly*. I intend to exercise regularly in the next 30 days.
• Exercise regularly, but have only begun doing so within the last 6 months.
• Exercise regularly, and have done so for longer than 6 months.

*Regular exericse = enough to meet the current ACSM recommendations.

The time taken to progress through the stages of change is variable, the 'set of tasks' which have to be accomplished at each stage are less variable.

Pre-contemplation

- There is no intention to become active in the foreseeable future. Many individuals in this stage are unaware of their problem (physical inactivity). Resistance to recognize the problem is the hallmark of precontemplators.
- Pre-contemplators need to acknowledge or take ownership of the problem, increase awareness of the negative aspects of the problem, and accurately evaluate self-regulation capacities.

Contemplation

- Serious consideration of problem resolution is central. Individuals need to convince themselves to begin to take action, otherwise contemplative behaviour becomes a habit.
- Contemplators need to take a firm decision to initiate physical activity, and engage in preliminary action to move to the next stage.

Preparation

- Individuals intend to take action immediately and have initiated small changes in their behaviour.
- Preparers need to set goals and priorities towards action. They are often already engaged in processes which would increase self-regulation and initiate behaviour change.

Action

- Individuals modify their behaviour, experiences and/or environment in order to meet the minimum levels of physical activity required for leading an active lifestyle.
- Actioners have to develop effective strategies to prevent lapses or slips from becoming a complete return to sedentary behaviours.

Maintenance

- Individuals work to prevent relapse and consolidate gains attained during action. This is not a static stage, rather a continuation of change. Being able to remain free of the chronic problem (inactivity) and/or to consistently engage in a new incompatible behaviour (i.e. sustained or regular participation in physical activity) for more than 6 months are the criterion for maintenance.
- Maintainers require sustained behavioural change for periods of time from 6 months up to 3 or more years after the initial action.

Progression through these stages was originally conceived as linear, as individuals were thought to progress from one stage to another in a simple discrete fashion. A linear progression—though possible—is extremely rare, especially in some chronic disorders. The model has now evolved to a spiral pattern.

In this pattern of change, each stage can be both stable and dynamic depending on the individual concerned. Individuals, for example, are thought to progress through the stages of change at different rates with some becoming stuck at certain stages, and others relapsing and sliding back to earlier stages.

Those that relapse may recycle into the model or alternatively, for a variety of reasons e.g. guilt, embarrassment, may return to precontemplation. Research shows that many relapsers return to the contemplation or preparation stage. Each time they recycle through the stages, they potentially learn from their mistakes and can try something different the next time around.

Clinical and community interventions to promote and support physical activity

Effective physical activity interventions should be systematically designed and evaluated.

Set an overall goal. Examples of outcomes generally include:
- Improvements in physical activity behaviour (e.g. increased time spent walking).
- Increases in selected fitness measures (e.g. increased aerobic capacity or other components of health-related fitness e.g. muscular strength and endurance).
- Decrease in sedentary behaviour (e.g. number of hours spent watching TV).

Set specific objectives, linked to your goal, based on the SMARTER principles (Specific, Measurable, Accepted, Realistic, Time bound, Enjoyable, Recorded).

Frameworks

Emphasis on individualism and lack of attention to the social and environmental factors that impinge on health, could in fact, increase rather than reduce the health gap in society.

King (1994)[1] provided an excellent framework for thinking about different interventions which aim to increase physical activity in the general population. There are four levels presented within this framework:
1. Personal.
2. Interpersonal.
3. Organizational or environmental.
4. Legislation or policy.

Level 1: personal approaches

The focus of level one is on individual change. Information is delivered through a variety of sources.

Face-to-face, one-on-one consultations offer intensive, individualized attention by a trained professional, and the opportunity for clients' behavioural prescriptions to be tailored to fit their needs. Office-based exercise consultations are an example of this type of intervention. A physician, exercise scientist, or health promotion professional generally conducts them. They have been shown to be very effective for clinical populations.

Mediated approaches include electronic (tv, radio, video) and/or print media (booklets, self-help kits, newspaper articles, newsletters). They provide advice and support to individuals on how to initiate, adhere to, and maintain an active lifestyle. They, similar to a consultation, target key strategies to support and assist individual behaviour change. They are very useful for those who cannot engage in face-to-face consultation.

Telephone plus mediated approaches are a combination. They include supervized home-based programmes. They allow greater flexibility and convenience in choosing time, location, and setting for the consultation, they are more cost effective, yet still provide support from a trained professional for encouragement, advice, and motivation to enhance physical activity levels.

The key ingredients for level one interventions are:
- Target the known determinants (e.g. benefits versus barriers, self-efficacy, exercise enjoyment and choice).
- Explore behavioural change strategies to effect change in these determinants (e.g. goal setting, personal monitoring).
- Teach problem-solving for maintenance of physical activity and to avoid relapse into sedentary behaviours.

Advantages
- Individualized advice.
- Face-to-face feedback.
- Professional support.
- Learn specific problem-solving skills.
- Learn relapse prevention.

Disadvantages
- Select few.
- Staff intensive.
- Expensive.
- Limited impact.
- Volunteer sample.
- Long-term effects are unknown.

Level 2: interpersonal approaches

Interpersonal approaches use social forces to produce change. They are the most popular format for delivering exercise programmes in clinical settings e.g. cardiac rehabilitation exercise programmes.

They are concerned with how leaders, teachers, and programme providers can create the most appropriate intra- and interpersonal climates, including various exercise choices, to encourage groups of people to increase or maintain activity.

They are primarily focused on the individual within the group setting. However, in order to be successful the emphasis should be on the how to build, strengthen, and maintain social networks that support and promote initiation and maintenance of physical activity.

The key ingredients include:
- Enhanced feelings of group affiliation.
- Public support systems.
- Group problem-solving.

Support from peers, family, friends, teachers, coaches, instructors, or co-workers are the hallmark of interpersonal interventions.

Advantages
- Large expert-to-client ratio.
- More cost-effective.
- Visual modelling.
- On-site supervision.
- Set location/time/structure.
- Face-to-face encouragement by instructor.
- Group affiliation and support.
- Group problem-solving.

Disadvantages
- Inconvenient.
- Limited variety of activities.
- Expensive.
- Normative rather than individual advice.
- Social costs such as embarrassment at exercising in front of others.
- Need to recruit participants continually.
- Challenge of being a new exerciser in an established group.
- Group leader effect.

Examples
- Structured exercise groups/classes.
- Physical education classes.
- Classroom-based education focusing on information and development of skills, and reducing sedentary behaviours.
- Family-based social support:
  - Family record-keeping of amount of physical activity undertaken by family members.
  - Family-oriented special events.
- Community-based social support:
  - Buddy systems.
  - Peer-led systems.

Level 3: organizational or environmental approaches

The organizational or environmental level of the framework is focused on how communities and organizations, such as workplaces and schools, can change aspects of their setting or environment in order to promote physical activity. It includes personal and interpersonal levels, but adds approaches focused on organizational and environmental change.

The key ingredients include:
- Physical and organizational structures rather than the individual.
- Influence organisational rules/policies.
- Increase availability of facilities for physical activity.
- Remove or minimize organisational or environmental barriers to undertaking physical activity.

Advantages
- Accessible and diverse population base.
- Convenience.
- Potential of group support.
- Systematic and organised format for promoting physical activity.

Disadvantages
- Short-term effects.
- Lack of a public health focus.

Examples
- Enhanced access to places for physical activity, combined with informational activities.
- Enhanced access to physical activity where we work, play, learn, and live. Workplaces, schools, day-care and residential care centres for older adults, hospitals, and places of worship are all community-based settings for exercise programmes.
- Re-evaluation of physical environment for physical activity.
- Point-of-decision prompts to encourage people to use the stairs rather than the lifts.
- Traffic planning to reduce the amount of traffic congestion.
- Provision of cycle paths, foot paths, speed control measures, and adequate lighting.
- Safe routes to schools initiatives.
- Specific community initiatives such as family activity days, fun-runs, charity walks.
- Mass-media approaches combined with community based initiatives.

Level 4: legislation or policy approaches
This level focuses on societal change. Its idea is to develop passive prevention strategies, ones that do not require action on the part of the individual in order to be effective. Physical activity is a participation behaviour and not a product (like alcohol or cigarettes), this makes it more difficult to develop passive prevention strategies. The key ingredients include:
- Policies to enhance physical activity participation.
- Legislative interventions that mandate changes to encourage and facilitate participation in physical activity, and/or remove barriers that restrict individual and community involvement.
- Institutionalization of programmes and strategies to affect change.

Examples
- Active transit policies that ensure people have a choice of, and access to, safe, clean, and adequately maintained cycling and pedestrian pathways.
- Policies that reinforce and support use of active transport modes (walking and cycling) over inactive modes.
- Urban planning approaches: zoning and land use, street and living design to promote activity.
- Policies for flexi-time to promote activity at work.
- Standard minimum qualifications/facilities and curriculum for physical education in schools.
- Standard qualifications for exercise specialists, for example the National Quality Assurance Framework for GP exercise referral schemes.
- Countryside access which provides legal entitlement to the general public to use the countryside for recreation.

- Making the provision of recreation facilities a legal requirement for local councils, and providing monetary incentives for adequate public facilities for physical activity.
- Strategic documents which influence practice, such as the 'Let's Make Scotland More Active: A strategy for physical activity' http://www.scotland.gov.uk/Topics/Health/NHS-Scotland/show

Our Vision is that:

People in Scotland will enjoy the benefits of having a physically active life.

Unfortunately we know very little about the effectiveness of level four interventions. There is an increasing body of evidence to support policies that promote and support active transit, and those that influence the involvement in utilitarian physical activity e.g. street and living design to enhance physical activity. However, we do not know what policies will be most influential. More research is needed.

Summary
- Levels 1 and 2 suggest that short term increases in physical activity are relatively easy to achieve if people are ready to change; long term adherence remains the challenge.
- Levels 3 and 4 perhaps offer best public health strategy (reach the most).
- Each level has major influence for increasing the effectiveness of an intervention.

The strongest intervention strategy is likely to include a multi-level approach. Using a combination of powerful personal strategies such as social support or self-efficacy in a community-wide initiative has the potential for substantial impact and change in physical activity behaviour.

The way forward
- Establish a comprehensive baseline of patterns of physical activity.
- Set realistic physical activity goals, objectives, and outcomes.
- Within key settings identify your partnerships for intervention—local government, private and public sectors, agencies—those focused on health, exercise, recreation, transport, schools, worksites,and political/legislative aspects of community.
- Guided by relevant exercise theories that explain the determinants of physical activity e.g. transtheoretical model of behaviour change.
- Be aware of the different levels of intervention required to get a population more physically active. Aim for a multi-level approach where appropriate.

Reference
King, A.C. (1994). Clinical and community interventions to promote and support physical activity participation. In R. K. Dishman (Ed.), *Advances in Exercise Adherence*. (pp. 183–212). Champaign, IL: Human Kinetics.

Epidemiology

Epidemiology is the study of research methodology in humans. Clinical epidemiology is the application of these methods in research studies.

Experimental studies

- Researcher allocates treatment of interest (exposure) to one group, and a comparison treatment (control) to another group.
- Studies can also test several interventions at once.
- The allocation of individuals to a treatment or control group can be randomized or non-randomized.

Randomization

- Randomization should ensure that neither the researcher nor the subject influences the group assignment for the subject.
- Often uses 2 different size blocks. If only blocks of 4 are used, researcher would know which group the 4th person would be assigned to.

Blinding

- Knowing that one is in the exposure group vs. control group may affect their response.
- The outcome evaluator should be blinded because most outcomes include a subjective component (e.g. ST depression on the EKG).
- In rehabilitation therapy, patient blinding is often not possible. One can sometimes (ethically) blind the patient to the study purpose.

Observational studies

- Exposure is not controlled by researcher (e.g. evaluating a new surgery) or subject (e.g. smoking).
- Several types of studies:
  - *Prospective cohort:* start with exposed and control groups and follow over time. Pro: good quality data. Con: requires time.
  - *Historical cohort:* use databases or chart reviews to determine exposed and control groups in past. Determine outcome today. Pro: immediate answer. Con: important data may be missing.
  - *Case-control:* categorize individuals as having the outcome or not. Then examine if they were exposed to the intervention or not. Pro: cost-efficient for rare disease. Con: difficult to choose appropriate controls, important data may be missing.
  - *Cross-sectional:* evaluate outcome and exposure of individuals at any one point in time. Pro: easy to obtain data. Con: unknown if exposure occurred before or after the outcome.
- The term prospective means that exposure and outcome data are obtained as they occur.
- The term retrospective means that the data was recorded in the past and the researcher is retrieving the data.
- Cohort and cross-sectional studies can be prospective or retrospective.
- Case-control studies are only retrospective.

Measuring outcomes in sports injuries

The type of outcome determines how data is analyzed. Outcomes are categorical (e.g. yes/no, mild/moderate/severe) or continuous (scale of 1–100).

Categorical outcomes

We are often interested in the risk of outcome (e.g. injury, re-injury). This is often measured as proportion of subjects injured (e.g. 10/20). The risk may be under- or overestimated when:
- Exposure is different for different individuals (e.g. one athlete plays 40min/game, another 2min/game).
- Follow-up is different between subjects (e.g. some subjects followed for 5 years post-surgery, others 2 years post-surgery).

Many studies examine person–time outcomes (e.g. 10 injuries/1000 hours playing). This assumes that following 100 people for 1000 hours is the same as 1000 people for 100 hrs. This is not true when risk varies over time, and the assumption should be checked for each study.

Survival analysis accounts for individual differences in follow-up and incorporates all the data on individuals during the time they are followed. Cox regression is used to adjust for potential confounders.

Sometimes we are interested in the severity of the outcome rather than if it occurred or not. The analysis is a little more complicated but in principle, one simply compares the risk between each category (e.g. severely injured, mildly injured, and not injured).

Continuous outcomes

Some outcomes are measured on a continuous scale (anterior-posterior displacement following anterior cruciate ligament repair).

It is important that one knows the error associated with any measure. There are many ways to assess this, but in general, it is done through comparing the results of testing the same individual multiple times:
- Single tester is intra-rater reliability.
- Multiple testers is inter-rater reliability.
- Inter-rater reliability is always less than intra-rater reliability.

The usual measures include standard deviation of differences, regression co-efficients, intra-class correlation, and others. Each provides different information and is appropriate under certain conditions.

Usual analyses include the following. Each item on the list is a specific situation of the item below it, i.e. the paired t-test is a special situation of the unpaired t-test, ANOVA, and multiple regression.
- *Paired t-test*: two groups, matched subjects.
- *Unpaired t-test*: two groups, subjects not matched.
- *ANOVA*: more than 1 comparison (>2 groups, 2 groups pre-post).
- *ANCOVA*: similar to ANOVA, but can adjust for other variables.
- *Multiple Regression*: include many exposures, adjust for confounders. More robust to missing data than ANCOVA.

When outcomes are highly correlated with each other, MANOVA is the analysis of choice.

Physiotherapy and rehabilitation

Stretching

Many people confuse stretching, flexibility, and mobility. Stretching is an intervention, flexibility is the limits of range of motion (ROM) due to muscle-tendon, and mobility is the limits of ROM due to capsule-ligaments. The effects of stretching depend on whether one is trying to affect the muscle-tendon, or the capsule-ligament. This topic focuses only on muscle-tendon.

Pre-activity stretching

- ROM is increased. Increases in ROM are superior if warm-up is done prior to stretching.
- The increase in ROM is partly due to decreased stiffness of the tissue, and partly due to a decrease in the sensation of pain associated with the stretch.
- A single bout of stretching decreases the strength of tissue in animal studies in the immediate post-stretch period.
- The results below are unchanged whether or not warm-up is done prior to stretching:
  - Decreases tests of performance for strength and jump height in every study (over 20). Running speed changes are conflicting across different studies but different methodologies prevent definitive conclusions.
  - No effect on overall injury rate when performed regularly.
    —Some authors suggest the risk for some injuries are reduced with stretching before exercise. If so, then other injuries must be increased as the total number of injuries is unchanged.

Daily stretching (not pre-activity)

- ROM is increased with daily stretching.
- The results below are unchanged whether or not warm-up is done prior to stretching:
  - Daily stretching increases strength of tissue in animal studies.
  - Three studies have shown an approximate 20% reduction in injuries with daily stretching, but 2 of these had small sample sizes and did not achieve statistical significance.
  - Tests of performance for strength, jump height, and running speed are improved with daily stretching.

Additional comments

If daily stretching outside periods of exercise is protective against injury, but stretching immediately prior to activity is not associated with a reduction in injuries, it must mean that stretching immediately prior to activity removes the protective effect of daily stretching, i.e. it is harmful. However, because the overall effect of importance to the subject is whether the risk is increased when they stretch vs. when they don't stretch, this is only an academic point.

Balance and proprioception

Over the last 40 years, we have recognized that balance and proprioception are important in the prevention and rehabilitation of injuries.

Definitions
- *Balance*: ability to maintain a given posture.
- *Proprioception:* (used interchangeably with kinaesthesia): control of movement and posture. There are 4 contributing sensations:
  - Limb position and movement.
  - Muscle effort, tension, heaviness, and stiffness.
  - Timing muscle contractions.
  - Body posture and size representation across more than one joint.

Many different physiological processes contribute to proprioception. These include afferent nerve fibres from:
- *Musculoskeletal*: muscle spindles, tendon organs, joints (ligaments, disks, and menisci).
- *Other*: cutaneous, pain fibers.

Biomechanics
The body sways to-and-fro in all directions. When the body's centre of pressure is not immediately over its centre of mass, the body moves. Resting muscle tone provides stiffness that prevents some motion. Muscles dynamically contract to restore position following perturbations.

Clinical research
Patient relevant outcomes include:
- Falls, and/or fall causing injury.
- Fear of falling: someone with poor balance may alter behaviour to avoid falls. This can have a dramatic impact on quality of life.

Role for primary prevention
Exercises designed to improve proprioception have been successful in the primary prevention of:
- Falls in the elderly.
- Anterior cruciate ligament tears in girls.
- In a recent study, proprioceptive exercises for the ankle reduced ankle injuries by 20% but the results were not statistically significant.

Role for secondary prevention
Many studies show proprioceptive exercises are effective in reducing re-injury rate following an ankle sprain. They may also be effective following anterior cruciate ligament reconstruction.

Other benefits
Proprioceptive exercises are effective in the elderly, frail elderly, those with Parkinson's disease, and patients post hip fracture. Despite the lack of research on other musculoskeletal topics, the basic science and theoretical evidence suggest that it is a promising intervention with very low risk.

Plyometrics

Purpose

Plyometrics train power. Power is the ability to generate force in a very short period of time (e.g. jumping, sprinting). One study suggested that plyometrics are used by 90% of USA Division I strength and conditioning coaches and another suggested they are used by 94% of National Football League coaches.

Definition

Plyometrics is a very specific type of exercise. Some basic terms:
- *Concentric exercise*: the muscle shortens as it generates force.
- *Eccentric exercise*: the muscle lengthens as it generates force because it is unable to overcome a greater force being applied to it.

Plyometrics refers to any exercise where the muscle goes through an eccentric contraction-concentric contraction cycle repeatedly at a fast rate. In physiological studies, it is also called the stretch-shortening cycle, but those studies often limit themselves to one cycle—plyometrics requires repetitions.

Plyometric examples
- Jumping up and down.
- Push-ups and clap hands when body is high.

Theoretical reasoning

- Plyometrics is based on the SAID principle. (Specific Adaptations to Imposed Demand).
- If one trains strength, strength is increased, but there are very small gains in power and endurance. Weightlifters are not marathon runners and marathon runners cannot lift large amounts of weight.
- Plyometrics should be used for jumping sports, or when acceleration is essential (sprint start).
- There are no meta-analyses or systematic reviews comparing plyometrics to other types of training. Some studies show it is superior and some show no difference. The opposing results may be due to differences in populations and/or required power output.

Safety

- Plyometrics represent a high intensity workout.
- As exercise intensity increases, the stress applied to muscles, tendons, and ligaments increases.
- If the stress applied to a tissue is greater than it can absorb, an injury occurs.
- As with all exercises, the best way to prevent injury is to start slow and increase gradually.

PNF

Definition

PNF means proprioneurofacilitation. There are both PNF stretching and strengthening exercises. The common use of the term is for stretching.

Theory

The theory behind PNF stretching is that an antagonist muscle contraction causes reflex inhibition of the agonist muscle (e.g. quadriceps inhibits hamstring), which would lead to greater increases in ROM. Some forms use a contraction of the agonist muscle as well.

Types of PNF stretching

For each of the examples, the hamstring muscle is being stretched. Different authors use different nomenclature for the same procedures. I have chosen the one that is sensible if one considers the hamstring as the agonist muscle and the quadriceps is the antagonist muscle. The subject is lying on the floor on their back.

- Contract–Relax (CR): the leg is lifted passively by a partner. The subject contracts the hamstring muscle for a short period (2–10secs.) and then relaxes the muscle. As the muscle is relaxed, the partner passively raises the leg higher to increase the stretch on the agonist.
- Contract–Relax–Antagonist–Contract (CRAC): this is the same as the CR method, but following the passive stretch, the quadriceps is actively contracted by the subject.
- Agonist–Contract–Relax (ACR): this is a confusing name. In fact, the subject contracts the antagonist (quadriceps/hip flexors) to stretch the agonist (hamstring), and the muscle is supported during the rest phase. A variation termed Hold–Relax (HR) is to contract the hamstring before resting.

Experimental evidence

Since being widely promoted in the mid-1970s, there have been several studies examining the effectiveness of PNF stretching. The results are:

- With respect to ROM, studies suggest ACR and CRAC (these two have not been directly compared) superior to CR, which is superior are HR, which is superior to static stretching.
- There is no inhibition of muscle reflex activity. In fact, the EMG of the stretched muscle is increased with PNF compared to static stretching. The mechanism for the increase in ROM remains to be determined.
- There is a change in the muscle visco-elasticity with PNF stretching for the immediate period following the stretch, but there are no long-term changes in visco-elasticity even though ROM increases. These changes are similar to those seen with static stretching.
- Taken together, the above suggests that PNF stretching has a greater analgesic effect than static stretching and this may be the reason for the increased ROM.

Taping and strapping

Taping and strapping refer to the use of bandage material wrapped around a joint with the objective of improving stability of that joint. Taping refers to the use of an adhesive tape and strapping refers to the use of non-adhesive wrap.

Background
- There is both static and dynamic stability of a joint.
  - Static stability (or mechanical instability) refers to passive mobility of a joint. Typically, this is tested by a second person while the subject's muscles are relaxed. Mainly ligaments provide stability.
  - Dynamic stability (or functional instability) refers to the mobility of a joint during active motion. Mainly muscles provide stability.
  - Example: the normal anterior-posterior movement observed in the knee with the Lachman's Test, or in the anterior cruciate ligament with the Anterior Drawer test, tests static stability. This movement does not occur during walking or running (i.e. dynamic stability).
  - Dynamic stability is more clinically relevant than static stability and measured by joint displacement following a sudden force (e.g. trap-door). Injury or re-injury rate is even more clinically relevant.

Effectiveness
- Most of our knowledge comes from ankle studies or anecdotal experience.
- For large joints, taping and strapping have lost 20–50% of their effect on static stability within 15–20 min. Whether this is true for small joints exposed to lesser forces remains to be determined.
- Taping and strapping appear to improve dynamic stability in most studies. This is associated with an increase in resting EMG, which results in increased stiffness of the joint (should protect against injury).
- Clinical trials suggest taping and strapping are effective in preventing ankle injuries.
- Anecdotal evidence suggests that they are useful to limit motion for injured small joints such as wrists, fingers, toes.
- Some clinicians will also tape acromio-clavicular joints, knees, and shoulders. The effectiveness for these joints is controversial and should be evaluated on an individual basis, i.e. tape the joint and if the patient feels it allows them to compete with less pain it is effective for that patient.

Potential deleterious effects
There are no studies on long-term effects. Probable potential deleterious effects include:
- Allergic reaction to the adhesive used in tape. Pre-wrap and hypoallergenic tape may reduce this problem.
- Tenosynovitis if tendon is superficial. Small foam pads placed over the tendons may reduce this problem (e.g. anterior tibialis and achilles tendons for the ankle).

Principles of rehabilitation

The principles of rehabilitation following any injury can be broadly classified into three phases—early, middle, and late. These stages are not mutually exclusive. Short- and long-term goals should be defined for each athlete and reviewed at appropriate time intervals, depending on the injury. Appropriate clinical markers should be used to define the progression of rehabilitation.

Athletes should not be allowed to progress until they have, ideally, completed each stage without difficulty. Rehabilitation ladders or recipes should be used only as guidelines and each athlete should have a customized sport-specific and individually-negotiated rehabilitation plan.

Aerobic fitness and sport-specific motor control and coordination must be maintained where possible throughout rehabilitation.

The plan should be designed around what the athlete can do rather than what they cannot.

Early phase (protection of the injured part)
- Strapping or bracing the injured part to prevent unwanted motion.
- Non-or partial-weight bearing with crutches may be necessary with lower limb injury and a resultant antalgic gait.
- Relative rest.
- Protect, rest, ice, compress, elevate (PRICE).

Middle phase
- Range of movement and flexibility: aim to restore full range of joint motion (physiological and accessory) and muscle length.
- Strength and conditioning (motor control and re-education, strength, power, and endurance).
- Proprioception: aim to restore normal kinaesthetic awareness to the injured part.
- Progression of proprioceptive exercises:
  - Static → dynamic.
  - Conscious → automatic.
  - Decrease the base of support.
  - Decrease visual input.
  - Functional.

Late phase

- Agility drills: shuttle and sprint drills, cone and ladder drills. Start with straight line work, progress to change of direction, cutting, and pivoting.
- Functional activities.
- Sport-specific skills.
- Power work.
- Plyometric training (where appropriate).
- Identification of a safe return to full training.

Determinants of outcome

- Age.
- Pre-injury activity level.
- Post-injury expectation.
- Motivation.
- Associated injury.

Sports-specific fitness tests

Cardiorespiratory fitness tests

Graded maximal exercise tests for aerobic capacity e.g. shuttle run or bleep test for VO_2 max.

Functional performance tests (FPTs)

Sporting activities require manoeuvres that demand a combination of vertical and horizontal force production. FPTs assess a variety of musculoskeletal parameters simultaneously:

- Joint laxity/mobility.
- Muscle extensibility (flexibility).
- Muscle strength and power.
- Proprioception.
- Neuromuscular control.
- Dynamic balance.
- Agility.
- Pain.
- Athlete confidence.

Functional tests can be done unilaterally or bilaterally, and progress may be measured (repetitions, time, distance). They may be used as baseline tests (pre-season), to monitor progress, or as an integral part of training. In rehabilitation they may be used to monitor progress or set targets for return to sport.

- One leg hop.
- Vertical jump.
- Triple hop.
- Side jump.
- Stair/slope running.
- Shuttle runs.
- Figure of 8.
- 6m hop.
- Crossover hop.
- Vertical squat jump.
- Drop jump.

Types of skeletal muscle fibre

Type I or slow oxidative fibres (SO)

These have a higher proportion of oxidative enzymes and mitochondria and a greater capillary density and greater aerobic capacity.

These fibres have a slow contraction time, are difficult to fatigue and good for prolonged, low-intensity work.

Type II

Larger diameter, higher proportion of glycolytic enzymes rather than oxidative enzymes and fewer mitochondria.

Greater anaerobic capacity.

Type IIa or fast twitch oxidative-glycolytic (FOG)

These fibres have a fast contraction time and have the capacity for both aerobic and anaerobic activity. They have the ability to maintain contractile activity for relatively long periods of time.

Type IIb or fast twitch glycolytic fibres (FG)

These fibres are able to generate a lot of tension but fatigue rapidly.

Features of skeletal muscle

Most muscles contain a mixture of fibre types. The nerve innervating the muscle determines the fibre type. Postural muscles tend to have more Type I fibres.

Functional unit is the motor unit—a single motor neuron and all muscle fibres innervated from it. The motor unit is the smallest part of a muscle that can contract independently. The number of muscle fibres forming a motor unit closely relate to the degree of control. Motor units show an all-or-nothing response.

The calling in of additional motor units in response to a greater stimulation of the motor nerve is known as recruitment.

The force a muscle can produce is dependent on the following:
- The length-tension relationship.
- The load-velocity relationship.
- The force-time relationship.
- Temperature.
- Pre-stretching.

Muscle training (isokinetic/isometric/isotonic)

During contraction, the force developed by muscle is known as muscle tension, and the external force acting on it is known as the load or resistance.

There are 3 types of muscle contraction:

- *Isometric*: tension is generated within the muscle without a change in muscle length.
- *Isotonic*: tension is generated within the muscle with a change in muscle length. During a concentric contraction the muscle shortens. During an eccentric contraction the muscle lengthens.
- *Isokinetic*: tension is generated within the muscle where the velocity of contraction remains constant.

Only isometric and isotonic contractions occur naturally. Greater tension can be generated by an eccentric contraction than a corresponding concentric contraction. Any isotonic contraction that results in a change in muscle length must initially have an isometric phase whereby enough tension is generated to overcome the load imposed.

Isokinetics can be used for training and assessment purposes. The ability of a muscle to contract depends on the availability of ATP. Fatigue occurs when the ability to synthesize ATP is insufficient to keep up with ATP breakdown during contraction.

Muscle adaptation to exercise

Physiological adaptations

- Neurogenic—start slow—activate more motor units.
- Myogenic—onset after 6–8 weeks—hypertrophy.
- Increase in muscle size, strength, and power.
- Alter the mechanical properties of other connective tissues and bone.

Age-related changes

As we become older we lose strength. There is debate about the effect of ageing alone or disuse. Muscle mass decreases by 1%/year after the age of 60. A decrease in the number of muscle fibres (preferentially type II), results in slower contractile properties. There is also a decrease in the number of motor units. Remaining units increase in size but the reduction in number compromises precision activities.

Principles of strength training

The fundamental principles of exercise training to optimize the response are: overload, specificity and reversibility. When a muscle adapts to a given stimulus, additional loads must be applied for further adaptation to occur (SAID).

The parameters of a training programme include speed, resistance, repetitions, frequency, and duration; the recovery time between bouts; the form of the exercise; and the range through which the muscle works.

Overload

Intensity

- The greater the load, the higher the intensity.
- Normally expressed as a % of the 1 repetition maximum (1RM).
- A resistance of 80–95% 1RM is the optimal to maximize strength gains for most sports.
- This equates to 3–8 RM set.

Volume

- Volume = sets x reps x load.
- In general as intensity increases, volume decreases.

Rest intervals and recovery

- The total rest time between reps, sets, and exercises for the specific muscle being trained.
- Relates to the intensity of the training 2–3 minute rest intervals between sets is common.

Frequency

- Strength can be maintained by 1 session per week.
- During rehabilitation when the emphasis is on regaining/maximizing muscle strength, this can be optimized by 2–3 sessions per week.

Mode

- Free weights.
- Resistance machines.
- Body weight.
- Variable resistance—sport cord, theraband.
- Isokinetic machines.

Specificity

The exercise chosen should target the specific muscle(s) with regard to its function during the specific activity/sport.

Reversibility

Any training adaptations will be reversed/reduced if training is stopped for 2–8 weeks.

Biomechanical assessment

Static

Observation while standing

- Posture type—kyphosis-lordosis, sway back, flat back, round back. Signs of scoliosis.
- From the front: ASIS levels, patella heights and orientation, femoral anteversion and tibial torsion, genu varum or valgum with feet together, forefoot to rearfoot relationship, position of first ray.
- From the side: pelvic position, signs of genu recurvatum.
- From the back: equal levels of PSIS and gluteal and knee folds. Heel position—everted or inverted. Too many toes sign—increased lateral hip rotation.

Leg length discrepancy

- Quick visual check: supine, flex knees, subject lifts and lowers pelvis, knees straightened, check levels of medial malleolus.
- Tape measure method: measure ASIS to medial malleolus. Discrepancy should be less than 1.5cm.

Range of passive movement

- *Hip*: internal and external rotation with the hip at 90° and 0°.
- *Knee*: hyperextension or fixed flexion.
- *Ankle*: dorsiflexion with the knee at 90° and 0°—a difference may indicate gastrocnemius tightness, anterior drawer test.
- *Subtalar*: assess ROM. In subtalar neutral assess forefoot/rearfoot positions and the eversion/inversion relationship.
- *First ray*: ROM and position in subtalar neutral and midtarsal pronation.

Dynamic

- Bilateral knee bend in standing—any compensatory movement in foot.
- Single leg knee bend—maintaining correct knee alignment and avoiding femoral internal rotation.
- Gait analysis—visual or video analysis.
- Performance specific—video analysis of training, competition, and specific sport techniques.

Orthotics

Indications for use
- Designed to correct abnormal foot/lower limb biomechanics.
- Have been shown to relieve symptoms where abnormal lower limb biomechanics are thought to be a causative factor, especially in overuse conditions e.g. ITB friction syndrome, patellofemoral pain, patella tendinopathy, plantar fasciitis.

How do they work?
- Shock absorption.
- Mechanical control of subtalar and midtarsal movement.
- Neural control—afferent feedback from cutaneous receptors.
- Muscle control—reduce muscle activation required to control the foot.

Different types
- Preformed—heel cups or insoles normally bought off-the-shelf. Generally made of less durable material and provide less control. Do not last as long.
- Custom made following biomechanical assessment and plaster cast taken of the foot. Generally made of more rigid material, provide more control, and last longer.

Choice of orthotics may depend on:
- Foot type.
- The sport played and the type of footwear used.
- The type of biomechanical problem.
- Weight of the patient.

Physiotherapy

Aims to restore normal function and return the athlete to their pre-injury activity level in the shortest possible time, using manual and exercise therapy and advice.

Manual therapy

- Joints can be mobilized passively or with active movement in their accessory or physiological range. Accessory mobilization is aimed at pain relief or restoring range of movement.
- Soft tissue techniques including massage and muscle energy techniques can be applied to muscles, tendons, ligaments, and fascia. They are used for pain relief by decreasing excessive tissue tension, stimulating large diameter fibres, and removal of substance P. Techniques that target myofascial trigger points are also be used for pain management. Other potential benefits include releasing adhesions or reducing excessive scar tissue, releasing tension and spasm and promoting normal tissue length (e.g. myofascial release and PNF techniques).
- Neural mobilization techniques can be used as part of the pain management programme in isolation or associated with other pathology such as sciatic involvement with hamstring lesions. Their involvement can be assessed using neural tension tests (e.g. Slump test, ULTTT) as appropriate.

Manipulation.

A small amplitude high velocity thrust normally performed on intervertebral joints at the end of the range. Normally performed where range of movement is limited by stiffness or in the acute locked neck. Care must be taken with cervical manipulation and vertebral artery screening should be conducted beforehand. Other contraindications include fracture, local malignancy or bony infection, *cauda equina*, RA of the C_0- C_1/C_1- C_2 joints, pregnancy during the last trimester, recent whiplash, haemophilia, spondylolisthesis, and children with open ephyiseal plates. Can be applied to peripheral joints.

Exercise therapy

- Motor control and re-education peripherally and centrally: centrally, the 'core' muscles are transversus abdominis, multifidus, diaphragm and the perineal muscles. Exercise programmes that enhance the timing and recruitment of these muscles under low and high load are widely employed as part of an athlete's regular training programme, as well as during rehabilitation. Central stabilization is essential for efficient control of the upper or lower limb. Peripheral exercises are aimed at those muscles primarily affected by the injury.
- Good biomechanical alignment: Appropriate joint loading and muscle recruitment relies on good biomechanical alignment. Intrinsic and extrinsic factors need to be considered.
- Good technique during specific sporting activity: technique needs to be evaluated, often done in conjunction with a biomechanist and/or coach.

Electrophysical agents

A variety of these modalities are frequently used as an adjunct to treating soft tissue injury. The aim is to deliver physical energy to the tissue to help the natural healing process. Each modality appears to be dose dependant.

Low level laser therapy

Output less than 60mW, therefore no thermal effects. Two types—the gallium arsenide (GaAs) and helium neon (HeNe). Thought to alter cellular mechanisms that increase collagen synthesis. Used for pain management and the promotion of healing.

Ultrasound

The application of high frequency sound waves (1–3MHz) which produce thermal (continuous application) and non-thermal (pulsed) effects. Thermal effects increase local blood flow, non-thermal doses are thought to create mechanical and chemical effects that influence cellular permeability via cavitation and acoustic streaming. Frequency choice relates to the depth of the target tissue, 1MHz 2–5cm, 3MHz 1–2cm. The intensity and pulse ratio vary depending on whether the injury is acute, sub acute, or chronic. For example, typical dose for an acute lateral ligament sprain 3MHz 1:4 (pulse ratio) $0.2W/cm^2$ (intensity) for 10 minutes.

Interferential

The application of 2 alternating medium frequency currents that creates a low frequency current where they 'interfere'. Thought to have 4 main effects: pain relief, increase in blood flow, reduction of oedema, and muscle stimulation. Frequency selected depending on the desired outcome. Frequency range for stimulation of selected structures:

Sympathetic nerve	1–5Hz
Smooth muscle	0–10Hz
Motor nerve	10–50Hz
Parasympathetic nerve	10–150Hz
Sensory nerve	90–100Hz
Nocioceptive nerves	90–150Hz

Combination therapy

The simultaneous application of ultrasound and electrical stimulation such as interferential. Little evidence to support any additional benefits compared to their application independently.

Injury prevention, screening, and prehab

The relationship between injury prevention, musculoskeletal screening and 'Prehab' (in contrast to rehabilitation), is complex.

Injury prevention

We may identify risk factors but eliminating these risk factors can only reduce the likelihood of injury and not completely eliminate injury. It may also be impossible to predict when an injury will occur.

Risk factors are commonly categorized into extrinsic and intrinsic risk factors:

Extrinsic risk factors include:
- Direct contact.
- Sport-specific skills.
- Level of competition.
- Shoes and equipment.
- Surfaces.
- Training errors.
- Overtraining.
- Environmental factors.
- Workplace design.

Intrinsic risk factors include:
- Movement dysfunction and muscle imbalance.
- Malalignment.
- Muscle weakness.
- Loss of flexibility.
- Poor proprioception.
- Intrinsic overload.
- Physical fitness.
- Age.
- Gender.
- Hydration and nutritional status.
- Inadequate warm-up.
- Previous injury.

Previous injury is the greatest predictor for a range of sports injuries. Thus, effective rehabilitation is essential in reducing recurrence.

Preventative strategies that address extrinsic risk factors include:
- Law change.
- Protective equipment.
- Better planning of training/competitive programmes.
- Athlete education.
  - Technique.
  - Preparation.
- Improve facilities.

Preventative strategies addressing intrinsic risk factors can be more difficult to implement and must be appropriate to the athlete and sport involved.

Screening/profiling

Musculoskeletal screening or 'profiling' is a detailed assessment of the athlete in an attempt to achieve the following aims:

- Identify predisposing factors to injury.
- Detect musculoskeletal impairments that may affect performance.
- Identify ongoing injuries, which may or may not be receiving treatment.
- Provide information to coaches on the management of ongoing injuries.
- Identify problems not responding to treatment.
- Follow-up to previous screening.
- Put in place appropriate measures to prevent injury and enhance performance.

Timing

Where possible, profiling should be carried out:

- Outside of the competitive season.
- As part of induction on entry to the elite athlete programme.
- At the end of the competitive season.
- On exit from the programme/club.

Personnel

Where possible, musculoskeletal profiling should be carried out by a chartered physiotherapist with:

- Sport specific knowledge.
- Experience in the management of musculoskeletal problems in sport.

Content

The profiling process should include the following elements:

- Personal details.
- GP contact details.
- Previous injury/illness history.
  - Nature.
  - Management/rehabilitation.
  - Recurrence.
- Anthropometric measures.
- Sports specific information.
  - Training.
  - Competitive cycle.
- Clinical tests to assess:
  - Posture (incl. alignment etc.).
  - Flexibility.
  - Range of motion.
  - Joint systems.
  - Muscle tightness/inhibition.
  - Neural systems.
  - Neurological assessment (where appropriate).
  - Specific pathology (where appropriate).

It is also important that profiling includes a number of functional tests to assess:
- Muscle strength.
- Neuromuscular control.
- Motor control stability.
- Physical fitness.

Examples of functional tests (depending on the sport) that may be used are:
- Single leg squat.
- Overhead squat.
- Lunge.
- Gait analysis.
- Small knee bend.
- Prone hip extension.

It is important that any tests included in the profiling protocol are:
- Relevant.
- Quick & simple to perform.
- Reliable (intra & inter-tester reliability).
- Valid.
- Provide quantitative and qualitative information.
- Ensure standardization of testing protocols and reporting mechanisms.

Example: selecting appropriate test to measure hamstring range
- Straight leg raise:
    - Indication of contracture of hamstring & other posterior hip tissues.
    - Does not give true indication of restrictions due to movement occurring at the pelvis and lumbar spine.
- Possible alternative:
    - Active knee extension test[1, 2].

Significance and consequence of findings
- Consider variations that exist within the normal population.
- Consider findings that may be advantageous to the relevant sport.
- Clinically relevant.
- Technically relevant.

Communication of findings
It is essential that the following people/groups are informed of profiling findings:
- Medical team.
- Coach.
- Sports science team.
- Governing body (where appropriate).

Following profiling it is necessary to formulate and implement an action plan to address issues identified. This should be carried out in conjunction with the multidisciplinary team and the following issues considered:
- How will the action plan be implemented? Consider:
    - The time of season.
    - Next competitive event.
    - Resources.

- Establish who is responsible for follow up?
  - Doctor.
  - Physiotherapist.
  - Coach.
  - Performance manager.
  - Athlete.
- How will implementation be monitored?
  - Identify person responsible.
  - Multi-disciplinary meetings.
- How will the results of intervention be assessed?

In order to ensure that the profiling process is beneficial the following potential problems should also be considered and avoided:
- Time intensive.
- Relevance of tests.
- Lack of follow-up.
- Lack of agreement between therapists regarding findings and interventions.
- Lack of communication with coaching staff.

'Prehab'

Exercise programmes that specifically address intrinsic risk factors in an effort to reduce the incidence of injury are commonly referred to as 'prehab'.

Prehab programmes should be based upon the findings of musculoskeletal profiling and should be tailored to the individual athlete and sport in which they are involved, and reflect the incidence of injury, the common injury mechanism, and probable causes of injury.

In sports, for example, where there is a high incidence of knee injuries, it is advisable to implement prehab programmes that focus on improving knee control and reducing the incidence of such injuries.

A number of prehab programmes have been shown to effectively reduce the incidence of knee, ankle and hamstring injuries.

Principles of prehab programmes

Technical components
- Correct technique is usually the biomechanically safest.
- Developing correct technique requires input from coaching staff e.g.
  - Correct lifting technique for weight training.
  - Correct toss of the ball for tennis serve.
  - Correct body position during rugby scrum.
  - Correct movement mechanics for volleyball player.

Strength training
- Ensure adequate strength to achieve and maintain correct technique for specific sport e.g.: strengthening of hip abductors and external rotators can reduce the incidence of lower limb injury in athletes who are deficient in this area.
- Eccentric strength training is particularly effective in reducing muscle and tendon injuries e.g.: Nordic (Norwegian) hamstring curls significantly reduce incidence of hamstring injuries: (Note: these are a high load eccentric exercise).

The athlete is in a kneeling position, with a therapist/training partner holding his/her feet. Maintaining a neutral lumbar spine and pelvis, the athlete drops forward, hinging at the knee joint, using eccentric hamstring control to slowly lower them down into a fully prone position. Initially, most athletes will need to use their upper body to cushion them onto the ground.

The athlete stops at various points through the range. Extra resistance is used by the therapist, acting to push the athlete into a prone position.

Eccentric patellar tendon loading may help to prevent patellar tendinopathy in jumping sports:
- Eccentric unilateral squats are performed on a decline slope of 25 degrees.
- Load is lifted concentrically using the contralateral limb and slowly lowered.
- 3 x 15 reps daily using a 10RM weight.
- Similar eccentric loading programmes can be used for shoulder external rotators and the achilles tendon.

Balance and neuromuscular control training
Can significantly reduce the incidence of ankle and knee ligamentous injuries. Exercises used may include the following:
- Single leg standing.
  - Throw/catch ball.
    —Vary type of throw e.g. underarm, overhead, side pass, chest pass.
    —Vary the direction of the pass receive e.g. In front, from side, overhead.
    —Vary type of ball e.g. tennis ball, medicine ball.
- Single leg standing on dynamic surface:
  - Folded towel.
  - Mini trampoline (rebounder).
  - Wobble board.
  - Balance pad.
  - Balance cushion.
  - Progress as for basic single leg stands.
- Manual perturbation from therapist/training partner.
- Pro-fitter exercises.
- Dynamic sport-specific drills with balance/control challenge included.

In order to reduce stresses on ligamentous structures, significant emphasis should be placed on dynamic movement control and the maintenance of correct limb alignment. Ensure that hip, knee, and foot are in correct alignment during movements such as:
- Hopping.
- Jumping and landing (bilateral and unilateral support).
- Lunging.
- Stepping.
- Planting and cutting drills.
- Sports-specific movements.

Flexibility

It is important to ensure that the athlete has adequate flexibility to enable them to complete the demands of their sport without placing excessive strain on the muscular system. Lack of flexibility will have been identified during the musculoskeletal profiling process.

Core stability

Appropriate core stability training is an important element of most pre-hab programmes. Core stability provides optimal control of the trunk, supporting the effort and forces from the extremities, which in turn can contribute to safe, efficient, and effective limb function.

Core stability training should incorporate the following elements:
- Appropriate recruitment patterns of stabilizing muscles to facilitate and stabilize the rest of the kinetic chain.
- Focus on improved postural awareness and control.
- Emphasize perfect form.
- Appropriate load for the ability of the athlete.
- Performed in biomechanically correct position for muscle function of the extremities.
- Functional progression.
- Increase complexity as ability permits.
- Sports-specific skills.

In addition to specific prehab exercises to prevent injury, it is important to ensure that athletes are appropriately aerobically conditioned to participate in the sport. Other intrinsic elements that may contribute to the prevention of injury include:
- Nutrition.
- Hydration.
- Psychological preparation.

References

1 Fredriksen H, Dagfinrud H, jacobsen V, Maehkum S (1997). Passive knee extension test to measure hamstring muscle tightness. *Scand J Med Sci Sports*, **7**(5), 279–82.
2 Gajdosik R, Lusin G (1983). Hamstring muscle tightness. Reliability of an active-knee-extension test. *Phys Ther*, **63**(7), 1085–90.

Hip and pelvis

Examination of the hip

History

The usual complaints are:

- Pain.
- Limp.
- Decreased walking/running distances.
- Snapping or clicking sensation of the hip.
- Stiffness.
- Deformity.

Look for evidence of asymmetry or biomechanical abnormality.

Inspection

- Scars.
- Sinuses.
- Swellings.
- Muscle wasting.
- Apparent limb length discrepancy is noted by measuring the distance from umbilicus to medial malleolus.
- Real limb length discrepancy is noted by measuring the distance from anterior superior iliac spine (or any ipsilateral fixed bony point) to medial malleolus after squaring the pelvis (unmask the fixed abduction or adduction deformity of the affected limb so that both anterior superior iliac spine and medial malleolus are leveled, and place the normal limb in similar position).

Examine gait, usually before the above sequence.

Palpation

- Skin temperature.
- Tenderness over the femoral head and greater trochanter.
- Palpate swellings if present.

Active and passive movements:

The pelvis must be squared and stabilized before hip movements are measured.

A normal hip has:

- Flexion range of 0–130°
- Extension of 0–10°
- Abduction of 0–45°
- Adduction of 0–40°
- Internal rotation of 0–30°
- External rotation of 0–60°

Pain at extremes of movements and restriction is noted. In early osteoarthritis, internal rotation is restricted. In advanced osteoarthritis, there is fixed flexion deformity with absent extension, decreased abduction, adduction, and external and internal rotation. All movements are associated with pain.

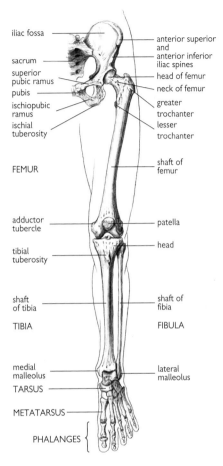

Fig. 5.1 Bones of the lower limb and pelvic girdle: anterior view. Reproduced with permission from Mackinnon P and Morris J (2005). *Oxford Textbook of Functional Anatomy Vol 1.* Oxford University Press, Oxford. ©2005.

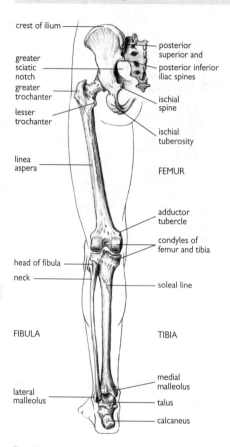

crest of ilium

posterior superior and

posterior inferior iliac spines

greater sciatic notch

greater trochanter

lesser trochanter

ischial spine

ischial tuberosity

linea aspera

FEMUR

adductor tubercle

condyles of femur and tibia

head of fibula

neck

soleal line

FIBULA

TIBIA

medial malleolus

lateral malleolus

talus

calcaneus

Fig. 5.2 Bones of the lower limb and pelvic girdle: posterior view. Reproduced with permission from Mackinnon P and Morris J (2005). *Oxford Textbook of Functional Anatomy Vol 1*. Oxford University Press, Oxford. ©2005.

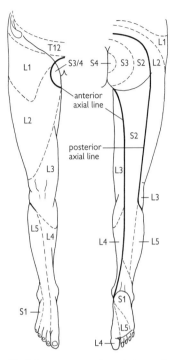

Fig. 5.3 Dermatomes of lower limb; note the axial lines. Reproduced with permission from Mackinnon P and Morris J (2005). *Oxford Textbook of Functional Anatomy Vol 1*. Oxford University Press, Oxford. ©2005.

Table 5.1 Hip joint: movements, principal muscles, and their innervation[1]

Movement	Principal muscles	Peripheral nerve	Spinal root origin	
Flexion	Psoas major	Ventral rami of lumbar nerves	L 1, 2, 3	
	Iliacus	Femoral nerve	L	2, 3
	Rectus femoris	Femoral nerve	L	2, 3, 4
	Pectineus	Femoral nerve	L	2, 3, 4
Extension	Gluteus maximus	Inferior gluteal nerve	L	5, S1, 2
	Hamstrings	Sciatic nerve (tibial component)	L	5, S1, 2
Adduction	Adductors longus, brevis, magnus, and gracilis	Obturator nerve	L	2, 3, 4
Abduction	Gluteus medius and minimus	Superior gluteal nerve	L	4, 5, S1
	Tensor fasciae latae	Superior gluteal nerve	L	4, 5, S1
Medial rotation	Tensor fasciae latae	Superior gluteal nerve	L	4, 5, S1
	Gluteus medius and minimus	Superior gluteal nerve	L	4, 5, S1
	Adductor longus	Obturator nerve	L	2, 3, 4
Lateral rotation	Obturator externus	Obturator nerve	L	2, 3, 4
	Sartorius	Femoral nerve	L	2, 3, 4
	Quadratus femoris	Sacral plexus	L	4, 5, S1
	Obturator internus	Sacral plexus	L	5, S1, 2
	Gluteus maximus	Inferior gluteal nerve	L	5, S1, 2

1 Reproduced with permission from Mackinnon P and Morris J (2005). *Oxford Textbook of Functional Anatomy Vol 1*. Oxford University Press, Oxford. ©2005.

Table 5.2 Main spinal nerve root supplying the movements of the lower limb[1]

	Movement	Main nerve roots	
Hip	Flexion, adduction	L 2, 3, 4	
Knee	Extension, abduction	L	4, 5, S1
	Extension	L	3, 4
Ankle	Flexion	L	5, S1
	Flexion (plantar flexion)	L	4, 5
Subtalar joint	Extension (dorsiflexion)	L	5, S1
	Inversion	L	5
Toes (long muscles)	Eversion	L	5, S1
	Flexion (plantar flexion)	L	5, S1, 2
Toes (small muscles of foot)	Extension (dorsiflexion)	L	S1, 2, 3
			S1, 2, 3

Because of the rotation of the lower limb, extension of the knee is supplied by higher segments.

1 Reproduced with permission from Mackinnon P and Morris J (2005). *Oxford Textbook of Functional Anatomy Vol 1*. Oxford University Press, Oxford. ©2005.

Special tests

Trendeleburg test
Helps to assess the integrity of the abductor mechanism of the hip. Patients are requested to stand on one leg, and the position of the pelvis is noted. If the pelvis drops, and patients sway to loaded leg, the test is positive. Pain on weight bearing, weakness of hip abductors, shortening of femoral neck, and dislocation or subluxation of the hip joint result in a Trendelenburg +ve test.

Thomas' test
Fixed flexion deformity of the hip can be masked by the pelvic tilt and exaggerating the lumbar lordosis. Therefore, this test helps unmask the fixed flexion deformity of the hip and measure the true range of hip flexion.

In supine position, both hips are flexed until the lumbar lordosis is obliterated (confirmed by examiner's hand). The normal (or contralateral) hip is kept flexed, and the affected hip is lowered to the maximum possible extent. The angle between couch and the lower limb is the fixed flexion deformity angle.

Tests for suspected labral tears
- Pain on flexion, adduction, and internal rotation of the hip joint occurs with anterior superior tears.
- Pain on passive hyperextension, abduction, and external rotation occurs with posterior tears.
- Pain moving the hip from a position of full flexion of the hip with external rotation and full abduction, to extension, abduction, and internal rotation occurs with anterior tears.
- Pain moving the hip from extension, abduction, and external rotation to flexion, adduction, and internal rotation occurs with posterior tears.

The above manoeuvres may also be accompanied by clicking and locking sensations.

Hip examination is completed by performing neurovascular examination of the lower limb and examining the contralateral hip and ipsilateral knee, joint, and spine.

Investigation
Plain radiographs, CT scan, MR scan, bone scan, and arthroscopy are helpful to confirm clinical diagnoses.

Femur: acute injury

Femoral shaft fractures follow a high energy injury, and associated injuries must be ruled out. Follow ATLS guidelines (airway with cervical spine control, breathing, circulation, disability assessment, and exposure) when managing such injuries. Secondary survey will help identify associated injuries. Fractures are usually closed, and if open, they are often within-out injuries. The mechanism of injury is usually a torsional stress causing a spiral fracture that may extend into the proximal or distal metaphysis. A direct force causes transverse or oblique fractures. Severe trauma results in comminuted/segmental fractures.

History and examination

- Severe pain, with obvious swelling and deformity.
- Unable to move the limb.
- Beware of hypovolaemic shock; up to 1.5 litres of blood may be lost into the thigh.
- Check and document the presence of distal pulses and the neurological status of the affected limb.

Investigation

- Radiographs to include both hip and knee joints. The incidence of ipsilateral femoral shaft and femoral neck fractures is 3%.

Treatment

- Manage shock:
  - Two wide bore venous cannulae (brown or grey coloured).
  - Hartmann's solution is preferred.
  - Urinary catherization.
  - Crossmatch 2–4 units of blood.
- Analgesia.
- Adequate splint (Thomas splint).
- Gold standard is early closed intramedullary nailing for closed fractures (<24 hours).
- Fix femoral neck first, if present.
- Open fractures need emergency debridement and stabilization.
- Paediatric femoral shaft fractures can be managed with traction.

Complications

- Fat embolism.
- Infection.
- Delayed union requiring dynamisation of interlocking nail.
- Nonunion may need reamed exchange nailing.
- Malunion (may need corrective surgery).

Growth plate injury

The growth plate (physis) can be injured in many ways. The most common cause of growth plate injury is trauma. Other causes, although less common, include: disuse, infection, tumour, vascular impairment, neural involvement, metabolic abnormalities, radiation, laser injury, electrical injury, burns, frostbite, chronic stress, and iatrogenic or surgical insults[1].

Physeal fractures

The physis is the weakest structure near a paediatric joint. They occur in a male:female ration of 2:1. In males, the peak incidence is at 14 years, and in females it is at 11–12 years. The most common sites of injury are the phalanges of fingers (37%) followed by the distal radius (18%). Children present with pain, inability to use the limb, and a possible deformity. AP and lateral radiographs of the affected part will usually confirm the diagnosis. Occasionally, stress views, tomograms, CT scans, MR scan, or a US scan can help detect growth plate injury.

Classification

The Salter-Harris classification of the physeal injuries is widely used.
1. Separation of the epiphysis from the metaphysis with disruption of the complete physis. Distal fibula is a common site.
2. Separation of part of the physis, with a portion of metaphysis attached to the epiphysis (Thurston-Holland sign). Finger phalanges and distal radius are common sites.
3. Fracture of the epiphysis extending into the physis. Finger phalanges and the distal tibia are common sites.
4. The fracture traverses metaphysis, physis, epiphysis and the articular cartilage. Lateral condyle of humerus, finger phalanges, and the distal tibia are common sites.
5. This injury is end-on crush of the physis. Diagnosis is retrospective as radiographs are normal at initial presentation.

Treatment

Immediate anatomical reduction either by gentle closed or open methods and adequate fixation by conservative or surgical methods will favour restoration of function and normal growth.

Complications

If the entire physis is affected, bone length is retarded. If a part of physis is affected, angular deformity may result.

Reference

1 Peterson HA (2001), Physeal injuries and growth arrest. In Beaty JH, Kasser JR, (eds), *Fracture in children*. Lippincott Williams & Wilkins, Philadelphia, pp. 91-138.

Femoral neck stress fracture

Stress fractures occur when bone cannot adapt quickly enough in response to the repeated traumatic strain from exercise. Long distance runners and dancers (especially females) are prone to femoral neck stress fractures. Predisposing factors include changes in the training programme with increase in intensity, frequency, and duration, changes in shoes, running on a different surface, nutritional deficiency, and in female athletes with abnormal menstrual cycles and hormonal imbalance due to relative osteoporosis.

History and examination

- Deep aching pain in the groin that may radiate to the knee.
- Pain is progressive, occurs with activity, and resolves with rest.
- Pain becomes constant if activities are continued without modification.
- May present with a limp.
- May be no specific site of point tenderness.
- Range of motion of the hip, particularly internal rotation, may be limited due to pain.
- Walking, static running, or hopping on the affected extremity often reproduces the pain.

The differential diagnosis includes infection, tumor, compartment syndrome, arthritis, ligamentous, or soft-tissue injuries.

Investigations

- Plain radiographs may be negative.
- MRI is more sensitive, specific, and accurate than a bone scan in identifying a femoral neck stress fracture.
- Femoral neck stress fractures are classified by Fullerton and Snowdy[1] as tension (type I—superior aspect of the femoral neck), compression (type II—inferior aspect of the femoral neck), or displaced (type III).

Treatment

- Tension (type I) and displaced (type III) fractures should be internally fixed and referred urgently to orthopaedic surgeons.
- Compression (type II) can be managed conservatively with non/partial weight bearing depending on pain and analgesia. Nonimpact activities are initiated once the patient has become pain-free.
- Internal fixation in athletes with stress fractures of the femoral neck aids early rehabilitation and return to sports.

Complications

- Avascular necrosis.
- Non-union (with conservative management).
- Varus deformity (with conservative management).
- Displacement (with conservative management).

Prognosis

Any of above complications lead to inability to return to pre-injury performance levels.

Prevention

A gradual progression in the intensity and duration of all conditioning activities is crucial in the prevention of stress fractures. A useful rule of thumb is that an increase in training volume (distance) or intensity should not exceed 10% per week.

Trochanteric bursitis

Inflammation of the greater trochanteric bursa. This bursa minimizes the friction between the greater trochanter and the iliotibial band, which passes over the bursa. Predisposing factors include a broad pelvis (female runners), training on banked surfaces or roads with a slope, and a recent increase in mileage, duration, or intensity of training.

History and examination

- Lateral hip pain, occasionally radiating along the distal lateral thigh.
- May be associated with snapping or clicking sensation.
- Point tenderness over the greater trochanter may be associated with crepitus on hip flexion and extension.

Provocative positions include external rotation and adduction.

The differential diagnosis includes:
- Stress fractures.
- Gluteus medius tendinopathy (dancers).
- Lumbosacral radiculopathy.
- Avascular necrosis.
- Osteoarthritis.

Investigations

Diagnosis is usually made by clinical examination.
- Radiographs may help rule out other conditions.
- The role of US and MRI is unclear.

Treatment

Most patients improve with conservative management which includes:
- Rest.
- Iliotibial band and tensor fascia lata stretching.
- Gluteal muscle strengthening.
- Anti-inflammatory drugs.
- Iontophoresis.
- Ultrasound.
- Injection of local anaesthetic (5ml of 1% lignocaine 10mg/ml) into the point of maximal tenderness.

Surgical management may be offered following failed conservative management. The iliotibial band is released by a cruciform incision with or without debridement of the trochanteric bursa. The iliotibial band may also be Z-lengthened or an ellipse of tissue can be excised.

Ilio-tibial band friction syndrome

The ilio-tibial band friction syndrome (ITBFS), an overuse injury, is characterized by pain on the outer aspect of the knee due to irritation and inflammation of the distal portion of the iliotibial band as it crosses the lateral femoral epicondyle. This is seen in long-distance runners, cyclists, and other endurance athletes.

Friction (or impingement) occurs predominantly in the stance phase, between the posterior edge of the iliotibial band and the underlying lateral femoral epicondyle. Downhill running predisposes the runner to iliotibial band friction syndrome because the knee flexion angle at footstrike is reduced. There is a higher incidence where long-distance running is the vogue, or where the climate is cool and running surfaces are slippery.

History and examination

Pain is usually poorly localized over the lateral aspect of the knee, is aggravated by running long distances or excessive striding, and is more severe running downhill. Pain may be relieved by walking with a stiff or a straight knee.

Point tenderness about 2cm above the joint line when the knee is flexed at 30° and palpated over the lateral femoral epicondyle.

- Flexion and extension of the knee may produce a crepitus.
- Pain is worse during weight bearing flexion and extension. Pain is typically worse at the 30° while flexion is occurring.

The differential diagnosis includes: knee pathologies including menisceal tears, ligament injuries, and loose bodies.

Investigations

Diagnosis is usually clinical and investigations including radiographs and MRI scan help in ruling out other pathologies but cannot positively confirm ITBFS.

Treatment

Conservative treatment is effective in most cases. It includes:

- Reduction of activity.
- Oral anti-inflammatories.
- Ice, heat, ultrasound, and/or electrical stimulation.
- Stretching exercises to address any excessive ITB tightness. Hip flexion tightness or contracture will need to be stretched before the ITB can be adequately stretched.

Physiotherapy in combination with analgesic/anti-inflammatory medication is the optimum combination and some recommend injections of local anaesthetic and corticosteroid (or aprotinin, a polyvalent inhibitor of proteolytic enzymes (6.25ml equivalent to 625,000 IU) repeated twice at two weekly intervals).

Surgery may be offered to patients who are resistant to conservative management. It is performed with the knee held in 30° of flexion and consists of cruciform incision of the iliotibial band or a limited resection of a small triangular piece at the posterior part of the iliotibial band covering the lateral femoral epicondyle. Prognosis is good with low morbidity, and quick return to sports.

Thigh contusion

Proximal thigh contusions are common athletic injuries, particularly in contact sports, as a result of direct trauma. The muscle is compressed between the external force and the subjacent femur. Severe injuries result in large haematomas that limit range of motion.

There is often significant haemorrhage and swelling.

History and examination

Classification[1]: (range of motion (ROM) assessed at 12 to 24 hours after the event).
- Mild thigh contusions—active ROM of the knee >90°.
- Moderate thigh contusions—active ROM of the knee 45–90°.
- Severe thigh contusions—active ROM of the knee <45°.

Treatment

The initial management for an anterior thigh contusion involves rest, immobilization with knee in flexion, ice, and compression to maintain motion and minimize haematoma formation.
- Weightbearing is limited until the patient regains good quadriceps muscle control and 90° of pain-free knee motion.
- Functional rehabilitation and non-impact sports are allowed when the range of motion has reached 120° and there is no residual muscle atrophy.
- Return to full activity: normal strength and range of motion (3 weeks). More severe injuries may have a longer recovery time.

Average disability time is 13 days for mild contusions, 19 days for moderate contusions, and 21 days for severe contusions.

If there is a major haematoma and if an athlete struggles to regain motion, refer to an orthopaedic surgeon or a radiologist for evacuation or aspiration of the haematoma. MRI or US scan will demonstrate the size and location of the haematoma. The aspiration can be performed under ultrasound guidance with aseptic technique. Protect the involved area with padding to avoid repeat injury.

Complications

- Myositis ossificans development depends on the severity of the initial injury. It is more likely with repeated trauma. This process may appear histologically similar to osteosarcoma, but the history is usually distinct and the periphery of a myositis ossificans lesion is mature. (□ Myositis ossificans).
- Loss of range of motion and loss of functional outcome.

Indomethacin may be useful for prevention of myositis.

☞ Monitor closely high-energy contusions for thigh and gluteal compartment syndromes in acute stages. Emergency fasciotomy may be rarely required, but serial examinations are an absolute requirement.

1 Ryan JB, Wheeler JH, Hopkinson WJ et al. (1991) Quadriceps contusions. West Point update. *AM J Sports Med* **19**(3), 299–304.

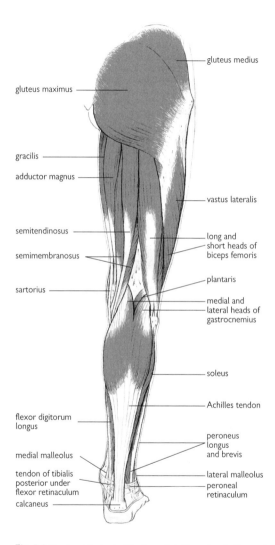

Fig. 5.4 Muscles at the back of the lower limb. Reproduced with permission from Mackinnon P and Morris J (2005). *Oxford Textbook of Functional Anatomy Vol 1.* Oxford University Press, Oxford. ©2005.

Myositis ossificans

This is usually a self-limiting condition in which a mass of heterotopic bone forms within the soft tissues. The term is a misnomer, as the muscle is not inflamed, and the process is not limited to muscle. Other descriptive terms include heterotopic bone formation, pseudomalignant osseous tumour of the soft tissue, extraosseous localized non-neoplastic bone and cartilage formation, myositis ossificans circumscripta, and pseudomalignant myositis ossificans.

The condition develops within one to two weeks of direct trauma to the area or unusual muscular exertion. A history of trauma cannot be elicited in 50% of patients. It is more common in adolescents and young males. Typical sites include the thigh (quadriceps femoris and adductor muscles), elbow (flexor muscles), buttocks (gluteal muscles), the shoulder, and the calf. The proximal portion of the extremity is more frequently affected than the distal part.

The pathological process includes muscle necrosis and haemorrhage after trauma. Histologically, there is marked proliferation of spindle cells with a well recognized zoning phenomenon.
- The least differentiated tissue lies in the central zone.
- In the middle or intermediate zone, the osteoid is more organized and separated by a loose cellular stroma.
- The outer zone is the most mature consisting of well formed bone which may form a shell around the entire lesion. Cartilage formation may also be present.

Soft tissue or bone sarcomas do not exhibit a similar zonal phenomenon.

History and examination

There is usually pain, swelling, and stiffness of the surrounding joints.
On examination, there is often a red, warm swelling, soft tissue tenderness and, in later stages, a hard mass is palpable.

Investigations

In the early stages, plain radiographs may be unremarkable except for non-specific soft tissue swelling. A periosteal reaction may be seen if the lesion is juxtacortical. By 2–6 weeks there is faint calcification and at 6–8 weeks, a lacy pattern of new bone forms around the periphery of the mass. Complete maturation is usual in 5–6 months.

A bone scan is highly sensitive because of the profuse osteoblastic activity and bone formation, and is non-specific, as soft tissue and bone tumours also show increased activity.

The MRI findings vary according to the stage of the disease.

The differential diagnosis includes soft tissue sarcoma and osteogenic sarcoma.

Treatment

Rest the part in a functional position until pain subsides. Gentle active movements may begin once pain improves. Oral biphosphonates, potent inhibitors of calcification are effective in modifying the process of heterotopic ossification.

Surgical resection is appropriate if the mass causes functional impairment and is best performed when the lesion has matured. Rapid recurrence occurs after resection of an immature lesion. If left alone, the mass may reduce in size with time, and, in some instances, disappear.

Osteoarthritis (OA) of the hip

A progressive degenerative joint disease of the hip. (Coxarthrosis: coxa is hip, arthrosis is degeneration of a joint. Osteoarthritis is a misnomer as inflammation is not the primary pathologic process). The incidence of idiopathic hip OA increases with age. (It rarely occurs before the age of 24 years. From 25–34 years 2%, from 35–44 years 4%, from 45–54 years 16%, from 55–64 years 31%, and 65+years 47%). Two million people in the UK suffer with osteoarthritis and, of those, 210,000 have moderate to severe osteoarthritis of the hips.

Ex-professional footballers had a significantly higher prevalence of OA of the hip than an age-matched group of radiographic controls[1]. A Finnish study of international competing athletes showed increased risk OA of the hip for all athletes, but those involved in endurance sports (long distance running, cross-country skiing) were admitted to hospital care for OA at a later age than those involved in power sports (boxing, weightlifting, wrestling, throwing) or mixed sports (soccer, hockey, basketball, track).

Regular cyclical loading of joints is required to maintain normal articular cartilage composition, structure, and function. Prolonged static loading, repeated sudden excessive loading, or the absence of loading may, however, cause degradation of articular cartilage.

Repetitive joint use, under abnormal loading conditions, is a risk factor for OA. This includes:
- Participation in heavy physical activity before 50 years of age.
- An elite level in high joint loading sports.
- Combination of heavy recreational physical activity with heavy occupational workload.
- Continued use of the joint after injury in sporting activity.

History and examination
Symptoms usually include pain, stiffness, deformity (late stages), and loss of mobility.

Clinical findings
- Muscle wasting.
- Tenderness.
- Deformity.
- Reduced range of motion (loss of internal rotation seen in early OA, normal range is 0°–40°).
- Crepitus.
- Alteration of gait.

Investigation
Plain radiographs demonstrate:
- Loss of joint space.
- Osteophyte formation.
- Subchondral cyst formation.
- Subchondral sclerosis.
- Erosion of bones, loose bodies and subluxed joint are characteristic of advanced OA.

Treatment
- Analgesia.
- NSAIDs.
- Physiotherapy: strengthening exercises, range-of-motion exercises, and functional training are beneficial.
- Oral chondroitin sulphate and glucosamine sulphate may help to alleviate pain in early OA of the hip.
- Osteotomy, total hip replacement, and hip resurfacing are the surgical options.

Osteotomy, if performed in the early stages, can delay the progression of OA of the hip due to redistribution of load on the articular cartilage. Eventually, patients who undergo osteotomy may require total hip replacement.

Metal-on-metal hip resurfacing has allowed many young patients, usually below 65 years with OA of the hip, to return to recreational sports like cycling, rowing, swimming, jogging, surfing etc. Competitive sports like sprints and gymnastics are not recommended. Hip resurfacing has inherent stability, which decreases the risk of post-operative dislocation of the hip.

Reference

1 GJ Shepard, AJ Banks, WG Ryan (2003). Ex-professional association footballers have an increased prevalence of osteoarthritis of the hip despite not having sustained notable hip injuries compared with age matched controls. *Br J Sports Med*, **37**, 80–1.

Osteitis pubis

Osteitis pubis is a degenerative condition of the pubic symphysis and surrounding muscle insertions. It is usually secondary to overuse or trauma. It occurs typically in sports with sprinting, kicking, and sudden changes of direction, such as running, basketball, soccer, ice hockey, Australian football, and tennis. Pelvic surgery and childbirth also predispose to osteitis pubis.

It occurs in almost any patient population, is self-limiting and usually improves within one year. It is recurrent in 25% of athletes.

History and examination
- Exercise-induced pain or pubic tenderness.
- Pain may also occur while walking, radiating to the perineal, testicular, suprapubic, or inguinal region, and can also develop in the scrotum after ejaculation.
- Clicking may indicate vertical instability.

Clinical findings
- Tenderness over pubic symphysis, aggravated by pelvic compression.
- Painful hip abduction.
- Wide based gait.

The differential diagnosis includes adductor sprains, a hernia, prostatitis in men. Sexually acquired reactive arthritis (SARA) can manifest as osteitis pubis. Osteomyelitis of the symphysis pubis can occur concomitantly with osteitis pubis. A biopsy and culture of the affected area is necessary to rule out osteomyelitis.

Investigations
- Radiographs are negative in the early stages. They may reveal widening of symphysis pubis, irregular contour of articular surfaces, and periarticular sclerosis in late stages.
- Flamingo views help demonstrate vertical instability of the symphysis.
- MRI, CT scan, bone scintigraphy can confirm osteitis pubis early.
- Blood investigations including WCC, ESR, and CRP may be abnormal and raised. Blood cultures are necessary to rule out infection.

Treatment
- Rest.
- Avoidance of pain producing activity.
- Analgesics.
- Adductor stretching and eccentric strengthening after symptomatic improvement of pain. Stretching is performed at least daily, with flexibility as the main focus of therapy. Aquatic conditioning may be begun at this time with the exception of frog kicking, which uses the adductors extensively. Sports-specific activities are added late in this phase, with offending motions added last.

Rarely, vertical instability of symphysis pubis can complicate osteitis pubis. This is surgically managed by arthrodesis with compression plating and bone grafting[1].

Prognosis is good if tackled early. In chronic cases, injection of the symphysis pubis under image intensifier guidance with aprotinin and local anaesthetic may be of some value before proceeding to surgery.

Reference

1 Williams PR, Thomas DP, Downes EM (2000). Osteitis pubis and instability of the pubic symphysis. When nonoperative measures fail. *Am J Sports Med* **28**(3), 350–5.

Sports hernia (Gilmore's groin)

Sports hernia (Gilmore's groin) is an overuse syndrome common in athletes participating in sports that require repetitive twisting and turning at speeds, e.g. field hockey, ice hockey, soccer, and tennis.

Hip abduction, adduction, and flexion-extension with the resultant pelvic motion produce a shearing force across the pubic symphysis, leading to stress on the inguinal wall musculature perpendicular to the fibres of the fascia and muscle. Pull from the adductor musculature against a fixed lower extremity can cause significant shear forces across the hemipelvis. Subsequent attenuation or tearing of the transversalis fascia or conjoined tendon can be the source of pain. Abnormalities at the insertion of the rectus abdominis muscle or avulsions of part of the internal oblique muscle fibres at the pubic tubercle, abnormalities in the external oblique muscle and aponeurosis, entrapment of the genital branches of the ilioinguinal or genitofemoral nerves have been suggested as sources of pain.

History and examination

Unilateral groin pain of insidious onset which occurs with exercise, and is aggravated by coughing and sneezing, may radiate laterally, across the midline, into the adductor region, scrotum, and testicles. Occasionally, athletes report a sudden tearing sensation.

Clinical findings

- Local tenderness over the conjoined tendon, pubic tubercle, and midinguinal region, or a tender, dilated superficial inguinal ring.
- Pain with resisted adduction, resisted sit-up, and reproducible with Valsalva manoeuvre.

The differential diagnosis includes osteitis pubis, adductor tendinopathy, symphyseal instability, osteoarthritis, and tumor.

Investigations

- Plain radiographs and bone scan can help rule out the above conditions.
- MRI may be useful to detect abnormalities within the muscles or pubic symphysis.

Treatment

Conservative management is occasionally effective for groin injuries, but results in a protracted clinical course. Surgery can be considered if conservative management fails after 6–8 weeks.

Conventional or laparoscopic herniorrhaphy is usually successful. Mesh reinforcement is often performed during these repairs. Return to sports within 6–12 weeks after specific rehabilitation targeted at abdominal strengthening, adductor muscle flexibility, and a graduated return to activity. If adductor muscle pain is present pre-operatively, adductor muscle release or recession is combined with herniorrhaphy.

Groin pain

A non-specific descriptive syndrome which is difficult to diagnose because of the complex anatomy and the possibility of co-existing injuries.

The overall incidence of injuries causing groin pain varies but it is prevalent (2–5%) in athletes participating in ice hockey, fencing, handball, cross country skiing, hurdling, high jumping, and soccer (5–7% of all soccer injuries). These sports involve side-to-side cutting, quick accelerations and decelerations, and sudden directional changes. The diagnosis may be unclear in up to 30% of cases.

History and examination

Acute onset of groin pain may be due to muscle contusion, sprain, or bony injury including fractures and dislocation of the hip joint. In muscle contusions and sprain, the athletes suffer swelling of the affected part, which may show bruising. In complete muscle tears, a gap may be palpable between the ruptured ends. In athletes with bony injuries, there is pain, swelling, deformity, and inability to bear weight on the affected limb.

In patients with chronic groin pain, a careful history including the onset, inciting event, and aggravating and relieving factors should be obtained. It is important to consider the age of the athlete, as different conditions affect groin and hip in adolescents and children in comparison with adults.

Children and adolescents presenting with groin pain and pain on weight bearing of the affected limb should be evaluated to exclude septic arthritis, avascular necrosis of the hip, Legg-Calve-Perthes disease, and slipped capital femoral epiphysis. Apophyseal avulsion fractures may present with acute groin or hip pain after an injury. Tendon lesions are rare in children and adolescents.

Clinical examination
- Adequate exposure of the groin and hip.
- Inspection of the symmetry and anatomic irregularity.
- Palpation of the affected area for tenderness.
- Assessment of the range of motion of the joints.
- Measurement for discrepancy of leg length (📖 Examination of the hip).
- Evaluation of gait, including the performance of sprints, jumps, and activities that exacerbate the athlete's pain.
- Neurological examination may reveal areas of numbness and motor weakness.

Investigations
- Plain radiographs may show fractures, avulsion fractures in adolescents, established osteitis pubis, later stages of stress fracture and osteomyelitis, slipped femoral epiphysis, or osteoarthritis.
- A bone scan can help demonstrate osteitis pubis, stress fracture, osteomyelitis, synovitis, avascular necrosis, sacroiliitis, tenoperiosteal lesion, or muscle tear.
- Sonograms may show a muscle tear, hematoma, inguinal hernia, or bursitis.

- Nerve conduction studies may demonstrate ilioinguinal neuropathy or obturator neuropathy.
- CT scans and MRIs may show the following: disc pathology; radicular lesions; osteitis pubis; and other bone and soft tissue.

Table 5.3 Common disorders producing groin pain in adults[1]

Acute onset:

Muscle strains

Contusions (hip pointer)

Acetabular labral tears and loose bodies

Proximal femur fractures

Insidious onset:

Sports hernias and athletic pubalgia

Osteitis pubis

Bursitis

Snapping hip syndrome

Stress fractures

Osteoarthritis

Other disorders:

Lumbar spine abnormalities

Compression neuropathies

Table 5.4 Disorders producing groin pain in children and adolescents

Acute onset:

Contusions (hip pointer)

Avulsions and apophyseal injuries

Proximal femur fractures

Insidious onset:

Avascular necrosis of the hip

Legg–Calve–Perthes disease

Slipped capital femoral epiphysis

Adductor tendinopathy rehabilitation

This is predominantly an overuse injury and therefore the time taken to return to sport is often difficult to predict. An athlete's return to full fitness may be affected by the duration of symptoms, and the nature of the sporting activity. Even athletes with a short history of problems may require 8–12 weeks of rehabilitation.

Symptomatic relief using electrotherapy, icing, and massage may be of benefit, but the most important aspect of management often involves progressive strengthening of the adductors.

Aims
- Assess intrinsic/extrinsic risk factors for injury.
- Begin isometric strengthening/loading of the adductors.
- Begin basic core exercises.

Risk factors

This is possibly the most important aspect of managing any overuse injury. Once the risk factors are identified, rehabilitation should be started as soon as possible.

Common intrinsic risk factors include:
- Weakness of hip adductors.
- Weakness of gluteal muscles.
- Decreased ROM of hip: in particular internal rotation, external rotation and extension.
- Reduced flexibility of hip musculature: in particular adductors/gluteals.
- Poor lumbopelvic control.
- Poor lower limb alignment.

Treatment

Massage
- Manual therapy usually focuses on the areas of muscle tightness—commonly the gluteus medius, piriformis and adductor muscle group.
- Deep transverse friction massage on the common adductor tendon should also be of benefit.

Electrotherapy
Various electrotherapeutic modalities can be used to promote healing and improve symptomatic relief.

Level 1 (weeks 1–2)

Core/adduction exercises
- Single leg standing: maintaining a neutral pelvis and lumbar spine. 45 seconds x 5. Athletes should record the number of touchdowns per set.
- Static adduction: in all cases, the athlete should be instructed to perform a static contraction at a pain free level.
  - Supine, hips (45°) and knees (90°) in flexion, feet on floor, squeeze ball between knees. (10 second holds x 8).
  - Supine, hips and knees in extension, ball between feet, squeeze ball between feet. (10 second holds x 8).

- Bent knee fall out: ensure that the pelvis stays in contact with the floor and the lumbar spine remains in a neutral position. Movement should be restricted to the hip joint.
- Supine alternate hip extension.
- Running man: stand on right leg, swing left leg and arms in running motion—add single leg squat as able. 30 seconds × 6.
- Lying on back, knees bent, back flat against floor—slowly straighten alternate legs keeping back flat. 3×10reps.
- Mini-squats (two legs) bend knee to 30° 3×20reps daily.
- Standing on one leg, throw ball against wall and catch, progress by standing on unstable surface.

Level 2 (weeks 3–8)

Core exercise

- Bent knee fall out—theraband.
- PNF long leg pattern. Start position: hip flexion, adduction, internal rotation.
- Static adductions knee to chest.
- Static adduction squats.
- Resisted adduction—pulley/theraband.
- Hip flexion (adduction theraband stabilisation).
- Worms.

The following exercises are directed towards the deficient tissues identified in initial assessment:

- Lunge walk—aim for thigh parallel to ground, keep knee in alignment with 2nd toe during lunge (no weight)—20m × 5 × 3 sets.
- Step-ups—approx 30cm step 3 × 20reps (no weight).
- Single leg mini trampoline:
  - Gently bounce for 1 min × 5 (to each leg).
  - Progress to throwing and catching ball.
- Lunge stabilisation:
  - Adopt ½ lunge position, throwing and catching a ball. 1 min × 3 to each leg.
  - Vary the knee position.
- Swiss ball ½ squat:
  - Swiss ball against the wall, in standing position, roll down to a ½ squat position, hold for 2 seconds, and up again. 6 × 3 sets.
- Step backs:
  - Step backwards off a low bench—keep movement as slow and controlled as possible. 8 reps to each leg × 3 sets.

Level 3 (weeks 8–12)

Progressive running

Running must be introduced gradually and be consistent with the ability of the athlete to perform without pain. Straight line running is commenced first, allowing sufficient time for gradual acceleration and deceleration. Once the athlete can run at 80% in a straight line without pain, directional changes should be introduced slowly to allow time for tissue adaptation.

Directional running may be introduced as follows:
- Long gradual snake runs.
- Side shuffles.
- Forward/backward running to fixed point.
- Figure of 8 runs—gradually reduce the size of the 8 and increase speed.
- Ladder drills.
- Cross overs/carioca runs.
- Cuts—begin with 45° cut to affected side (i.e. stepping off unaffected limb) and progress by stepping off affected side. Once this can be performed without pain, progress to 90° cuts and eventually to 180° turns.
- Side stepping drills—begin with sideways running between cones and progress to add some movement through the sagittal plane. Further progression to include stepping around cone at speed and eventually adding a dynamic target (opponent).

Kicking drills
Progressive kicking programme:
- It is easier and less stressful for the tissues to begin kicking a ball that is moving away from you. This can be progressed by kicking a ball that is moving in various directions, followed by kicking a ball from hand and eventually kicking a dead ball.
- Focus on maintaining accuracy and technique. When kicking, pre-tense the abdomen to maintain a solid base and try to maintain good alignment.

Only carry out exercises after a good warm-up and some close ball skills training, do not attempt to kick dead ball when 'cold'.

Begin with longer kicks of a moving ball—in various directions.

Session 1
- 20m x 10
- 30m x 5
- 40m x 5

Session 2
- 30m x 10
- 40m x 5
- 50m x 5

Session 3
- 30m x 10
- 40m x 10
- 50m x 5

Session 4
- 30m x 10
- 40m x 10
- 50m x 5
- 50m x 5

To progress kicking increase until doing 10 reps at each distance and then concentrate on increasing force and speed.

When the above sessions can be completed without pain, carry out the kicking at the end of at the following drills:
- Cutting at 45 and 90°.
- Snake runs.
- Snake runs with cut.
- Lateral running with sudden change of pace and direction.

Advanced strengthening and control exercises should also be introduced at this stage, as follows:

Abdominal strengthening programme

Exercise 1: prone bridge.
- In a face down position, balance on the tips of your toes and elbows while attempting to maintain a straight line from heels to head.
- Hold for as long as you can without pain.
- Repeat for set of 4–3–2.

Exercise 2: isometric hold.
- Try to maintain body in horizontal.
- Hold until onset of pain.
- Repeat for set of 4–3–2.

Exercise 3: eccentric lowering.
- Start in position 1 shown below, slowly and in controlled manner lower upper body to position 2.
- Pull self back to position 1 using arms and repeat controlled lowering.
- Repeat 3sets × 10reps.

Exercise 4: extension control in standing.
- Stand upright with spine in neutral position.
- Hold pole with theraband attached above head.
- Slowly and in controlled manner extend backwards keeping arms and legs straight—make sure you control the position of the back.
- Go as far as you can control.
- Return to starting position and repeat 3 × 10reps.

End stage rehab

Introduce sudden changes of pace and direction in all the above exercises e.g. introduce sudden change from sideways running to straight sprint followed by high speed snake run and kicking a dead ball.

Once this can be done without pain, introduce competition altering the following variables as appropriate to the sport and individual:
- Distance covered.
- Pace and intensity.
- Patterns of movement (falling, direction changes, spinning, getting up etc.).
- Space limitations.
- Feet action (quick, fast, powerful).
- Use of ball (no carry, carry, receiving/giving pass).
- Contact.

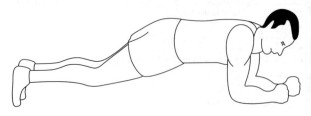

Fig. 5.5 Prone bridge.

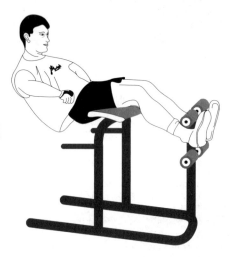

Fig. 5.6 Isometric hold.

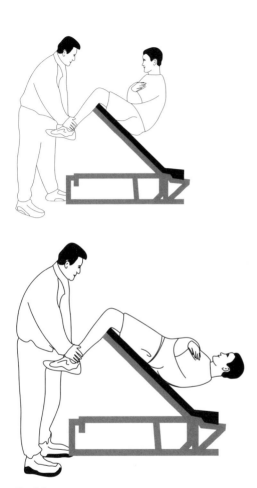

Fig. 5.7 (a), (b) Eccentric larening.

Avulsions around the ilium

The relative weakness of the growth plate at the apophysis of skeletally immature athletes predisposes them to a variety of avulsion fractures. Usually, they result from a violent eccentric muscle contraction.

Avulsion fractures of the anterior superior iliac spine (ASIS) are usually due to:
- Avulsion of the sartorius origin.
- Avulsion of the tensor fascia lata origin.

Avulsion of sartorius is usually due to sprinting. The fragment is smaller and displaced anteriorly. Tensor fascia lata avulsion is due to twisting injury. The fragment is much larger and displaced laterally.

Avulsion of anterior inferior iliac spine results from forceful flexion of the hip by the rectus femoris. Avulsion of the ischial tuberosity results from forceful contraction of the hamstrings.

History and examination
- Severe, sudden-onset, and well-localized pain over anterior superior iliac spine.
- Localized tenderness, swelling, and eventual ecchymosis.
- Posture that reduces tension on the involved muscle.
- Resisted contraction or stretch of the involved muscle worsens the pain.

Investigations
Plain radiographs, including comparison views, can usually identify the injury if the fragment is visible.

Treatment
Conservative:
- Rest.
- Analgesia.
- Comfortable positioning with protected weightbearing and gradual return to activity.
- Strengthening is begun after full, pain-free range of motion is achieved.

The periosteum and surrounding fascia often limit severe displacement. Reported disadvantages include a reduction in strength, function, and, in some patients, the formation of a painful callus.

Surgery is preferred to conservative management if:
- The size of the fragment is large enough to hold metal work.
- Displacement of the fracture fragment is ≥2cm.

Return to play
Patients should not return to competition until full strength and motion are restored.

Piriformis syndrome

The sciatic nerve exits the pelvis below the piriform muscle, and above the short external rotators. Entrapment of the nerve at this point causes piriformis syndrome[1]. In piriformis syndrome, patients usually describe cramping or aching in the buttock and/or hamstrings. The causative factors include an abnormal tenseness or spasticity of the piriformis caused either by trauma and overuse, or by muscle and nerve anomaly. In 6.2% of the population, the sciatic nerve passes through the piriformis muscle. Tumours, vascular anomalies and changes of gluteal muscles and nerves can predispose to piriformis syndrome. Post-traumatic piriformis syndrome may occur secondary to a contusion in the gluteal area. It occurs in middle-aged recreational athletes playing tennis, running, and cross country skiing.

History and examination
- Pain located maximally at the middle-upper part of the buttock during and after physical exercise.
- Pain radiates to posterior thigh, calf, outer leg, ankle, and heel. May be night pain.
- The leg may be held in semiflexion and in external rotation.

The differential diagnosis includes entrapment of the gluteal nerves, hamstring pain from entrapment of the posterior cutaneous nerve of the thigh, sciatica.

Clinical findings:
- Pinpoint tenderness on palpation at the upper middle gluteus, resisted internal-external rotation tests with straight leg may be positive.
- SLR test negative.
- Reflexes, motor functions and sensations are usually normal.
- Piriformis stretching is positive.
- Local anaesthetic infiltration test positive: pain disappears.

Investigations
- MR scan demonstrates the size and thickness of piriformis muscles, side difference, and anomalies.
- ENMG-examination may demonstrate distal radiculopathy or changes of proximal, but not lumbar nerve roots. H-reflex (A monosynaptic reflex elicited by stimulating a nerve) may be delayed in piriformis syndrome, when measured with hip in flexion, abduction and internal rotation.

Treatment
Conservative management
- Muscle relaxation.
- Stretching every 2–3 hours in either a supine or standing position with the involved hip flexed and passively adducted/internally rotated.
- Pelvic posture correction, core stabilization, hip and sacroiliac joint mobilization, strengthening of the gluteal and pelvic musculature.

- Refer to orthopaedic surgeon or pain specialist. Local anaesthetic and a steroid injection into the piriformis muscle can be useful if physiotherapy fails. Important to avoid sciatic nerve.
- Results from injection and physiotherapy may be as effective as surgical treatment.

Surgical management

- Offered after failure of conservative management.
- Piriformis muscle is divided and sciatic nerve is released.
- Light training in one month. Intensive training in 2 months.
- The results are good or excellent in 50–85% of a cases.

Technique of injection of piriformis

This injection should only be undertaken by a specialist. The description of the technique is given only to help the reader understand the anatomy. The painful piriformis muscle can be identified by palpating the buttocks or by palpating transrectally in males and transvaginally in females. A spinal needle or 25-gauge 1.5-inch needle is directly aimed at the examining finger. The location is usually through the sciatic notch and inferior to the bony margin; the most common trigger point is 1 inch lateral and caudal to the midpoint of the lateral border of the sacrum.

Reference

1 Yeoman W (1928). The relationship of arthritis of the sacro-iliac joint to sciatica. *Lancet*, ii, 1119–22.

Snapping hip syndrome

Audible snap or click that occurs on flexion and extension of the hip (coxa saltans—coxa is Latin for hip, and saltans means jumping; is a term to describe the feeling of the popping or snapping hip).

- External causes include snapping of the iliotibial band or gluteus maximus over the greater trochanter.
- Internal causes are snapping of the iliopsoas tendon over the iliopectineal eminence, over the femoral head, or over the lesser trochanter.
- Intra-articular causes include acetabular labral tear, and intra-articular loose body.

External

History and examination

This is more common than other causes of snapping hip. It occurs more often in females.

- Audible, painless snapping with a sensation of hip jumping out of place or giving way. The thickened posterior border of iliotibial band or anterior border of gluteus maximus muscle near its insertion catch the superior margin of the greater trochanter as the hip is flexed, adducted, or internally rotated causing snapping.
- Reproducible by passive hip flexion in an adducted position with the knee in extension.

Treatment

- Reassure that the hip joint is not subluxing or dislocating.
- Conservative management with rest, analgesics, NSAIDs, ice, ultrasound, phonophoresis, iontophoresisis is usually successful.
- Stretching and strengthening exercises of iliotibial band.
- Refer to orthopaedic surgeon for surgical release or Z-plasty of iliotibial band if conservative management fails.

Internal

History and examination

A less common cause of snapping hip. Snapping sensation localized to the anterior part of the groin.

- May reproduce the snapping by extending and adducting the hip from a flexed and abducted position. The iliopsoas tendon shifts from lateral to medial over the iliopectineal eminence and/or the femoral head when the hip is brought from flexion into extension.

Investigation

- Ultrasonography during hip motion may demonstrate the tendon subluxation.
- MRI scan will help demonstrate thickened tendon, and fluid in the iliopsoas bursa.
- Bursography may reproduce the symptoms associated with abnormal movement of the iliopsoas tendon and is diagnostic of internal snapping hip syndrome, but is invasive.[1]
- Local anaesthetic injection (5ml of 1% lignocaine 10mg/ml) into the iliopsoas bursa and/or around the tendon may be diagnostic.

Treatment
- Conservative management with rest, analgesics, NSAIDs, ice, ultrasound, phonophoresis, and iontophoresisis is usually successful.
- Stretching of the hip flexors and rotators, then strengthening and gradual return to sport.
- Symptoms refractory to physical therapy may be relieved by surgical lengthening of the iliopsoas tendon.

Intra–articular

History and examination
- Trauma, or synovial chondromatosis may predispose to intra–articular loose bodies.
- Labral tears may cause groin pain. Incidence is high in patients with dysplastic hips.

Investigation
- Plain radiographs help rule out bony pathology.
- MR arthrography can help confirm diagnosis.
- Arthroscopy of the hip joint may be both diagnostic and therapeutic in these patients, and is considered the gold standard.

Hamstring injury

The hamstring muscle group is prone to strains, which mostly occur near the proximal musculotendinous junction. Hamstring injuries account for 30–40% of lower limb injuries sustained in sports. The recurrence of hamstring strain is 33%. Such injuries occur commonly in sports that require rapid active knee extension (e.g. sprinting, track and field, jumping, football, rugby) and in sports where there is muscle contraction at a position of maximal muscle lengthening (e.g. martial arts, dance, water-skiing). The mechanism of injury is usually a passive stretch or a protective eccentric action (muscle develops tension while lengthening) to the hamstring muscles decelerating the lower leg. Predisposing factors for hamstring injuries include:

Extrinsic factors
- Warm up.
- Fatigue.
- Fitness level and training modalities.

Intrinsic factors
- Eccentric strength deficits (muscle unable to develop tension).
- Flexibility.
- Age.
- Joint dysfunction.
- Immobilization and rehabilitation of injured muscle.

History and examination
There may be sudden onset of sharp posterior thigh pain. This may be associated with an audible pop, resulting in immediate disability.

On examination, there may be bruising on the posterior thigh localized to the site of injury, or it may be more diffuse. There is tenderness on palpation, and muscle spasm over the hamstring musculature. In complete proximal ruptures, a palpable defect is present proximally, and the muscle belly is prominent distally.

Investigation
- Plain radiograph (to exclude bony avulsion from ischial tuberosity).
- US scan (dynamic method, useful for diagnosis and follow-up).
- MRI (better details).

Treatment
Conservative
- Rest the limb to prevent further injury.
- Ice: apply as soon as possible as it helps prevent further bleeding, swelling, and alleviates pain. Apply ice for ≤20 minutes for every 2 hours for first 48–72 hours.

Avoid direct contact of ice with skin to prevent ice burns. Crushed ice in a plastic bag, commercial cold packs, wrapping the ice in a damp towel, or bags of frozen peas are different suggested modes of applying ice.
- Compression.
- Elevation helps reduce the haematoma formation and limits tissue damage.

- Active range of motion exercises within limits of pain tolerance after 1–5 days depending on the severity of injury.
- Mobilize using crutches until pain free.

Inflammation is essential for the process of healing. NSAIDs, by their anti-inflammatory effect, may delay healing. No additive effect on healing of acute hamstring injuries was found when meclofenate or diclofenac was added to standard physiotherapeutic modalities in a double-blind placebo controlled trial[1]. Therefore, NSAIDs are not recommended in the management of acute hamstring injuries.

Physiotherapy

- Early immobilization is suggested to accelerate the formation of a granulation tissue matrix and can hasten healing.
- Prolonged complete immobilization will result in muscle atrophy, loss of strength and length, and inelastic scar formation (to be avoided).
- In the first 4 weeks following injury, physical therapy is focused on strengthening, improving range of motion (ROM), and flexibility:
  - Passive static stretching is begun.
  - Warm up the muscle tissues prior to stretching and exercising.
  - Strengthening exercises initiated by an expert therapist, within the available pain-free range of motion.
  - Later, concentric exercises with resistance, increasing gradually as tolerated.
  - The next stage is the inclusion of high-speed, low-resistance isokinetic exercises.
  - Resistance is increased gradually, while exercise speed is decreased.
  - The patient then progresses from concentric to eccentric strengthening exercises.
- After 4 weeks, stretching and strengthening exercises are continued to maintain flexibility and an adequate hamstring–to–quadriceps strength ratio (Strength testing can be performed using isokinetic exercise equipment).

A rehabilitation programme consisting of progressive agility and trunk stabilization exercises is more effective than a programme emphasizing isolated hamstring stretching and strengthening in promoting return to sports and preventing injury recurrence in athletes suffering an acute hamstring strain[2].

Surgical management

The indication for surgery in an acute hamstring strain is a complete rupture at or near the origin from the ischial tuberosity, or distally at its insertion. These should be identified clinically by a large defect or from an ischial tuberosity bone avulsion with displacement by 2cm on radiographs. In such cases, reattachment is indicated.

In chronic cases, tendinopathy results from scarring and abnormal healing. The diagnosis is clinical and confirmed by imaging (MRI). Surgical management is by longitudinal tenotomy of the tendinopathic hamstring tendon close to the insertion. The surgical results are usually good.

Return to play

- When the strength of the injured hamstring reaches 90% of the strength of the unaffected hamstring and when the patient has a full ROM.
- At least a 50–60% hamstring-to-quadriceps ratio is desired.
- Prior to return to play, sports-specific training maximizes recovery and minimizes chances for additional injury.
- Return to competition can be allowed after 20±7 days for I grade lesions, after 36±15 days for II grade lesions and after 45±14 days for III grade lesions[4].

Prevention

- Pre-exercise stretching.
- Adequate warm-up.
- Avoid block drills too early in the training season.
- Thermal pants may help reduce risk of recurrent hamstring injury[3].

Identification of the factors leading to injury and the development of appropriate preventative strategy to avoid re-injury is crucial.

Pre-season screening may identify athletes at risk due to deficits in skills, aerobic and anaerobic capability, general health, or musculoskeletal function, as these may predispose to hamstring injuries.

References

1 Reynolds JF, Noakes TD, Schwellnus MP, *et al.* (1995). Non-steroidal anti-inflammatory drugs fail to enhance healing of acute hamstring injuries treated with physiotherapy. *S Afr Med J,* **85**(6), 517–22.

2 Sherry MA, Best TM (2004). A comparison of 2 rehabilitation programs in the treatment of acute hamstring strains. *J Orthop Sports Phys Ther,* **34**(3), 116–25.

3 Upton PA, Noakes TD, Juritz JM (1996). Thermal pants may reduce the risk of recurrent hamstring injuries in rugby players. *Br J Sports Med,* **30**(1), 57–60.

4 Creta D, Nanni G, Vincentelli F (2004). Injuries of the hamstrings. The Rehabilitation of Sport Muscle and Tendon Injuries—International Congress 2004. Available at: http://www.isokinetic. com/pdf_attivita/2004/2004_02.pdf

Management of hamstring injury

Early stage hamstring injury management is the key to successful rehabilitation. Controlled mobilization should be performed within the limits of pain as soon as possible. If the early stage goals are not met, then accelerated rehabilitation may be contraindicated.

Early stage: days 1–3
Key aims
- Minimize inflammation.
- Prevent scarring.
- Minimize muscle spasm.
- Progressive loading.
- Assess risk factors.

Risk factors
Often the athlete may have one or more intrinsic risk factors, which have predisposed to hamstring injury. These should be assessed at an early stage. Common risk factors include:
- Poor general conditioning.
- Hamstring weakness/fatigue.
- Poor recovery strategies.
- Poor training periodization/inappropriate training.
- Decreased lower limb flexibility.
- Decreased neural mobility—lumbosacral plexus.
- Decreased hamstring strength/endurance.
- Poor running style:
  - Running styles that place a high load on the hamstring can cause early fatigue and an increased chance of injury.
- Poor lower limb alignment e.g. anterior rotation of pelvis:
  - Tight hip flexors.
  - Decreased strength/activation gluteal muscle.
  - Overactivity of erector spinae muscles.

General exercises
- Active knee flexion/extension: sitting off the end of a bed, keeping the pelvis in a neutral position, the athlete actively bends and straightens the knee. This exercise should be pain free. Perform 30 repetitions x 6 per day.
- Slump stretching/mobilization. This should take place within the pain free range of movement.
- Massage: lighter effleurage techniques may help minimize protective muscle spasm.
- Electrotherapy: low-level laser therapy, electrical stimulation.
- PRICE regimen.

- Cryokinetics:
  - Active hamstring movements are performed with simultaneous cryotherapy. Aim for 5–10 minutes cryotherapy, whilst performing slow and controlled active knee flexion/extension as described above. Note this exercise should be pain free.

Middle stage: days 3–14

Key aims
- Begin isometric/concentric loading.
- Begin to address/correct risk factors.
- Begin cardiovascular conditioning.

General exercises
- Isometrics: prone position, the athlete uses the uninjured leg to resist active knee flexion. This exercise should be pain free. Begin with 10 second holds x 10. Perform at the inner/middle and outer ROM.
- Concentrics: prone position, the athlete uses the uninjured leg to resist active knee flexion through the full ROM. Use the maximum amount of resistance without causing pain.
  - To progress: use therapist resistance, ankle weights, dynabands.
- Step-ups: leading with the injured leg, the athlete steps up onto a height (approx knee height), holds for a few seconds, before slowly lowering down. This movement should be performed slowly, maintaining lumbo-pelvic control at all phases.
- Lunges: leading with the injured leg. Progress to multidirectional lunges.
- Gluteal exercises:
  - Bridging. Progressing to single leg.
  - Superman/bird dog.
    —Four point kneeling, maintaining a neutral pelvis and lumbar spine, the athlete simultaneously extends the hip and knee joint of the injured leg.
    —To progress, the contralateral shoulder is simultaneously elevated through flexion.

Cardiovascular
- Cross trainer.
- Bike.
  - Aim for a progressive increase up to pre-injury heart rate/RPM levels.
    —Jogging: build to 10 minutes jogging, up to 50%.

NB. Jogging should be performed at a slow steady pace. At no stage should the athlete accelerate sharply. Jogging must be stopped immediately in the event of even mild tightness or apprehension.

Late phase: days 14–28

Key aims
- Increase eccentric loading.
- Continue to address risk factors.
- Continue with gluteal/core training.
- Begin progressive running.

Progressive loading
- Nordic (Norwegian) hamstring curls:
  - Note: these are a high load eccentric exercise. To begin with 3 sets of 4 reps may be sufficient.
  - The athlete is in a kneeling position, with a therapist/training partner holding his/her feet. Maintaining a neutral lumbar spine and pelvis, the athlete drops forward, hinging at the knee joint, using eccentric hamstring control to slowly lower themselves down into a fully prone position. Initially, most athletes will need to use their upper body to cushion them onto the ground.
  - To progress:
    —Athlete stops at various points through the range.
    —Extra resistance is used by the therapist, acting to push the athlete into a prone position.
- Hamstring flicks:
  - In a prone position, with the knee in full flexion, the athlete quickly extends the knee; the hamstrings should be activated just prior to full extension (ie. preventing locking or hyperextension at the knee).
- Wobbles:
  - In a prone position, holding the knee at 90 degrees of flexion, the athlete performs small oscillations into flexion and extension. Repeat at inner and outer ROM.
- Leg swings:
  - Standing on the uninjured side, the athlete flexes and extends the hip joint. Ensure good lumbo-pelvic control, isolating the movement to the hip. To progress, increase the speed of movement, up to 60 reps/minute.
- Leg speed/technical running drills:
  - Hip drives. Standing on the uninjured side. Maintaining good lumbo-pelvic control, the athlete quickly flexes the hip of the injured side (to 90–110 degrees flexion), with the knee in flexion and ankle in dorsi flexion. Return slowly to a neutral position.
  - Hip drive—hip extensions. As above, except from full hip flexion/knee flexion/ankle dorsiflexion, the athlete drives back into hip extension/knee extension. Again good lumbo-pelvic control is encouraged.
- Dynamic lunges.
- Single leg good mornings.

Progressive running

It is recommended that a coach/therapist/practitioner is present during all running sessions. Any deviations from normal running gait, differences in leg cadence, or subjective complaints of apprehension or tightness are indications for immediate cessation of the running session.

All sessions should begin with a 10-minute warm up:
- Progressive running:
  - Acceleration 40m maintain, 20m deceleration 40m—8 repetitions.
  - To progress the acceleration distance should be decreased with the maintenance distance increased.
- Snake/curved running: progressed as above.
- Backwards running.
- Shuttles.
- Figure of eights.
- Pick-ups/fartleks.
  - For example: From a 70% run, the athlete slows to 50%. On command (visual/verbal) they must then accelerate gradually back up to 70%, initially a long acceleration distance (e.g. 30m) is used; this distance can be decreased as the athlete progresses.
    —To progress: add defender/opposition/competition.
- Running to catch/control ball:
  - To progress:
    —Catches are more demanding, requiring faster reaction/greater leg speed.
    —Multidirectional.
    —Add competition/opponent.
  - Add decision making or a tactical component to the drill.

Return to play

Prior to beginning full training, the athlete must have achieved all preset rehab goals. In all cases the following objective measures should be equal to the contralateral side and/or preinjury data.

These should include:
- Appearance/general tone.
- Slump.
- Straight leg raise.
- Lower limb (hamstring) flexibility
- Eccentric strength:
  - Isokinetic assessment.
  - Nordic hamstring curls (number of repetitions/lumbo-pelvic control during exercise).

Field-testing
- 10m/20m/30m.
- 150's/shuttles.
- T–shuffles/agility drills.
- Vertical jump.

Obturator nerve entrapment

History and examination

The obturator nerve (L2–4) is formed in the psoas muscle and descends within the muscle, emerging from the medial border at the brim of the pelvis. The obturator nerve divides at the obturator notch into anterior and posterior divisions in the obturator foramen. The anterior division supplies the hip joint and adductor longus, brevis, and gracilis, with a sensory branch to the medial thigh. The posterior division supplies obturator internus and adductor magnus.

Entrapment of the nerve may occur within fascia as it leaves the pelvis, or by an obturator hernia or intra-pelvic mass. There is usually pain and dysaesthesia in the medial thigh, together with weakness of the adductor group, worsened by activity. Examination is often normal although there may be reduced cutaneous sensation over an area of skin along the middle of the medial thigh and/or weakness of adductors.

Investigations

Specialized neurophysiological tests or nerve blockade may confirm the diagnosis.

Treatment

Surgical release of the fascia overlying the nerve in the obturator foramen will release the entrapment. Neurolysis along the length of the nerve from the obturator foramen to the fascia between pectineus and adductor longus is required to ensure release.

Dislocation and subluxation of the hip joint

History and examination

Dislocation of the hip occurs only with considerable trauma, but subluxation may occur in adolescents with congenital hyperlaxity syndrome (or more rarely in those with significant neuromuscular impairment). Patients may describe a clunking, snapping, or popping in the groin followed by aching. Examination may be normal although usually there is hypermobility and poor pelvic girdle muscle strength.

Treatment

Reassurance, strength, and stability exercises. Thermal capsular shrinkage of the hip may be considered.

Stress fractures of the pubic rami

History and examination

Pelvic stress fractures, most frequently involving the pubic rami, account for 1–2% of stress fractures, and can be serious. They may arise due to overuse (fatigue fractures) or subnormal bone strength (insufficiency fractures).

Patients usually describe a severe, deeply felt pain in the groin and possibly the perineum, of gradual onset. The symptoms may follow an increase in training load or, occasionally, with minimal or no trauma during a long distance race, in an osteoporotic individual. Weight bearing is painful, and pain occurs at rest and at night. A sudden worsening may indicate a completion of the fracture. The patient must be advised to rest and the problem investigated urgently.

Investigations

The most common stress fracture is of the pubic rami. As with all stress fractures, the diagnosis can be made by plain X-ray after 3 weeks, but earlier on technetium bone scan or MRI scan.

Management

Rest is essential, in the expectation that the fracture will heal without complication. Patients should be non-weight bearing with crutches while symptoms persist. Athletes can participate in non-weight bearing sports when the stress fracture has settled sufficiently to allow walking.

Calcific tendinopathy of the hip

History and examination

Calcification at the site of origin of one or more muscles of the thigh, most commonly the rectus femoris, gluteus maximus, or vastus lateralis, is rare.

There may be severe groin pain and limitation of movement (due to pain), without a history of trauma. On examination, there may be pain induced global limitation of movement and/or pain on resisted testing of affected muscle groups.

Investigation

Confirmation on X-ray or ultrasound.

Treatment

Relative rest, analgesics or NSAIDs, ultrasound, shock wave therapy, and if necessary image guided local corticosteroid injection.

Acetabular labral tears

History and examination

The acetabular labrum is a thick rim of dense fibrous tissue which provides extra stability. The labrum can degenerate and tear, producing a flap which can interfere with the joint and give a deep, painful clunk during a range of activities. There is an association between labral lesions and adjacent acetabular chondral damage, and labral disruption and degenerative joint disease are frequently part of a continuum of joint pathology. On examination there may be impingement on internal rotation.

Investigations

Radiograph may show lateral marginal sclerosis in long standing cases. MR arthrography of the hip may be helpful, particulalry with lesions of the superior labrum.

Treatment

Arthroscopic trimming/repair.

Ischial (ischiogluteal) bursitis

History and examination

This may occur after a direct blow to the ischial tuberosity and cause localized pain and tenderness.

Investigation

Confirmed with ultrasound.

Treatment

Relative rest, ice, anti-inflammatories, and cushioning are usually effective. A local guided injection of corticosteroid may be necessary. Surgical excision of the bursa is rarely necessary.

Sacro-iliac joint (SIJ) disorders

History and examination

The SIJ is very stable with little joint movement. There is no single fixed axis of motion, with flexion/extension, translation, and rotation. While walking and running, the SIJs and ligaments absorb and dissipate stresses developed by twisting of the pelvis from flexion of one hip and extension of the other. Loss of mobility may cause stress fractures. There is debate as to whether the SIJ causes lower back and buttock pain in the absence of a true inflammatory sacroiliitis.

There may be joint strain or dysfunction following a direct blow to the joint, forceful torsion of the pelvis when rising from the crouched position, or sudden strong contraction of the hamstrings and/or abdominal muscles. But, beware as 'sacroiliac strains' are often subsequently found to be due to other pathologies. Forces on the sacroiliac ligaments are more likely to result in injury to the lumbosacral ligaments.

Pain may be felt in the buttock, groin, or thigh with activity and, in severe cases, at rest. Stress tests may exacerbate the pain.

Investigations

- Radiographs of the SIJ are often normal in the absence of an inflammatory process.
- Bone scans can demonstrate sacroiliitis and stress fractures at the ridges of joint surfaces.
- Where sacroiliitis is shown, it is important to look for the cause including seronegative arthropathy or pyogenic infection.

Treatment

Muscle imbalance affecting the muscles of the thigh and abdomen and coexisting abnormalities in the lumbar spine, should be addressed. Manipulation may help. A sacroiliac belt can provide some symptomatic relief. Sacroiliitis, if part of an inflammatory arthritis, should be treated with analgesics, anti-inflammatories, physiotherapy, other approaches indicated for the systemic condition, and, where necessary, image-guided local corticosteroid injection.

Injuries in children

Perthes' disease

Aetiology
- Avascular necrosis of the femoral head of unknown aetiology.

History and examination
- Presents at age 3–10, most commonly at 5–6 years.
- Boys > girls in ratio 4:1.
- May have hip, groin, or sometimes knee pain, although pain is not a feature after the early stages.
- May present with a painless limp.

Investigations
- Radiographs changes depend on the stage of disease.
- In early stages, widening of the joint space may be the only sign. This is followed by patchy sclerosis, flattening, fragmentation, and collapse of the femoral capital epiphysis.
- Bone scanning is useful in early cases, when radiographs are normal.

Treatment
- Should be referred to a paediatric orthopaedic surgeon for management.
- Treatment varies according to the amount of the femoral head involved and the age at presentation.
- Includes modifying activity, use of braces and, in severe cases, femoral osteotomy.
- Bisphosphonates may be useful in early stages.

Prognosis
- Depends on multiple factors, including age at presentation and amount of surface area involved.
- The younger the presentation(<5) the better the prognosis.
- Risk of osteoarthritis depends on irregularity of joint surface.

Slipped upper capital femoral epiphysis

- Posterior displacement of the upper femoral epiphysis on the femoral neck. It occurs in 1–3/100,000 Caucasian patients, two times more frequently in Afro-Americans, and four times more frequently in Polynesians. The male to female ratio is 2.5:1 and it occurs in girls at 11–13 years of age and in boys at 13–16 years of age. It is bilateral in 20–40% of patients and the contralateral slip occurs within 18 months of index slip. The predisposing factors include obesity, growth spurt, and endocrine abnormalities (hypothyroidism, renal rickets, pituitary def, GH def).
- Displacement of the epiphysis before skeletal maturity.
- Associated with delayed maturation and growth-plate stress (secondary to obesity).
- Hormonal factors may also play a role.

Classification
- Based on physeal stability:
  - *Stable*: able to weight bear with or without crutches.
  - *Unstable*: unable to weight bear, fracture-like symptoms.
- Based on duration:
  - *Acute*: <3 weeks (follows trauma).
  - *Chronic*: >3 weeks.
  - *Acute or chronic.*
- Based on displacement:
  - Mild.
  - Moderate.
  - Severe.

History and examination
Sudden or insidious onset of pain and limp. At rest, the lower limb is held in external rotation. On further flexion, the lower limb goes into further external rotation. Internal rotation is restricted.
- Boys > girls (2:1).
- Overweight pubertal boy with pain and a limp.
- Pain localized to the hip, groin, or knee.
- Onset of pain usually gradual but may be acute.
- Limitation of hip abduction, flexion, and internal rotation.

Investigations
- Radiographs demonstrate slip, which is graded from 1–3. AP and frog leg lateral views. The severity of the slip is graded by the head-shaft angle on frog leg lateral views. A mild slip is <30°, moderate is 30°–60°, and severe is >60°. Subtle changes seen on radiographs before slip occurs include widening and irregularity of epiphysis.
- CT scan: assesses the posterior displacement of the epiphysis and is useful for planning osteotomies.
- MRI helps early detection of avascular necrosis of the femoral epiphysis.

Treatment
- Orthopaedic referral for consideration of open reduction and stabilization is required.
- Primary goal is to prevent further slip and promote closure of the physis. *In situ* pinning for mild and moderate slip. Osteotomy for severe slip. Various techniques are described.

Complications
- Chondrolysis.
- Avascular necrosis.
- Subtrochanteric fracture.
- Osteoarthritis.

Prognosis
- Good if condition treated promptly with surgical stabilization.
- If untreated, may result in avascular necrosis or premature osteoarthritis.

Irritable hip

Unknown aetiology but thought to be a transient synovitis, which may have viral or autoimmune precipitant.

History and examination

- Child (usually aged 2–8) presents with pain or limp lasting from a few days to one week.
- Restricted hip ROM due to pain.
- Hip quadrant test (adduction, internal rotation and compression with hip and knee flexed) positive.

Investigations

- Diagnosis of exclusion.
- Radiographs, bone scans, and MRIs are normal.
- FBC usually normal—may show mild elevation of WCC and ESR.
- Important to exclude other more serious conditions such as Perthes' disease, slipped upper capital femoral epiphysis and septic arthritis.

Treatment and prognosis

- Rest and analgesia.
- May recur.
- Prognosis is good, with no known long-term complications.

Avulsion fractures

- Result of acute traction episode of the involved apophysis (by rectus femoris, hamstrings, or iliopsoas).
- Same injury mechanism in adult would produce muscle tear.

History and examination

- History of sudden onset of pain associated with a rapid eccentric contraction of the involved muscle-tendon unit, eg, sprinting in the case of rectus femoris, or hurdling in the case of the hamstrings.

Investigation

Radiographs of involved apophysis is diagnostic.

Treatment

- Depends on amount of separation and the site involved.
- Stretching and a graduated strengthening program combined with local physiotherapy.
- Graduated return to sport when symptoms have resolved.
- Surgical reattachment usually not necessary unless the bony fragment is displaced more than 2cm.
- Good prognosis with adequate rehabilitation.

Traction apophysitis of the ischial tuberosity

- Aetiology is similar to other traction apophysitis.
- Repetitive traction of the hamstrings tendon at its origin at the ischial tuberosity.

History and examination

12–16-year-old athlete involved in activities requiring forced hip flexion such as dancing, soccer, hurdling, and long-jump.

Investigations
- Clinical.
- No tests required unless avulsion fracture suspected.

Treatment and prognosis
- Same management principles as traction apophysitis in other regions.
- Prognosis is good.

Knee

History

If acute
- Mechanism of injury—e.g. twisting or in contact.
- Degree of pain and disability—able to weight bear/continue.
- Audible 'pop' or 'crack' at time of injury.
- Swelling—site and speed of onset—e.g. immediate or the next day.
- Site of symptoms.
- Symptoms since—pain, giving way, instability or locking.
- Referral of pain.
- Past injury history.

If insidious
- Specific location of pain.
- Aggravating factors—e.g. stairs or sitting for long periods.
- Night pain.
- Associated crepitus or clicking.
- Locking, swelling, or giving way.
- Past injury history.
- Past medical history.
- Any other joints affected.

Examination

Inspection

The knee consists of two joints:

- Tibio-femoral.
- Patello-femoral.

In standing

Look for evidence of asymmetry or biomechanical abnormality, e.g.:

- Leg length.
- Scoliosis—symmetry of body creases.
- Squinting patellae or malalignment.
- Weight held equally through both lower limbs.
- Muscle wasting—especially quadriceps.
- Scars or bruising.
- Loss of contour around patella, suggestive of effusion.
- Hyperrecurvatum of knees.
- Pronation/supination of feet.
- Swelling in popliteal fossa.

Functional tests

Whilst standing, functional tests such as squatting, lunging, hopping, stepping, or eccentric exercises can be assessed in an attempt to reproduce symptoms.

Palpation

In supine

- Assess for evidence of effusion, using fluid shift technique.
- Patella—assess position, angulation, freedom of movement, retropatellar crepitus, discomfort, and apprehension.
- Medial and lateral retinaculum for tenderness.
- Quadriceps muscles, tendon, and patellar tendon for tenderness or thickening.
- Tibial tubercle, check for swelling and any posterior sag compared to the other side.
- Fat pad.
- Medial and lateral tibio-femoral joint lines.
- Medial and lateral collateral ligaments.
- Lateral femoral condyle, including ilio-tibial band.
- Head of fibula and superior tibio-fibular joint.

In prone

- Hamstrings.
- Popliteal fossa for evidence of cyst.
- Medial head of gastrocnemius.

Active and passive movements

- Range of active movements should be −5° to 140° (i.e. hyperextension to full flexion).
- Apply gentle pressure at the end of range of active movement to assess joint 'end-feel' and passive joint movement. Note any hardness or unnatural springiness, as well as any discomfort.

- Assess hamstring flexibility at 90° of hip and knee flexion.
- Assess the subject's hip joints and straight leg raise to eliminate any possibility of referred pain, particularly in adolescents, where slipped upper femoral epiphysis should always be considered.
- If hyperrecurvatum of the knees is noted in standing or excessive hyperextension in supine, consider checking for more generalized hypermobility syndrome.

Resisted movements

- Check for pain and/or weakness on resisted knee extension (rectus femoris and quadriceps).
- Check for pain and/or weakness on resisted knee flexion (hamstrings).

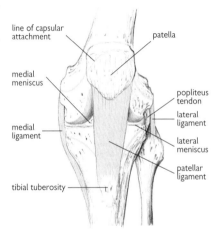

Fig. 6.1 Knee joint: anterior view showing capsule attachments and ligaments. Reproduced with permission from MacKinnon P and Morris J (2005). *Oxford Textbook of Functional Anatomy Vol 1*. Oxford University Press, Oxford. ©2005.

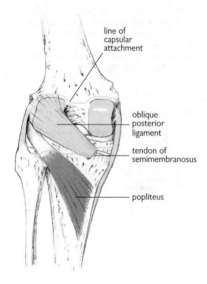

Fig. 6.2 Knee joint: posterior view showing oblique posterior ligament and attachment of popliteus. Reproduced with permission from MacKinnon P and Morris J (2005). *Oxford Textbook of Functional Anatomy Vol 1.* Oxford University Press, Oxford. ©2005.

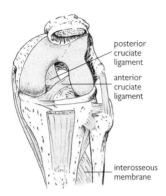

Fig. 6.3 Cruciate ligaments, anterior view. Reproduced with permission from MacKinnon P and Morris J (2005). *Oxford Textbook of Functional Anatomy Vol 1.* Oxford University Press, Oxford. ©2005.

Special tests

Medial and lateral collateral ligaments

- Resist inward (medial) and outward (lateral) movements at the knee.
- Ligaments are taut in full knee extension and are best assessed by valgus and varus forces applied by the examiner whilst the leg is supported in approximately 30° of knee flexion.

Ligament injury grading

- Grade 1 pain felt on stressing ligament but no laxity.
- Grade 2 (partial tear) pain and some laxity at site of injury, but a solid 'end-feel' at the limit of range.
- Grade 3 (complete tear) pain and laxity with no 'end-feel' at limit of range of movement. Clinically it may be difficult to distinguish between grades 2 and 3 due to pain-induced muscle spasm.

Anterior and posterior cruciate ligaments

The Anterior cruciate ligament (ACL)

- Prevents the tibia from extending forward from the femur and helps control pivoting movements.
- Often injured in twisting or hyperextension movements.

The Posterior cruciate ligament (PCL)

- Less commonly injured than the ACL.
- Limits backward movement of the tibia on the femur.

ACL and PCL can be assessed clinically in two ways:

Anterior and posterior draw tests

- Subject sits with knees bent at 90°.
- Posterior sag is excluded by examiner inspecting tibial tubercle from the side, to check for any loss of prominence, which may suggest a lax PCL.
- The examiner sits on the foot of the subject on the side to be tested. The hamstrings must be relaxed to allow the ACL to be stressed.
- Gentle traction is applied to the tibia forward (to assess ACL, called the anterior draw test). The tibia can then be gently pushed backwards (to assess the PCL, posterior draw test).
- Laxity and 'end-feel' are again important factors.
- If indicated, the posterior draw test can be repeated with the foot externally rotated. This will test for any evidence of postero-lateral corner disruption.

Lachman's test

- A useful test as a positive result is less reliant upon the subject not having any hamstring contraction as at the time of the draw tests.
- The subject sits on the couch and the examiner holds the thigh firmly, and flexes the knee to approximately 15°. The tibia can then be drawn forward or backward to assess cruciate integrity.

Many sports people have well-developed quadriceps musculature. If the examiner finds that Lachman's test is difficult to perform because if this, then the examiner's knee can be placed under the thigh of the subject to support the knee in 15° flexion and allow the tibia to be drawn to and fro.

Pivot shift test

- The knee is held in full extension and the tibia internally rotated.
- As the knee is flexed, a valgus force is applied to the joint.
- This tests for a deficient ACL.
- A positive test will reveal a 'clunk' as the lateral femoral condyle (dislocated in internal rotation in an ACL deficient knee) relocates.

Menisci

Medial and lateral meniscal injury will often be suspected from the history. There are several methods of meniscal assessment, but one of the more reliable is:

McMurray's test

- A flexion-rotation test, with the knee being flexed fully and extended, whilst internal and external rotation pressure is placed upon it.
- Positive tests are obtained with pain and/or palpable internal 'clinking' felt by the examiner's hand on the joint line.

Ilio-tibial band (ITB)

Can be assessed for tightness by:

Ober's test

- The subject lies on their side with the lower leg flexed at the hip. The upper leg is then extended at the hip with the examiner's hand resting on the pelvis to keep that neutral. The examiner then adducts the extended hip and the subject's knee should comfortably reach the couch. If the ITB is tight, the pelvis will move out of neutral or the knee will extend before it reaches the couch.
- Tightness of the ITB can be confirmed on modified Thomas' test when the relaxed leg falls into external rotation at the hip.
- ITB friction syndrome can be diagnosed by pressure from the examiner's thumb over the subject's lateral femoral condyle while the knee is repeatedly flexed and extended from 0–30°.

Investigation of knee injuries

Plain X-ray

Acute to exclude fractures:
- Tibial plateau.
- Patellar stress.
- ACL avulsion.
- Osteochondral.

Skyline views can be obtained to assess the retro-patellar surface.

Non-acute:
Osteoarthritis (weightbearing).

MRI scan

If suspected:
- Meniscal pathology.
- ACL/PCL tear.
- Articular cartilage damage.
- Patellar tendinpathy.

'Bone bruising' may be seen on MRI scans after significant knee injuries. Findings are sub-chondral bone oedema in the affected part.

Ultrasound

- Invaluable to assess patellar tendon pathology, particularly if degeneration (shows as areas of hypoechogenicity) or tear is suspected.
- Also useful to assess popliteal cysts or bursitis.

Arthroscopy

Still sometimes used to confirm a clinical diagnosis, but less so since the advent of MRI.

Medial collateral ligament (MCL)

History and examination

- MCL is a strong band of tissue on medial aspect of knee.
- Resists valgus strain.
- Often injured in football, rugby, and skiing.
- Mechanism of injury—any forceful movement of the lower leg outward at the knee or a hard blow to the outside of the lower thigh, which causes the knee to buckle.
- MCL is closely associated with the medial meniscus and the two structures are often injured in combination.
- Any forceful rotational element, in addition to a valgus strain can rupture MCL, medial meniscus, and anterior cruciate—a severe injury described as O'Donoghue's Triad.
- Symptoms include pain, mild to moderate swelling on the medial aspect of the knee, joint effusion (not immediate) and feeling of instability (like a 'wobbly' table leg).
- Injuries to MCL are graded 1 to 3 according to severity (see 'Knee examination').

Treatment

Most MCL injuries are treated by rehabilitation after initial 'PRICE' management. MCL injuries that occur in association with meniscal or cruciate damage are more likely to require surgical repair.

Rehabilitation after medial collateral ligament sprain (grade 2)

Time to return to function: 4–6 weeks.

Early stage: days 1–7
Key aims
- Maintain ROM—flexion and extension.
- Prevent vastus medialis (VM) inhibition/weakening/atrophy.
- Encourage heel-toe gait pattern.
- Early mobilization.

Strengthening/recruitment
- Static quads (with focus on activating VM).
- Simultaneous ankle dorsiflexion/glut recruitment may aid in activating the VM.
- Straight leg raise.
- Inner range quads:
  - With a ball under knee, the athlete moves his/her knee into full extension.

Mobility/stretching
- Heel slides:
  - Athlete flexes and extends the knee joint though the full pain free ROM.
- Static hamstring stretching: often the most comfortable position post medial ligament injury is 10–15° flexion, therefore regular hamstring stretching is important to minimize the degree of secondary hamstring tightness.

Proprioception/gait
- Weight transfers:
  - In standing, the athlete slowly transfers weight on to the injured leg.
- Heel-toe gait:
  - In the initial stages (days 1–5) crutches may be needed.
- Hydrotherapy:
  —Water at level of sternum:
  —Walking using heel-toe gait.
  —Weight transfers (as described above).
  —Single leg standing.
  —Mini squats.
  —Knee flexion and extension in standing.

Electrotherapy
- Electrical stimulation: the VM is stimulated using low frequency electric current.
- EMG biofeedback: reserved for cases of extreme VM inhibition.
- PRICE regimen should be initiated immediately after injury.
- Before moving onto the middle stages of rehabilitation the athlete must have reached all goals during week 1. The key milestones that MUST be reached by the end of week one are:
- Good quads recruitment with minimal inhibition of the VM.

- Ability to comfortably transfer weight onto the injured side.
- Full knee extension.

Middle stage: weeks 2–3

Key aims
- Enhance joint positional sense/proprioception.
- Increase strength/ROM/mobility.
- Progress cardiovascular exercises.

Mobility/strengthening/proprioceptive exercises
- Weight transfers: standing on both feet, with weight predominantly on the uninjured side. Within the limits of pain, he/she transfers weight on to the injured side. This should progress, until it is comfortable to stand solely on the injured side.
- Single leg standing/balance: standing on the injured side, the athlete balances, minimizing the number of touch downs. Progress to eyes closed.

Once the athlete is able to stand comfortably on one leg with his/her eyes closed, more advanced proprioceptive training can begin.

Single leg standing
- Throw/catch ball.
- Vary type of throw e.g. underarm, overhead, side pass, chest pass.
- Vary the direction of the pass received e.g. in front, from side, overhead.
- Vary type of ball e.g. tennis ball, medicine ball.

Sprinting action (upper body)
- Keeping control through the pelvis, the athlete drives arms forward and back as if he/she were running. To progress, the speed of the arm drives is increased, whilst maintaining balance.
- Upper body mirroring: athlete must match the upper body movements of therapist.
- Increase complexity/speed of movements.

Dumbbell raises
- Progress from basic movements (bicep curl) to multijoint movement patterns (sword draw).
- Bodyblade drills.
- With light manual perturbation from therapist/training partner.
- Fitter exercises.

Single leg standing on dynamic surface e.g. mini trampoline (rebounder), wobble board, balance pad/cushion, folded towel.

Progress as for basic single leg stands.

Progressive strengthening
This requires near full ROM, in particular through DF.
- Mini squats:
  - Ensuring an equal distribution of weight, the athlete should perform a 50% squat (to 45° knee flexion)

- Drop squats:
  - As for a mini squat, except the speed is increased whilst maintaining control.
- Single leg squats.
- Lunges:
  - Progress to multidirectional lunges.

All these exercises can be progressed by increasing the demand on the neuromuscular system e.g. the athlete must perform a single leg squat on a dynamic surface.

Testing
Strength
A measurement of isokinetic knee flexion or extension might be the gold standard, at this stage. However there are a number of simple tests that can act as a good benchmark.
- Number of heel raises/min (compare to uninjured leg).
- Number of calf raises/min (compare to uninjured leg).

Balance/proprioception—as for ankle rehabilitation
- Single leg stand.
- Single leg stand with eyes closed.
- Single leg stand with eyes closed and neck extended.
- Wobble board.

If the athlete looses balance during the test they must tap the ground with the uninjured foot. The number of touch downs/minute are recorded.

Cardiovascular
Bike/cross trainer/upper body ergometer.

End stage: weeks 3–6
To progress to the end stages of rehabilitation, the athlete must have full painfree knee flexion, a good baseline of strength through knee flexion and extension, be able to perform complex proprioceptive exercises in a pain free state and have good lumbopelvic/lower body control and alignment during squatting/advanced proprioceptive exercises.

As for ankle rehabilitation, the end stages of rehabilitation, the focus should become less joint specific and more sports specific.

Strength and conditioning
This may be progressed as follows:
- Squat.
- Deadlift.
- Hang clean.
- Clean.
- Snatch.

Ideally, the athlete should begin using the bar bell only. Their form and alignment should be monitored by a training partner or strength and conditioning coach. The weight should be increased accordingly, building to their pre-injury levels.

Running

Prerequisites:
- Full ankle ROM.
- Subject able to perform march walks/advanced proprioception with good control in a pain free state.
- Straight line running:
  - Light jog, building from 30%–50%.
    —Build up to 10–30 mins.
  - Begin progressive running:
    —This should be done on a flat surface, with cones dividing acceleration/maintenance/deceleration stages.
    —For the first session: athletes should accelerate from a standing start, up to 60% over the first 30m. They should then aim to maintain this pace over the next 30m, before decelerating slowly to a complete stop).
    —Build to 90%.
    —This can be progressed by decreasing the acceleration distance, and increasing the maintenance distance. For example:

Acceleration	Maintenance	Deceleration
20m	40m	20m
10m	30m	20m
10m	40m	20m

- Curved running.
- Figure of eight running.
- Shuttles (doggies).
- Run stops:
  - From a 60% run the athlete must come to a complete stop within 5 steps:
    —To progress increase the speed of the run/minimize the number of steps.
- Run to lunge:
  - From a 60% run the athlete must come to a complete stop in a lunge position.
- 45° cuts.
- 90° cuts.
- Spins:
  - Running at 50% the athlete must spin 360° without slowing down.
- T shuffles.
- Ladder/cone agility drills.

Plyometric exercises

Throughout all plyometric exercises, the athlete is encouraged to keep a 'soft' knee, using hips, knees, and ankles to cushion the impact. The athletes ability to avoid 'corkscrewing' by keeping good pelvic, hip, knee, and toe alignment will act as a good guide for their progress.

- 2–1 (two legs to one).
  - Standing in a stationary position the athlete jumps vertically to land on the injured side.
- Hop scotch:
  - This involves multiple 2–1's, whilst moving forwards.
- 90°/180°/270°/360° rotations:
  - From a stationary position, the athlete jumps vertically and turns 90° clockwise/anticlockwise before landing.
- Jump–land (from height).
  - Using two foot landing.
  - Athlete rotates 45° in air before landing.
    —Add 90°/180° rotation.
  - Single leg landing.
  - Landing on dynamic surface.
  - Immediately catching a ball on landing.
  - Therapist adds a light perturbation on landing.

Field testing

If available, field test results should be compared with pre season, or normative data. Useful test might include:

- 10m/20m/30m sprint times.
- 150 test.
- T-shuffle agility drill.
- Vertical jump.
- Standing broad jump:
  - Jumping forward from two feet to land on two feet.
  - Jumping forwards from injured foot landing on two feet.
  - Jumping forwards from injured foot/landing on injured foot.
- Lateral broad jump:
  - Jumping laterally R or L and progress as for standing broad jump.

Lateral collateral ligament (LCL)

History and examination

- Thinner than the MCL, a cord-like structure on the lateral aspect of the knee.
- Resists varus strain.
- LCL is separate from the lateral meniscus and the two are not so often injured in combination as on the medial aspect.
- LCL can be injured in combination with cruciate ligaments.
- Mechanism of injury—varus loading of knee and hyperextension.
- Postero-lateral complex* injury can produce significant functional impairment and instability.

Treatment

- LCL can be repaired or augmented, but this is usually in association with surgery to the other damaged tissues.

---

* Postero-lateral complex consists of the LCL, arcuate ligament, lateral head of gastrocnemius, biceps femoris tendon, and musculo-tendinous junction of popliteus muscle.

Anterior cruciate ligament (ACL)

History and examination

- ACL is the primary restraint for anterior movement of the tibia on the femur.
- Also acts to stop antero-lateral rotation of the knee.
- Mechanism of injury is valgus force with a twisting motion (pivoting) or hyperextension of the knee.
- Injury usually occurs in contact situations, but non-contact ACL is frequently reported, particularly in females.
- Females are thought to be particularly prone to non-contact ACL injuries. Women playing basketball and soccer are 2–6 times more likely than men to sustain ACL rupture.
- Theories as to why women are so at risk include:
  - Women having a smaller intercondylar notch and ACL than men.
  - Lower limb mechanics.
  - Hormonal variations.
  - Joint laxity.
- Collateral ligament and meniscal damage often also occurs at time of cruciate injury.
- Symptoms of ACL rupture include immediate swelling of the knee joint due to haeamarthrosis, and a 'pop' which may be heard at the time of contact.
- Haemarthrosis is very painful. With the above history, there is a 90% chance of an ACL tear.
- Clinically, there will be reduction of extension, and signs of ACL laxity (see p.212).Pivot shift test is often positive, but may be difficult to perform on an injured athlete. Medial joint line tenderness may suggest medial meniscus injury.
- ACL laxity on clinical examination (see p.212) does not mean that the knee is necessarily unstable.
- Recurrent episodes of instability will increase the risk of developing accelerated osteoarthritis of the knee.

Treatment

ACL repair

Most individuals involved in sports which involve pivoting, will require surgical reconstruction of a torn ACL, if they wish to continue in their sport.

Repair of an ACL tear is indicated if:
- There is associated meniscal or MCL tear.
- High level athletes (especially in pivoting sports).
- Lower level participants who wish to pursue sports which involve pivoting.
- Children/adolescents (giving way can cause significant damage to the joint).
- The knee remains unstable (i.e. gives way) after completion of rehabilitation protocol.
- Occupational factors (e.g armed forces or police).

The aim of surgery to repair a torn ACL is to mimic the functional anatomy of the ligament. ACL repair can be undertaken using many techniques, although primary repair is not usually successful and currently the most commonly used reconstruction techniques involve harvesting the:

- Semitendinosus and gracilis tendons.
- Middle third of the patellar tendon.
- The method of choice varies between specialist knee surgeons, and results appear to be very similar, although patellar tendon repairs have a higher incidence of post-operative anterior knee pain.
- The optimum time for ACL reconstruction is thought to be approximately 3 weeks post-injury, unless earlier repair is indicated by the clinical condition.
- There is no evidence that ACL repair reduces the long term incidence of osteoarthritis of the knee.

ACL rehabilitation

- Standard protocols for ACL reconstruction post surgery, or as a conservative treatment approach have changed significantly over recent years.
- Early mobilization with brace protection allows commencement of strengthening and proprioceptive exercises within days, rather than the original periods of weeks or even months.
- With modern rehabilitation, return to sport is now usually possible (90%+) at 6 months post-operatively.

Posterior cruciate ligament (PCL)

History and examination

- Less common than ACL injuries.
- PCL tears constitute less than 2% of acute knee injuries.
- PCL is the primary restraint for posterior movement of the tibia on the femur.
- Also acts as restraint of external rotation.
- Mechanism of injury involves falling on a bent knee, hyperextension of the knee, or torn with the ACL via a violent twisting movement.
- Postero-lateral complex may be involved in PCL tears.
- Usually minimal swelling on examination. Posterior sag of the tibia may be seen.

Treatment

- Isolated PCL tears can generally be managed conservatively using a predominantly quadriceps strengthening programme.
- Surgical reconstruction is indicated if there is associated postero-lateral complex damage (rotatory instability).
- PCL tears usually lead to long term osteoarthritis.

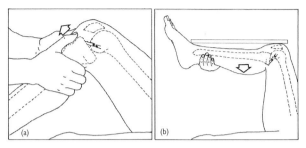

Fig. 6.4 (a) Anterior 'drawer' test; (b) 'sag' test.

Meniscal injuries

History and examination

- Mechanism of acute injury involves a violent rotation of the knee.
- Tears may also occur without significant trauma due to repeated small injuries to the cartilage or degeneration of the tissue in older patients.
- Medial meniscus often injured in combination with MCL.
- Lateral meniscus is more likely to be damaged in isolation from the LCL, and is prone to degeneration secondary to biomechanical abnormalities.
- Meniscal tears are typically associated with pain along medial or lateral joint line of the knee.
- Mild to moderate joint effusion is noted.
- Symptoms of clicking, catching or locking of knee (the latter in extension rather than flexion) may be present.
- Knee may tend to give way.
- History often strongly suggestive of diagnosis.
- Cystic swelling of meniscus may be present at joint line.

Articular cartilage injury

History and examination

- Can occur in association with cruciate or MCL tears, patellar dislocation, post menisectomy or in isolation.
- Medial femoral condyle often affected in ACL tears.
- Lateral tibial condyle and retro-patellar surface also commonly affected areas.

Investigations

- Diagnosed on MRI scan or at arthroscopy.
- Pain and swelling are usually acute symptoms.

Treatment

Articular cartilage receives its blood supply from sub-chondral bone. Healing is therefore slow and treatments include:

- Microfracture (drilling or using a curved awl to encourage healing with fibrocartilage from the sub-chondral area).
- Chondrocyte implantation.

Success of these procedures is greatly aided by correction of any existing biomechanical abnormalities.

Anterior knee pain

This is one of the commonest presenting symptoms in sport and exercise medicine. A precise diagnosis may be difficult and the term anterior knee pain describes symptoms without a specific cause identified.

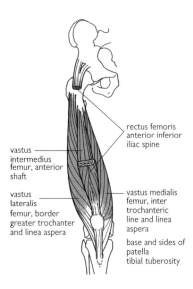

rectus femoris
anterior inferior
iliac spine

vastus
intermedius
femur, anterior
shaft

vastus
lateralis
femur, border
greater trochanter
and linea aspera

vastus medialis
femur, inter
trochanteric
line and linea
aspera

base and sides of
patella
tibial tuberosity

Fig. 6.5 Quadriceps femoris. Reproduced with permission from MacKinnon P and Morris J (2005). *Oxford Textbook of Functional Anatomy Vol 1.* Oxford University Press, Oxford. ©2005.

Patellar dislocation

History and examination
- Usually a lateral displacement onto the lateral femoral condyle.
- Often traumatic and associated with haemarthrosis.
- Also in young girls with predisposing factors such as lower limb malalignments and generalised hypermobility.

Treatment
- Treatment aims to reduce the risk of recurrence with vastus medialis strengthening, although recurrent episodes will require surgery.

Hoffa's syndrome

History and examination
- Also known as fat pad impingement.
- Very painful, especially either side of the patellar tendon.
- Mechanism is usually a hyperextension injury.
- Haemarthosis often present.

Treatment
- Treat to reduce inflammation and taping if inferior tilting of patella is present.

Ilio-tibial band friction syndrome (ITBFS)

History and examination
- Also called 'runners'knee'.
- Caused by friction of the ilio-tibial band (ITB) on the lateral femoral epicondyle (usually at less than 30° of knee flexion.
- Causes pain over lateral aspect of knee during a run, especially on a cambered course.
- Tightness of the ITB may be present on Ober's test.
- Abnormal biomechanics (e.g. leg length discrepancy), excessive training load, downhill and distance running are other predisposing factors.
- Usually associated with bursitis at the site of pain.

Investigation
Diagnosis usually on clinical findings.

Treatment
- Non steroidal anti-inflammatory drugs (NSAIDs).
- Myofascial tension massage to ITB.
- ITB stretching.
- Corticosteroid injection if bursitis present.
- Correction of biomechanical abnormalities/training errors.

Patello-femoral pain (syndrome)

- Often misnamed chondromalacia patella.
- Usually insidious onset, but can occur acutely.
- Vague, aching pain over anterior aspect of knee.
- Aggravated by activity especially distance running, squatting, lunging, going up or down stairs, or sitting for long periods.
- Patient may describe 'clicking' or 'grating' behind the patella on knee movement.
- Knee may give way due to pain and quadriceps inhibition.
- Clinical features may include tenderness in the retro- or infra-patellar areas, a small effusion, crepitus and stiffness of patellar movement, and wasting of vastus medialis obliquus (VMO).
- There may be signs of squinting patellae, hyperrecurvatum, tibial torsion, or hyperpronation in standing.
- Usual causes are:
  - Overuse (excessive loading of patello-femoral joint—PFJ).
  - Lower limb malalignment—squinting patellae and femoral anteversion, hyperpronation (↑ PFJ forces).
  - Patellar maltracking (↓ PFJ contact area).

Patellar tracking

- During knee flexion, the patella moves from lateral to medial to travel within the intercondylar notch of the femur at end of range.
- The movement of the patella is dependent upon passive and active restraints.
- Any imbalance of these restraints is most likely to cause the patella to track more laterally, and during episodes of loading, patello-femoral symptoms may arise as a result.
- Some typical causes of this so-called patellar maltracking are:
  - Tightness of passive restraints (ITB, lateral retinaculum).
  - Weakness of active restraints (VMO).
  - Weakness of gluteus medius muscles, leading to increased internal rotation at the hips.
  - Muscle tightness—hamstrings and quadriceps.

Note: if patello-femoral pain occurs on sitting, then it is unlikely to be caused by maltracking. Retro-patellar pressure is more likely.

The 'Q' angle

- Refers to the angle at the junction between two lines drawn from the anterior superior iliac spine to the middle of the patella and a line drawn to the same point from the tibial tubercle. (Normal is less than 20° and is increased in femoral anteversion).
- A greater than normal angle is associated with patellar maltracking.
- Females tend to have a greater 'Q' angle than males, which will also predispose them to patellar maltracking, and therefore patello-femoral pain.

Investigation
Diagnosis usually on clinical findings.

Treatment

Primary aim is to attempt to correct any abnormal biomechanics:

- Manual treatment and stretching of ITB, hamstrings, gastrocnemius and rectus femoris.
- Patellar taping to correct any malposition/tilt—can reduce pain by up to 50%.
- VMO strengthening (± biofeedback).
- Gluteus medius strengthening.
- Orthotics to correct hyperpronation.
- Proprioception.
- Modification of training regime to avoid overuse.
- Surgery for patello-femoral pain syndrome is not common due to improved rehabilitation techniques.

Patellar tendinopathy

History and examination

- Also known as 'jumper's knee'.
- Overuse injury.
- Underlying pathology is a degenerative tendinosis, not an inflammatory tendonitis.
- Commonest site is at the deep part of the tendon attachment to the inferior pole of the patella.
- Main complaint is of anterior knee pain aggravated by jumping, bounding, or hopping.
- Insidious onset usually, but tears can present acutely.
- Eccentric contraction usually reproduces symptoms.

Investigations

Ultrasound and MRI scanning are both very effective at confirming diagnosis.

Treatment

- Often very prolonged.
- Physiotherapy—transverse frictions and progressive strengthening to include eccentric exercises.
- Correction of biomechanical abnormalities/training errors.
- Surgery is rarely indicated and should only be considered after intensive rehabilitation.

Osgood–Schlatter disease

History and examination
- Commonest traction apophysitis.
- Affects tibial tubercle.
- Boys > girls (4:1).
- Presents between ages 10 and 14 (earlier in girls).
- Insidious onset of anterior knee pain (sometimes bilateral) in child involved in running and jumping sport.
- Pain worse during and after activity.
- Difficulty kneeling.

Clinical findings
- Tenderness ± localized swelling over tibial tubercle.
- Quadriceps may appear wasted, depending on the duration of the symptoms.
- May be some restriction in knee flexion.
- Pain may be reproduced by resisted knee extension from the flexed position.
- May be associated biomechanical factors contributing to the condition, such as hyperpronation or lateral patella tilt or subluxation.

Investigations
- Not usually required.
- If performed, X-ray will show overlying soft tissue swelling (diagnostic) and may demonstrate fragmentation of the tibial tubercle apophysis.
- Only indications for X-ray in this group of children are:
  - If the diagnosis is in doubt.
  - If symptoms persist and calcification is suspected.
  - If an avulsion of the tibial tubercle is suspected.

Treatment
- Depends on the stage at presentation.
- Child who has pain with daily living activities will need to avoid running and jumping until the pain subsides.
- Children with minimal symptoms may be able to continue some running and jumping activities at a reduced level.
- Quadriceps flexibility program to ↓ traction force on TT.
- Biomechanical abnormalities such as hyperpronation and patella malalignment should be corrected with exercise programme, patella taping, and orthotics.
- Quadriceps strengthening.
- Gradual resumption activity.

Prognosis
- Usually very good.
- In about 5% of cases, calcification can develop adjacent to the tibial tubercle, which causes persistence of symptoms and inability to kneel and may require surgical resection.
- Important to reassure child and parents that this condition does not cause long-term disability but can be troublesome over one or two seasons during periods of rapid growth.

Sinding–Larsen and Johannson disease ('jumper's knee')

History and examination

- Traction apophysitis affecting inferior pole of the patella.
- Less common than Osgood–Schlatter disease but similar presentation.
- Pain localized to inferior pole of the patella.
- Gradual onset of anterior knee pain exacerbated by activities that load the flexed knee, such as running and jumping.
- Focal tenderness inferior pole of the patella.
- Swelling rarely present.
- Resisted knee extension from flexed position usually reproduces the pain.
- Biomechanical factors such as hyperpronation, femoral anteversion and patellar misalignment may be present.

Investigation

Not required.

Treatment

- Similar to that in Osgood–Schlatter disease.
- Prognosis is good.

Juvenile osteochondritis dissecans

- Probably results from combination of minor repetitive trauma and microvascular compromise affecting the subchondral bone and articular cartilage.
- Bone becomes sclerotic, fragmented, and loose bodies may form.

History and examination

- More common in boys than girls.
- Average age at diagnosis of 13.
- Present with knee swelling ± pain.
- May or may not have history of injury.
- May give history of locking secondary to loose body.
- A differential diagnosis is inflammatory arthropathy.

Clinical findings

- Effusion.
- Tenderness usually localized to medial joint line.
- Quadriceps wasting if symptoms prolonged.

Investigations

- X-ray—look for irregularity. Medial femoral condyle 75%, lateral femoral condyle 20%, patella and trochlear groove 5%.
- May also see loose body.
- If X-ray is normal but clinical history suggests OCD an MRI should be performed to confirm the diagnosis.

Treatment

- Conservative treatment appropriate if articular cartilage intact.
- If loose bodies present, arthroscopy and removal or reattachment of the loose body is indicated.

Prognosis

- Depends on site and size of the defect and age at presentation.
- Closer to skeletal maturity child is, poorer the prognosis.

Bipartite patella and patellofemoral pain syndrome

- Bipartite patella results when secondary ossification centres at supero-lateral aspect of the patella fail to unite.
- May result from excessively tight lateral patellar retinaculum.

History and examination

- Commonly asymptomatic.
- Can sometimes be palpated.
- May present with patellofemoral pain syndrome, i.e. anterior knee pain exacerbated by climbing stairs, squatting, and prolonged sitting.
- May present with localized pain over superolateral aspect of the patella, where fibrous union between ossification centres lies.
- Trauma may precipitate the pain.

Investigation

PA X-ray will demonstrate bipartite fragment.

Treatment

- Strengthening vastus medialis oblique.
- Lateral retinacular releases.
- Trial of medial patella taping.
- If pain persists at the superolateral border of the patella, lateral retinacular release with or without excision of the bipartite fragment may be required.
- Bipartite patella rarely causes long-term disability.

Discoid lateral meniscus

When the lateral meniscus is D-shaped rather than normal C-shape, it is predisposed to tearing.

History and examination
- May present with a painless clunking in the knee.
- May present after a twisting injury, when child complains of lateral joint pain, swelling, clicking, and sometimes locking.
- Examination unremarkable if no tear has occurred.
- If associated with lateral meniscal tear, effusion is often present and restricted range of motion.
- There may be a positive lateral McMurray's sign.

Investigations
- X-ray may demonstrate subtle widening of lateral joint space.
- MRI will confirm diagnosis but is not usually necessary.

Treatment
- Not required if condition is asymptomatic.
- If discoid meniscus is torn, usually requires excision of the torn lateral meniscal fragment and conversion of the meniscus to a C-shape.
- Discoid lateral menisci may be bilateral.
- After partial lateral meniscectomy, prognosis is favourable.

Ankle and lower leg

Examination of the ankle

Inspection

The ankle contains three joints
- Talocrural joint.
- Inferior tibiofibular joint.
- Subtalar joint.

With the feet in a symmetrical position the subtalar joint is in neutral—neither pronated or supinated. Pronation consists of eversion, dorsiflexion, and abduction of the foot. Supination consists of inversion, plantarflexion, and adduction of the foot.

Look for evidence of abnormal biomechanics:
- Excessive pronation.
- Excessive supination.
- Forefoot varus.
- Forefoot valgus.
- Rearfoot varus.
- Rearfoot valgus.
- Ankle equines.
- Genu varum.
- Genu valgum.
- Leg length.

When:
- Standing.
- Walking.
- Supine.
- Prone.

Palpation

Anterior structures
- Ankle joint.
- Antero-inferior tibio-fibular ligament (AITFL).
- Talus.

Lateral structures
- Distal fibula.
- Lateral malleolus.
- Lateral ligaments (ATFL, CFL, PTFL).
- Peroneal tendons.
- Sinus tarsi.
- Base of fifth metatarsal.

Medial structures
- Medial ligament.
- Tibialis posterior.
- Flexor hallucis longus.
- Sustentaculum tali.
- Navicular tubercle.
- Midtarsal joint.

Posterior structures
- Achilles tendon.
- Retrocalcaneal bursa.
- Posterior talus.
- Calcaneum.

Active and passive movements
- Ankle dorsiflexion (10–20°).
- Ankle dorsiflexion can be restricted by inflexibility of gastrocnemius and soleus.
- The minimum range of ankle dorsiflexion for normal locomotion is 10°.
- Ankle plantarflexion (45–50°).
- Dorsiflexion and plantarflexion take place between the talus and tibia and fibula.
- Subtalar inversion (10–20°).
- Subtalar eversion (5–10°).
- Inversion and eversion take place at the talocalcaneal, talonavicular, and calcaneocuboid joints.
- Inversion is usually double that of eversion.

Resisted movements
- Plantarflexion.
- Gastrocnemius (knee extended).
- Soleus (knee flexed).
- Flexor digitorum longus, flexor hallucis longus (flex the toes against resistance).
- Dorsiflexion.
- Tibialis anterior (dorsiflex the foot against resistance).
- Extensor digitorum longus (dorsiflex the toes against resistance).
- Extensor hallucis longus (dorsiflex the big toe against resistance).
- Inversion.
- Tibialis posterior (invert the foot against resistance).
- Eversion.
- Peroneus longus and brevis (evert the foot against resistance).

Special tests

- *Anterior draw test*

A positive anterior draw test in plantarflexion implies injury to the ATFL. It is performed by holding the heel and pulling the foot anteriorly while applying a posterior force to the tibia. A positive anterior draw test in neutral suggests additional injury to the CFL and possibly the PTFL.

- *Talar tilt test*

The talar tilt test examines for CFL instability. It is performed by holding the calcaneum and inverting the talus on the tibia. A talar tilt of 15° or 5° more than the opposite ankle is positive.

- *Tinels test*
- *The squeeze test*

Is positive when compression of the proximal tibia and fibula precipitates distal pain suggesting an injury to the syndesmosis.

- *Biomechanical examination*

Functional tests

- Proprioception
- Lunge
- Hop
- Jump.

Ankle sprains are classified as:
- Grade 1: is painful without instability.
- Grade 2: demonstrates mild instability.
- Grade 3: complete rupture.

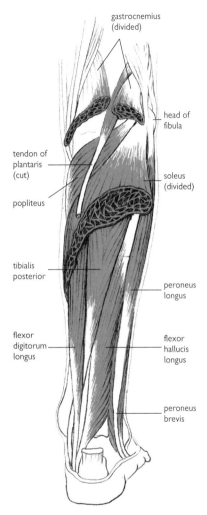

Fig. 7.1 Deep muscles of the calf (plantaris may or may not be present).
Reproduced with permission from MacKinnon P and Morris J (2005). *Oxford Textbook of Functional Anatomy Vol 1.* Oxford University Press, Oxford. ©2005.

Persistent painful ankle

Pain, swelling, and impaired function may persist for four to six weeks after an acute injury. Secondary injuries may be overlooked at the time of the original injury. With persistent symptoms one should look for occult injury in addition to acute ankle sprain. Functional instability resulting from inadequate rehabilitation is the commonest cause. Other possible causes include:

Osteochondral injuries
- Initial radiographs may appear normal. Repeat radiographs or MRI are required for diagnosis.
- Osteochondral injuries occur most commonly at the following sites:
  - Superomedial talus.
  - Superolateral talus.
  - Tibial plafond.

Fractures
- Initial radiographs may appear normal. Follow-up radiographs or MRI may be required for diagnosis.
- Lateral talar process.
- Anterior calcaneal process.
- Posterior talar process.
- Os trigonum fracture.
- Avulsion fracture base of fifth metatarsal.

Impingement syndromes
- Anterior impingement syndrome.
- Anterolateral impingement syndrome.
- Posterior impingement syndrome.
- Capsular injury resulting in synovitis can present with anterior impingement on dorsiflexion.
- Synovium or ruptured ATFL becomes trapped between the lateral malleolus and talus provoking anterolateral impingement.
- Posterolateral process fracture or os trigonum injury may require CT or MRI to confirm the diagnosis.

Tendon dislocation and rupture
- Peroneal tendons.
- Radiographs may demonstrate a small bone chip.
- Resisted eversion in dorsiflexion precipitates tendon subluxation.
- Tibialis posterior tendon.
- Occurs with ankle dorsiflexion and inversion.
- Subluxation may be demonstrated by resisted plantarflexion.

Sinus tarsi syndrome
- Small osseous canal anterior and inferior to the lateral malleolus.
- Pain from subtalar ligament injury and fat-pad necrosis.
- Diagnosis confirmed by a local anaesthetic injection into the sinus tarsi.

Other causes
- Anteroinferior tibiofibular ligament (meniscoid lesion).
- Synovitis or ATFL scar tissue produces a meniscal lesion that impinges between the lateral talus and lateral malleolus.
- Post-traumatic synovitis.
- Calcaneocuboid ligament sprain.
- A bony fleck may be seen adjacent to the cuboid.
- Peroneal nerve or sural nerve injury.

Acute ankle sprain

History and examination

Acute ankle sprains can occur in any sport but are most common in sports that involve a change of direction or jumping e.g. football, rugby, basketball, netball, and volleyball. The lateral ligament includes the anterior talofibular ligament (ATFL), calcaneofibular ligament (CFL) and posterior talofibular ligament (PTFL). The medial or deltoid ligament is composed of four bands—three superficial and one deep. The interosseous ligaments include the anterior tibiofibular ligament, posterior tibiofibular ligament, and interosseous ligament.

The mechanism of injury is important, an inversion injury suggests lateral ligament sprain, an eversion injury medial ligament sprain. Compression may suggest an osteochondral injury.

- Inversion injuries account for 70–85% of all ankle injuries. They occur when the foot is plantarflexed and inverted. Inversion injuries lead to sprains of the lateral ligament complex including the anterior talofibular ligament (ATFL), calcaneofibular ligament (CFL) and posterior talofibular ligament (PTFL).
- The ATFL is most susceptible to injury. The CFL is injured in 40% of ATFL injuries. Complete tears of the ATFL, CFL and PTFL result in ankle dislocation and are associated with a fracture.
- The location of pain and swelling normally indicates the ligaments injured, most commonly the anterolateral aspect of the ankle involving the ATFL.
- Ability to weightbear after the injury suggests a sprain and not a fracture.
- Clinical examination includes palpation of the ligaments, tendons, and also the lateral and medial malleoli, base of the fifth metatarsal, and proximal fibula to consider collateral injuries.

Investigations

- Radiographs are required if the patient cannot weightbear or has point tenderness, particularly over the malleoli, tarsal navicular, base of the fifth metatarsal, or proximal fibular.
- Repeat radiographs should be considered if there is no improvement or progress is delayed.
- Radiographs should include the base of the fifth metatarsal to exclude avulsion fracture.
- Anteroposterior, lateral, and mortise views are required. Fractures including osteochondral injuries to the medial and lateral talar dome are excluded. Mortise views assess the distal tibial syndesmosis.
- If symptoms persist four to six weeks after an apparently simple ankle sprain an MRI is indicated to exclude an osteochondral injury.

Treatment

- Initial treatment consists of rest, ice, compression, and elevation (RICE).
- Analgesics or NSAIDs for pain.
- Compression and elevation help reduce swelling.

- Adequate rehabilitation is required to prevent functional instability and injury recurrence.
- Restore range of movement.
- Strengthen dynamic ankle stabilizers (ankle evertors and dorsiflexors).
- Proprioception e.g. wobble board, mini-trampoline.
- Functional exercises e.g. jumping, hopping, twisting.
- Return to sport. Athletes can return to sport when they can perform sport specific actions without pain or instability.
- Functional bracing or taping may be required to prevent recurrence.

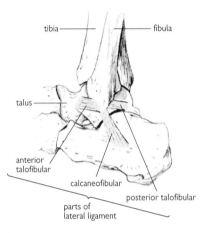

Fig. 7.2 Ligaments of ankle joint, lateral view. Reproduced with permission from MacKinnon P and Morris J (2005). *Oxford Textbook of Functional Anatomy Vol 1.* Oxford University Press, Oxford. ©2005.

Rehabilitation after ankle sprain (grade 2)

Time to return to sport is based largely on the quality of early management.

Early, intermediate, and late rehabilitation objectives should be highlighted immediately after diagnosis. It is not possible to move on to the later stages of rehabilitation until all early stage goals are achieved. The athlete should be aware that progressive rehabilitation is necessary to minimize the chances of recurrence.

Anticipated time to return to sport: 3–6 weeks.

Early stage: days 1–7

Key aims
- Minimize swelling.
- Maintain range of movement and general ankle mobility.
- Prevent achilles tendon stiffness/shortening.
- Begin controlled loading.
- Begin isometric strengthening.
- Enhance joint positional sense/proprioception.
- Maintain upper body strength.

General exercises
- The athlete should be encouraged to weight bear or partially weight bear within the limits of pain. The use of crutches may be useful, but should not be to excess. A heel-toe gait pattern should be encouraged at all times. This will prevent the development of a toe-tap gait and minimize shortening of the achilles tendon.
- The RICE regimen should be used as soon as possible after injury:
  - The use of horseshoe or focal compression around the maleolus is most effective at preventing swelling accumulating around the healing ligaments.
  - Focal compression should be removed before cryotherapy is initiated, in order to prevent a barrier effect which can reduce the effectiveness of cooling.
- Gentle mobility exercises should be encouraged as soon as pain allows. Range of movement through dorsiflexion and plantar flexion (ankle pumps) should be followed by light circling exercises.
- The athlete may perform alphabet exercises—this involves using ankle movements to trace each letter of the alphabet in the air. This becomes more challenging with closed eyes and acts to improve the athletes' awareness of where their ankle is in space.
- Cryokinetics is a technique that involves performing mobility exercises immediately after or during cryotherapy. The pain relieving effect of cooling reduces muscle spasm and inhibition, thereby facilitating the exercises.

- The athlete should begin static stretching of the achilles tendon as soon as pain allows. Decreased dorsiflexion is a risk factor for ankle sprain, and in many cases athletes may have already been tight through this range prior to injury.
  - Stretching can be performed in a non weight bearing position initially. For example with the athlete in high sitting, using a towel wrapped around his foot, to pull it into dorsiflexion.
- If pain allows, gentle calf stretching can be performed in standing.
- Static strengthening can be performed through all movements. The non-injured foot can be used to provide counter pressure initially. This can be progressed to counter pressure coming from the therapist.
- Electrotherapeutic modalities: the use of low level laser therapy and/or electrical stimulation can act to enhance healing and minimize pain at this stage.
- Massage: this will have a role to play even at this early stage of management. Light finger kneading around the injured area can help disperse swelling. Deeper soft tissue release around the achilles tendon will be of value, especially if used in conjunction with mobility and stretching exercises.
- Mobilization: light mobilizations into the accessory and physiological range can be of value, especially with the less compliant athlete.
- Hydrotherapy/pool rehab: the buoyancy of the water reduces the impact on the joints, and may be used to aid rehabilitation.
  - Athletes with greater levels of pain on weight bearing may benefit from pool walking; again a heel-toe gait is encouraged.
  - The pool environment may also facilitate basic weight transfer or single leg standing exercises.
- Upper body strength and conditioning:
  - Athletes should be able to perform any upper body exercises that require them to lie (eg. bench press) or sit (shoulder press).

Middle stage: weeks 2–3

Key aims
- Enhance joint positional sense/proprioception.
- Increase strength/ROM/ankle mobility.
- Progress to cardiovascular exercises.

Mobility/strengthening/proprioceptive exercises
- Weight transfers: standing on both feet, with weight predominantly on the uninjured side. Within the limits of pain, he/she transfers weight on to the injured side. This should progress, until it is comfortable to stand solely on the injured foot.
- Single leg standing/balance: standing on the injured side, the athlete trys to balance, minimizing the number of touch downs. Progress to eyes closed.

Once the athlete is able to stand comfortably on one leg with his/her eyes closed, more advanced proprioceptive training can begin.
- Single leg standing
  - Throw/catch ball:
    —Vary type of throw e.g. underarm, overhead, side pass, chest pass.
    —Vary the direction of the pass received e.g. in front, from side, overhead.
    —Vary type of ball e.g. tennis ball, medicine ball.
  - Sprinting action (upper body):
    —Keeping control through the pelvis, the athlete drives arms forward and back as if he/she were running. To progress, the speed of the arm drives is increased, whilst maintaining balance.
  - Upper body mirroring: athlete must match the upper body movements of therapist:
    —Increase complexity/speed of movements.
  - Dumbbell raises:
    —Progress from basic movements (bicep curl) to multijoint movement patterns (sword draw).
  - Bodyblade drills.
  - With light manual perturbation from therapist/training partner.
  - Fitter exercises.
- Single leg standing on dynamic surface e.g. mini trampoline (rebounder), wobble board, balance pad/cushion, folded towel.
  - Progress as for basic single leg stands.

Strengthening
Manual/PNF patterns. These require aid from a training partner or therapist. Athlete is in long sitting with foot in a neutral position off the end of a bed/plinth. Therapist/training partner applies manual pressure into DF/PF/inv/ev or combinations of movement. To progress, the athlete must close their eyes and fire up the appropriate muscles based on the tactile stimulation.
- These can progress to long or short leg PNF patterns.
- Heel to toes: the athlete rocks from heel to toe. This requires good ROM though DF and PF with a good baseline of balance. This will begin initially with two legs.
  - To progress: single leg heel to toes with upper body support.
  - Single leg only.
- Walking on heels/toes. Forwards/backwards/side to side.
- March walk: this is an excellent prerequisite to jogging.

Progressive strengthening
This requires near full ROM, in particular through DF.
- Mini squats.
  - Ensuring an equal distribution of weight, the athlete should perform a 50% squat (to 45° knee flexion).
- Drop squats:
  - As for a mini squat, except the speed is increased whilst maintaining control.

- Single leg squats.
- Lunges:
  - Progress to multidirectional lunges.

All these exercises can be progressed by increasing the demand on the neuromuscular system.
  - E.g. the athlete must perform a single leg squat on a dynamic surface.

Testing
Strength

A measurement of isometric eversion strength or isokinetic dorsiflexion/plantar flexion might be the gold standard, at this stage. However there are a number of simple tests that can act as a good benchmark.
- Number of heel raises/min (compare to uninjured leg).
- Number of calf raises/min (compare to uninjured leg).

Balance/proprioception
- Single leg stand.
- Single leg stand with eyes closed.
- Single leg stand with eyes closed and neck extended.
- Wobble board.

If the athlete loses balance during the test they must tap the ground with the uninjured foot. The number of touch downs/minute are recorded.

Cardiovascular
Bike/cross trainer/upper body ergometer.

End stage: weeks 3–6

To progress to the end stages of rehabilitation, the athlete must have full ankle ROM, a good baseline of strength through all ankle movements, be able to perform complex proprioceptive exercises in a pain free state and have good lumbopelvic/lower body control and alignment during squatting/advanced proprioceptive exercises.

In general, as the athlete progress through the later stages of rehabilitation, the focus should become less joint-specific and more sport-specific.

Strength and conditioning
This may be progressed as follows:
- Squat.
- Deadlift.
- Hang clean.
- Clean.
- Snatch.

Ideally, the athlete should begin using the bar bell only. Their form and alignment should be monitored by a training partner or strength and conditioning coach. The weight should be increased accordingly, building to their pre injury levels.

Running
Prerequisites
- Full ankle ROM.
- Subject able to perform march walks/advanced proprioception with good control in a pain free state.

Straight line running
- Light jog, building from 30%–50%.
- Build up to 10–30 mins.

Begin progressive running
- This should be done on a flat surface, with cones dividing acceleration/maintenance/deceleration stages.
- For the first session athletes should accelerate from a standing start, up to 60% over the first 30m. They should then aim to maintain this pace over the next 30m, before decelerating slowly a complete stop).
- Build to 90%.

Progress by decreasing the acceleration distance, and increasing the maintenance distance. For example:

Functional running exercises
- Curved running.

Acceleration	Maintenance	Deceleration
20m	40m	20m
10m	30m	20m
10m	40m	20m

- Figure of eight running.
- Shuttles (doggies).
- Run stops:
  - From a 60% run the athlete must come to a complete stop within 5 steps. To progress increase the speed of the run/minimize the number of steps.
- Run to lunge:
  - From a 60% run the athlete must come to a complete stop in a lunge position.
- 45°cuts.
- 90°cuts.
- Spins:
  - Running at 50% the athlete must spin 360° without slowing down.
- T-shuffles.
- Ladder/cone agility drills.

Plyometric exercises
Throughout all plyometric exercises, the athlete is encouraged to keep a 'soft' knee, using hips, knees, and ankles to cushion the impact. The athletes ability to avoid 'corkscrewing' by keeping good pelvic, hip, knee, and toe alignment will act as a good guide for their progress.

- 2–1 (two legs to one):
  - Standing in a stationary position the athlete jumps vertically to land on the injured side.
- Hop scotch:
  - This involves multiple 2–1s, whilst moving forwards.
- 90°/180°/270°/360° rotations:
  - From a stationary position, the athlete jumps vertically and turns 90° clockwise/anticlockwise before landing.
- Jump–land (from height)
  - Using two foot landing.
  - Athlete rotates 45° in air before landing:
  - Add 90°/180° rotation.
  - Single leg landing.
  - Landing on dynamic surface.
  - Immediately catching a ball on landing.
  - Therapist adds a light perturbation on landing.

Field testing

If available, field test results should be compared with pre-season, or normative data. Useful test might include:

- 10m/20m/30m sprint times.
- 150 test.
- T-shuffle agility drill.
- Vertical jump.
- Standing broad jump:
  - Jumping from two feet/landing on two feet.
  - Jumping from injured/landing on two feet.
  - Jumping from injured/landing on injured.

Back to play.

Medial ligament injuries

- The medial or deltoid ligament is injured as a result of an eversion injury, commonly external rotation of the tibia with the foot planted.
- The medial ligament is stronger than the lateral ligament and more often accompanied by additional injuries including fractures e.g. medial malleolus, distal fibula, and talar dome.
- Radiographs are mandatory and widening of the ankle mortise (more than 2mm between the talus and tibia) represents an unstable ankle and requires surgery.
- Treatment of medial ligament injuries is similar to that of lateral ligament injury, however, recovery is much longer—often six to twelve weeks.

Syndesmosis sprain

- The anterior tibiofibular ligament is injured as a result of external rotation.
- Tenderness and swelling are maximal superomedial to the lateral malleolus.
- Provocation tests including the squeeze test and external rotation test (foot externally rotated on a fixed tibia) are positive.
- Treatment is similar to that for lateral ligament sprains but recovery can take six to eight weeks.
- This injury may lead to diastasis of the ankle joint.

Fractures

- A fracture of the lateral, medial, or posterior malleoli is known as a Pott's fracture.
- Specialist orthopaedic opinion is required.
- Medial ligament injuries or medial malleolar fractures extending through the interosseous membrane and associated with a fracture of the proximal fibula are called Maisonneuve fractures. Palpate the proximal fibula to avoid missing this potentially unstable ankle injury.

Lateral ankle pain

Peroneal tendinopathy

History and examination

The peroneus longus and brevis muscles dorsiflex and evert the ankle to provide functional lateral ankle stability. An injury often complicates an acute lateral ankle sprain. The patient may attend with an acute injury or a longer history of chronic subluxation. Rupture of the peroneal retinaculum may lead to subluxation of the peroneal tendons.

Diagnosis is confirmed by demonstrating subluxation of the tendons over the lateral malleolus, by everting the foot against resistance. Initial treatment is rehabilitation.

Investigation

Diagnosis is usually on clinical findings.

Treatment

Surgery is often needed.

Chronic tendinopathy

History and examination

- This is the commonest cause of lateral ankle pain. Examination confirms tenderness and swelling posterior to the lateral malleolus, and passive inversion and resisted eversion reproduces symptoms.
- Precipitating factors include: rearfoot varus (supination), a history of ankle ligament sprains, a plantar-flexed first metatarsal, overpronation, and overuse e.g. jumping sports.

Investigation

Diagnosis can be confirmed by musculoskeletal ultrasound or MRI.

Treatment

Resisted eversion exercises in plantarflexion to strengthen the peroneals.

Sinus tarsi syndrome

History and examination

A small osseous canal anterior and inferior to the lateral malleolus runs between the talus and calcaneum. It is part of the subtalar joint containing the subtalar ligaments. It may be injured in an acute inversion injury or by repetitive damage from excessive subtalar joint pronation. Athletes present with diffuse lateral ankle pain after an acute injury or of gradual onset. Symptoms result from subtalar ligament injury, synovial hypertrophy, peroneal nerve entrapment, or degenerative OA.

The symptoms include:
- Lateral ankle pain.
- Pain worse in the morning.
- Pain aggravated by eversion.
- Local tenderness over the sinus tarsi.
- Pain induced by forced passive inversion.

The clinical findings may include subtalar instability and a positive Tinel's test. The diagnosis is confirmed by injection of local anaesthetic.

Investigation
The diagnosis is based on clinical findings above, but the athlete will often have had an ankle X-ray and other investigations.

Treatment
- NSAIDs.
- Local injection.
- Rehabilitation.
- Biomechanical assessment.

Anterolateral impingement

History and examination
This usually results from an acute ankle sprain or recurrent ankle sprains. The patient complains of chronic pain or with pain and catching at the anterior aspect of the lateral malleolus. The pain is usually worse on dorsiflexion. There is synovitis, soft tissue thickening, and scar tissue developing from the injured capsule and anterior talo fibular ligament. A meniscoid soft tissue lesion often develops.

Investigation
- Clinical assessment better than MRI.

Treatment
- Injection.
- Arthroscopic surgery.

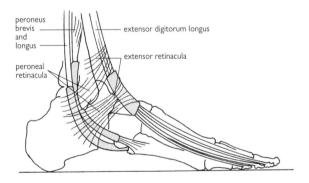

Fig. 7.3 Tendons, synovial shealths, and retinacula on the lateral side of the ankle and foot.

Medial ankle pain

Tibialis posterior tendinopathy

History and examination

Medial ankle pain most often over the retinaculum postero-inferior to the medial malleolus although the patient may also complain of medial midfoot pain at the site of insertion of the tendon. The pain is exacerbated by resisted inversion and passive eversion. It may be associated with excessive pronation (rearfoot valgus).

Rupture of tibialis posterior presents with posteromedial tibial pain extending around the medial malleolus to the navicular tubercle. Clinical examination reveals swelling and an inability to raise the heel. Immediate flattening of the medial arch may not be present.

Investigation

Ultrasound or MRI confirms the diagnosis.

Treatment

- Assess biomechanics as orthotics may be required.
- Rupture of tibialis posterior requires surgical repair.

Flexor hallucis longus tendinopathy

There is usually pain over the posteromedial calcaneum and sustentaculum tali with pain on plantarflexion. This pain is exacerbated by resisted flexion of the first toe with pain on passive extension of the first toe. It is associated with posterior impingement syndrome.

Tarsal tunnel syndrome

History and examination

- The posterior tibial nerve becomes trapped in the fibro-osseous tarsal tunnel around the medial malleolus. This compression may be as a result of trauma, an inversion injury, overuse, excessive pronation, footwear, or chronic flexor tenosynovitis.
- The patient has medial ankle pain radiating into the arch of the foot, heel, and occasionally the toes. The pain is aggravated by prolonged standing, walking, and running. There is rarely paraesthesia and numbness over the sole of the foot.
- Examination confirms local tenderness and a positive Tinel's sign.

Investigations

- Radiographs may demonstrate an os trigonum which compresses the tibial nerve.
- Consider nerve conduction studies.

Treatment

- Footwear, orthotics.
- Injection.
- Surgical decompression.

Also see p.294.

Medial plantar nerve entrapment (Also see p.296)

History and examination

There is pain over the inferomedial calcaneum and this pain may radiate to the arch of the foot. Running aggravates the symptoms and it may be associated with pronation. Recently acquired orthotics can provoke symptoms. A branch of the posterior tibial nerve passes close to the calcaneonavicular ligament.

Examination confirms tenderness and a positive Tinel's sign is positive.

Investigation

Nerve conduction studies confirm the diagnosis.

Treatment

Modification of abnormal biomechanics, injection, or surgical decompression.

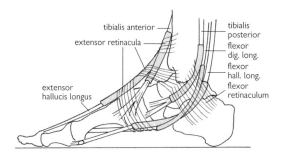

Fig 7.4 Tendons, synovial sheaths, and retinacula on the medial side of the ankle and foot. Reproduced with permission from MacKinnon P and Morris J (2005). *Oxford Textbook of Functional Anatomy Vol 1.* Oxford University Press, Oxford. ©2005.

Anterior ankle pain

Extensor tendinitis

History and examination

Tibialis anterior tendinopathy causes pain over the anterior ankle and midfoot. This pain is exacerbated by dorsiflexion of the foot. It is an overuse injury associated with excessive hill running and may be precipitated by poor footwear. The athlete is tender over the anterior ankle joint and the pain is exacerbated by resisted dorsiflexion.

With tendonitis of the extensor hallucis longus there is pain on resisted dorsiflexion of the first toes and of extensor digitorum, there is pain on resisted dorsiflexion of the toes.

Treatment

Management is conservative.

Anterior impingement ('footballer's ankle')

History and examination

Repetitive forced dorsiflexion and plantarflexion of the ankle produces traction osteophytes at the margin of the joint capsule and exostoses develop on the anterior tibia and talus. It also occurs in basketball, triple jump, long jump, and dance and may follow from ankle instability.

There is pain on running, lunging, or kicking with diffuse anterior ankle joint pain and swelling after activity. The pain is caused by impingement of soft tissues. Examination confirms local tenderness and pain on dorsiflexion. Anterior impingement test positive (active dorsiflexion with the heel on the ground).

Investigation

X-ray.

Treatment

- Physiotherapy, NSAIDs, and corticosteroid injections can improve symptoms.
- Surgery may be required.

Posterior ankle pain

History and examination

Impingement of the os trigonum or posterior process results from forced plantarflexion of the ankle. This produces posterior ankle joint pain deep to the achilles tendon. Ballet dancers, jumpers, and fast bowlers are at risk.

Investigations

- Radiographs demonstrate the ossicle or talar process.
- Isotope bone scan or MRI can confirm the diagnosis.

Treatment

- Management is conservative including rest, physiotherapy, and occasionally corticosteroid injections.
- If symptoms persist surgical excision of the ossicle or posterior spur.

Shin splints

A patient may tell you they have shin splints but it is not a diagnosis. It is a general term used to describe shin pain and describes a group of symptoms due to a variety of causes. The most common are:

- Stress fractures.
- Medial tibial stress syndrome.
- Compartment syndromes.
- Popliteal artery entrapment.

Stress fracture

- These are micro-fractures associated with repetitive stress.
  The bones are unable to adapt and breakdown is greater than repair.
- The history is of a crescendo type pain.
- The pain increases in severity with the duration of exercise.
- As the condition progresses the pain begins earlier in exercise.
- Night pain is a symptom of a severe stress fracture.
- Stress fractures occur most commonly in weight-bearing activities such as running or dancing, although may occur in the ribs of rowers or weight lifters.
- Stress fracture of the femoral neck is serious and most often occurs in female runners.

Medial tibial stress syndrome

- Exercise induced leg pain.
- Pain is felt at the middle to lower 1/3 of the medial side of the tibia.
- The medial edge of the tibia may be swollen and tender.
- When symptomatic there is often a periostitis due to traction with repetitive stress.
- The initial treatment is rest although surgery with release of the fascia may be required.

Compartment syndromes

- Exertional pain.
- Swelling in the anterior compartment.
- Pain on dorsiflexion of the ankle.
- There may be tenderness in the muscle on palpation with hypertrophy.
- There may be increased anterior compartment pressure.
- The initial treatment is rest with alter fasciotomy.

Other compartment syndromes include posterior compartment syndrome where there is pain during and after running in the posterior compartment. Peroneal compartment syndromes have also been described.

Investigations

- X-ray may show some changes with increased callus formation or simply resorbtion at the edges of the fracture.
- Bone scan may show a hot spot. CT scan and MRI may also be helpful in identifying the lesion.

Prevention

- Lower limb stress fractures associated with running may be prevented by looking at the impact and biomechanics.
- Impact may be reduced by running on a forgiving surface. Grass is best. Footwear which gives adequate shock absorbtion.
- Biomechanical anomalies such as hyperpronation of the foot or increased 'Q angle' may increase impact stress.

Treatment

- Alter training to reduce impact.
- Run on a forgiving surface.
- Lose weight.
- Wear good supportive running footwear.
- Orthotics may improve biomechanics.

Achilles tendinopathy

History and examination

The Achilles tendon is formed by the insertion of the soleus and gastrocnemius. Plantaris inserts into the achilles tendon. The tendon is surrounded by a paratenon. At first, there is gradual development of pain and stiffness after rest which may occur, for example, in the morning. In the early stages the symptoms usually improve with exercise. As the condition progresses, there may be pain after exercise and, finally, pain during exercise. On examination, there is local tenderness and swelling. Predisposing factors include overpronation, lack of calf flexibility, and restricted dorsiflexion. Footwear may also contribute. Other contributory factors include a change in training pattern with increased exercise and reduced recovery.

Investigation

The diagnosis may be confirmed by ultrasound or MRI.

Treatment

- Relative rest, ice, and elevation. An eccentric exercise programme is most effective. The next stage is of functional and sport-specific rehabilitation. It is important to correct predisposing factors. With delayed recovery some suggest ultrasound-guided steroid injection or Aprotinin injection. Finally, surgery remains an option.

Achilles tendon rupture

History and examination

- The achilles tendon is the most frequently ruptured tendon.
- The patient has a sudden acute pain in the achilles tendon with an audible snap or tear which is often described as 'like being hit or kicked in the back of the leg'.
- On examination there is swelling and a palpable defect.
- There is reduced function with an inability to plantarflex the ankle.
- Simmond's calf squeeze test positive.
- With a partial tear there is acute onset of pain, tenderness, and swelling but examination confirms no defect and normal function.

Investigations

Ultrasound or MRI confirms the diagnosis.

Treatment

- Surgery. Either open or percutaneous repair. Surgery is probably the treatment of choice for physically active young adults.
- Non-operative. Rehabilitation is prolonged.

Retrocalcaneal bursitis

History and examination

Inflammation of the bursa between the achilles tendon and the calcaneum causing symptoms similar to achilles tendinopathy. The patient is tender over achilles tendon insertion. Retrocalcaneal bursitis can coexist with achilles tendinopathy. Haglund's deformity consists of Achilles tendinopathy, and retrocalcaneal bursitis associated with retrocalcaneal exostosis, or prominent calcaneum.

Treatment
- Physiotherapy, NSAIDs, and injection of corticosteroid.

Chronic exertional leg pain

- Chronic exertional compartment syndrome.
- Medial tibial stress syndrome.
- Stress fracture.

Anterior compartment syndrome

History and examination

This affects the anterior compartment which includes tibialis anterior, extensor digitorum longus, extensor hallucis longus and peroneus tertius. The patient may describe exercise induced discomfort or dull aching cramp-like pain lateral to the anterior border of the tibia. The symptoms develop within 10–30 mins of exercise and are often associated with an increase in the intensity. The athlete may describe a feeling of tightness. The symptoms are often reproducible, bilateral (50–60%), and resolve slowly on stopping exercise. As the syndrome becomes more severe, symptoms take longer to resolve but are usually gone by the next day. There may be numbness on the top of the foot and weakness of ankle dorsiflexion suggesting nerve compression. It occurs most often in repetitive loading sports such as running, football, and cycling.

Clinical examination is often normal. There may be tightness of the anterior compartment. Muscle herniation is sometimes seen in the distal third of the anterior compartment where the superficial peroneal nerve exits the compartment. Examination after exercise may demonstrate fullness of the compartment with discomfort on passive stretching.

Posterior compartment syndrome

History and examination

The lateral compartment consisting of peroneus longus and brevis and the superficial compartment of gastrocnemius and soleus are less frequently affected.

The patient may describe a cramp-like discomfort of the calf and medial border of the tibia and a tightness that increases with exercise. There may be associated weakness and paraesthesia. Examination is often normal or there may be tenderness over the medial border of the tibia. Occasionally small muscle hernias are present.

Investigations

Compartment syndrome consists of increasing pressure in the limited myofascial compartment which causes reduced tissue perfusion and abnormal neuromuscular function.

- Intracompartmental pressure studies: a catheter is inserted into the relevant compartment and the muscles exercised to reproduce the pain. Normal compartment resting pressures are between 0–10mmHg. The diagnosis of chronic compartment syndrome is supported by a preexercise pressure >15mmHg, maximum pressure during exercise >35mmHg and a resting post-exercise pressure >25mmHg.
- Plain radiographs may demonstrate a stress fracture.
- Isotope bone scan may reveal increased linear uptake consistent with medial tibial stress syndrome or focal uptake indicative of a stress fracrture.

Treatment

Conservative treatment includes activity modification to avoid symptoms. Physiotherapy often includes stretching and deep massage. Assessment includes the correction of biomechanical abnormalities.

If conservative treatment fails then surgery is indicated. Surgical fasciotomy relieves symptoms and allows the athlete to return to previous levels of activity.

Foot

Fracture of the calcaneus

History and examination

Acute fractures usually occur as the result of a fall from height and are therefore uncommon in sports.

Investigation

X-ray.

Treatment
- Generally treated conservatively with a period of bed rest in the acute stage, followed by non-weight bearing on crutches, progressing to full weight bearing as tolerated.
- Fractures of the anterior process of the calcaneus can complicate an acute ankle sprain and, if displaced, may require open reduction and internal fixation.

Fracture of the metatarsal bones

History and examination
- Fractures occur commonly in many sports.
- May be caused by direct trauma (e.g. a kick in football) or a twisting injury (usually resulting in a spiral fracture).
- Avulsion fractures of the base of the 5th metatarsal may complicate acute ankle sprains.
- See also Jones fracture of the 5th metatarsal (p.300).

Investigation
X-ray.

Treatment
- Generally respond well to conservative measures—strapping or use of a walking cast for a period of two or three weeks, followed by a return to sport in approximately six to eight weeks.
- Complications are rare—see Jones fracture of base of 5th metatarsal.
- Fitness should be maintained through non-weight-bearing activities such as cycling, aqua jogging, or swimming.

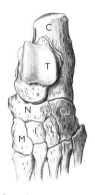

C = calcaneus
T = talus
N = navicular
Cu = cuboid
M = medial cuneiform
I = intermediate cuneiform
L = lateral cuneiform

Fig. 8.1 Tarsal bones: dorsal view. Reproduced with permission from MacKinnon P and Morris J (2005). *Oxford Textbook of Functional Anatomy Vol 1.* Oxford University Press, Oxford. ©2005.

Lisfranc fracture: dislocations

History and examination

- Occurs at the tarsometatarsal joints and are rare in sports.
- Usually occur as the result of an acute plantar flexion injury.

Investigations

- Plain X-ray appearances are subtle and may be missed. A diastasis and occasionally a bone fragment between the base of the first and second metatarsal may be present.
- CT or MRI scan is very helpful in making the diagnosis.

Treatment

- Aimed at restoring the exact anatomical alignment and may be conservative for minor (grade 1 and 2 sprains) injuries or pinning of more severe, unstable injuries.

Fat pad contusion

History and examination

- Occurs either as a result of landing from a jump directly onto the heel, or due to repetitive heel strike on hard surfaces (especially in heavy individuals or those wearing inadequate footwear).
- Fat pad atrophy may be precipitated by steroid injection (e.g. for plantar fasciitis) and is irreversible.
- Tenderness is felt more proximally than with plantar fasciitis.

Investigations

- Not necessary.
- Diagnosis based on clinical findings.

Treatment

- Includes the use of shock absorbing heel cushions, taping, and modification of training surfaces.
- Footwear with a firm heel counter should be worn to prevent splaying of the heel pad.

Midtarsal joint sprains

History and examination

- Sprains may occur as a result of an acute injury or due to repetitive stress in an individual with an overpronated gait. They generally involve the calcaneonavicular ligament.

Investigations

Diagnosis based on clinical findings, although X-ray may be undertaken to exclude other causes of mid-foot pain.

Treatment

- Conservative treatment with electrotherapeutic modalities and taping/orthotic supports.
- Occasionally a cortisone injection is required if there is a persistent synovitis of one of the midtarsal joints.

Turf toe

History and examination

- An acute dorsiflexion sprain injury of the first metatarsophalangeal joint.
- Common on artificial surfaces where the traction between the surface and the shoe is great.
- Severe injuries may result in dislocation of the first meta-tarsophalangeal joint, but most are typical sprain injuries.

Investigation

X-ray to exclude a fracture.

Treatment

- Managed conservatively with ice, analgesics, rest, and taping to limit joint movement on return to sport (generally after two to four weeks).
- These injuries can result in persistent discomfort on return to running.
- Choice of footwear is important in preventing these injuries, with a rigid insole limiting excessive movement at the first MTPJ (especially in those with hallux limitus).

Hallux rigidus (footballer's toe)

History and examination

- Occurs after repeated minor injuries to the 1st MTPJ resulting in early degenerative changes and restricted movement, especially dorsiflexion.
- Very common in sports such as soccer where repetitive stress occurs during kicking and sprinting.
- This condition may cause the athlete to change his normal gait pattern to push off on the lateral border of the forefoot rather than at the hallux.

Investigation

X-ray will demonstrate osteophyte formation and joint space narrowing.

Treatment

- Very difficult—NSAIDs and corticosteroid injection can give temporary relief.
- Referral to a podiatrist is indicated as orthotics can be used to unload the joint.
- Surgery to remove the osteophytes is employed in more severe cases.
- The term hallux limitus is used to describe less severe cases of this condition.

Normal walking

- The normal gait cycle consists of heel strike (usually towards the lateral border of the heel with the foot slightly supinated), stance phase and toe off with the gait cycle completed by the swing phase leading to heel strike once more.
- During distance running this gait cycle is maintained.
- In sprinting the stance phase tends to consist of a midfoot or forefoot rather than a heel strike (i.e. sprinters tend to run more on their toes).
- Following heel strike, the foot pronates (see below) to allow full contact with the ground, subsequently supinating to form a rigid lever to allow toe off to occur.
- The subtalar joint is responsible for the conversion of the rotatory forces of the lower limb and is important in dissipating shock following foot strike. Stiffness of the subtalar joint will reduce the ability to absorb shock.

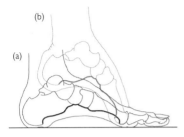

Fig. 8.2 (a) Medial longitudinal arch of the foot when standing. (b) Change in medial arch and dorsiflexion of metatarso-phalangeal joint when standing on tip-toe and at the start of locomotion. Reproduced with permission from MacKinnon P and Morris J (2005). *Oxford Textbook of Functional Anatomy Vol 1.* Oxford University Press, Oxford. ©2005.

Pronation

- Pronation is a tri-planar movement occurring at the subtalar joint.
- Pronation is a normal component of the gait cycle.
- Pronation consists of eversion, dorsiflexion, and abduction of the foot.
- Pronation should not occur past the latter stages of midstance, as the normal foot should then supinate in preparation for toe off.
- Excessive (over) pronation may contribute to, or be a consequence of, biomechanical anomalies elsewhere in the kinetic chain, placing abnormal stresses on other structures. (e.g. will cause internal rotation of the lower limb and place abnormal stress on the medial structures of the foot and ankle).
- Overpronation or hyperpronation has been implicated as a causative factor in the development of many lower limb problems, including achilles tendinopathy, plantar fasciitis, metatarsalgia, sesamoiditis, tibialis posterior tendinopathy, medial tibial periostitis and stress fractures, patellofemoral pain, and iliotibial band friction syndrome.
- Overpronation can be corrected by the use of orthoses placed in the individual's shoe.
- Orthoses can be either preformed or (preferably) custom-cast to suit the individual athlete.
- Many asymptomatic athletes overpronate—there is little or no evidence for the use of orthoses to correct this as a preventative measure.

Supination

- Supination also occurs at the subtalar joint and normally occurs towards the end of the midstance phase of the gait to allow the foot to form a rigid lever in preparation for toe off.
- The supinated foot is plantar flexed, inverted, and adducted.
- Typically these individuals have a cavoid (high arched), rigid foot with poor shock absorption which predisposes to metatarsal stress fractures.
- Excessive supination may also contribute to the development of iliotibial band friction syndrome.
- Supination is much more difficult to correct with orthoses—individuals should buy shoes with maximum shock absorption.

Footwear

- Different sports require different footwear and individuals also have different footwear requirements.
- Shoes consist of an upper (the part covering the foot) and sole (consisting of inner sole, mid-sole, wedge, and out-sole). The mid-sole is the main shock absorber and can be made of various materials with different inserts. The out-sole is designed for both traction and shock absorption while the wedge increases heel height and aids shock absorption.
- The upper should have a toe box providing adequate room and a firm heel counter to stabilize the subtalar joint and help prevent excessive pronation.
- The shape of the shoe can be straight or curved—a straight last shoe provides more stability.
- Board lasting and slip lasting describes the way the upper of the shoe is attached to the sole. In board lasting the upper is attached to a hard inner sole board and is heavier and more stable.
- Those with a tendency to overpronate require a running shoe providing more control—a straight (rather than curved) last construction, a combined last inner sole (i.e. board last to metatarsals, allowing more flexibility at the forefoot) with added medial support and a firm heel counter.
- Tennis and other court shoes are generally constructed to provide more control and will be of a full board last construction.
- Running shoes are not designed to allow sudden changes of direction and are unsuitable for sports involving a lot of twisting.
- A high heel tab should generally be avoided as this may cause impingement on the achilles tendon when the ankle is fully plantarflexed.
- Shoes should be individual and sport-specific—those designed for distance running should provide stability and shock absorption, while those aimed at sports involving sudden changes in direction should provide good traction between the foot and the playing surface to avoid slipping.
- Running shoes lose their shock absorbing qualities after about 500 kilometres, and should be changed frequently. Using worn out footwear may lead to injury.
- Football boots should allow the player to 'feel' the ball. Boots with 'blade' type cleats may increase the likelihood of some lower limb injuries, in addition to causing tibial lacerations.
- Shoes designed for aerobic classes become worn after approximately 100 hours of activity.

Gait analysis

A detailed description of the techniques used in formal gait analysis is beyond the scope of this book. However, from the above discussion it is clear that the physician should have some understanding of the normal biomechanics of walking and running, and should be able to recognize abnormal gait patterns and refer appropriately for more detailed podiatric assessment.

Pronation is a normal component of the gait cycle and there is no evidence supporting the prescription of foot orthoses as a preventative measure in asymptomatic athletes who 'overpronate'—these are generally individuals who have adapted and learnt to cope with their 'abnormal' gait and the introduction of orthoses into their shoes may cause considerable secondary problems.

- Athletes should first be assessed standing from the front and then the posterior aspect.
- Alignments such as persistent femoral anteversion will be obvious, producing a 'squinting patellae' appearance.
- A pelvic tilt may be due to a leg length discrepancy—this can be formally measured from the anterior superior iliac crest to the medial malleolus with the athlete supine.
- From the posterior aspect, the shape of the longitudinal arch and the angle between the achilles and the calcaneus can be assessed— athletes who overpronate will tend to have a flat footed appearance with valgus heel position, producing the 'too many toes' sign.
- The athlete should be asked to perform a half squat with the heels flat—this will reproduce the position of the foot in the mid stance phase of running and will demonstrate any tendancy to overpronate.
- The athlete should be observed walking in bare feet and if possible treadmill running in normal training shoes.
- The athlete who supinates excessively will typically have a rigid high arched foot with rearfoot varus alignment.
- Core stability should be assessed, for example by asking the athlete to perform a one leg squat and observing the degree of pelvic tilt and twisting that occurs during this manoeuvre.
- Any abnormal gait patterns identified in a symptomatic athlete should prompt referral to a podiatrist for more formal gait analysis.
- Several different types of orthoses are available, with the most appropriate usually being made from a cast of the athlete's foot taken in the 'subtalar neutral' position.

Plantar fasciitis

History and examination

- Plantar fasciitis is a chronic overuse injury resulting from repetitive traction on the plantar fascia attachment to the calcaneus.
- It is often found in individuals with *pes planus* or a tendency to overpronate, and may be initiated by wearing sandals or soft shoes.
- Older or middle aged athletes are more commonly affected.
- The classical symptom is heel pain and stiffness which is worse in the mornings—individuals report that they have to walk on their toes for the first few strides, with their symptoms improving as they 'warm up'.
- Pain may be present during the day if walking long distances or after a period of sitting.
- Patients with plantar fasciitis have point tenderness at the plantar fascia attachment to the calcaneus anteromedially. They may also experience tenderness at the plantar fascia origin when the great toe is dorsiflexed.
- The differential diagnosis includes calcaneal stress fracture, tarsal tunnel syndrome, medial or lateral plantar nerve entrapment, Reiter's disease, and lumbar radiculopathy.

Investigations

- X-ray often reveals a calcaneal spur in asymptomatic individuals (approximately 15% of the general population will have a heel spur) and the presence of a spur is not related to the development of pain.
- There is an association with inflammatory conditions such as gout, RA, ankylosing spondylitis and Reiter's syndrome (especially if heel pain is bilateral), so further investigation may be appropriate.

Treatment

- A tension night splint is very useful in relieving morning pain and stiffness.
- Stretches for the calf/achilles tendon and plantar fascia should be advised and heel cups or orthoses to correct abnormal foot biomechanics are indicated.
- Strapping techniques to support the plantar fascia are very useful in providing short term symptomatic relief. Taping begins at the level of the metatarsal heads and continues to the heel, forming a fan to support the plantar fascia. It is quick and easily applied by the patient and may also be used on return to impact activities.
- Intrinsic foot exercises should be advised—easily performed using a towel on the floor and instructing the athlete to pull this towards him using his toes.
- Extracorporeal shock wave therapy has recently been reported as being a promising treatment option.
- Electro-therapeutic modalities are usually ineffective.

- Cortisone injections may be useful but can cause rupture of the plantar fascia or fat pad atrophy which may lead to permanent heel pain. The preferred technique is to use a medial approach rather than inject directly through the heel pad which has a plentiful nerve supply. Injection is usually reserved for patients who have failed to respond to other conservative measures.
- Surgery is occasionally required for refractory cases (i.e. at least twelve months duration)—results are generally good, although long term problems following surgery have been reported.

Extensor tendinopathy

History and examination
- Overuse of the extensor tendons can be caused by uphill running, and in some cases an acute peritenonitis can occur, causing crepitus and swelling.
- Pain can also arise from ill-fitting shoes or laces tied too tightly.

Treatment
- Attention to footwear; soft padding may prevent excessive pressure.
- Steroid injection along the tendon sheath is often helpful in cases of peritenonitis.
- Referral for physiotherapy, including eccentric strengthening exercises is indicated.
- Surgery is very rarely necessary.

Tarsal tunnel syndrome

(Also see p.266.)

History and examination
- This describes an entrapment of the posterior tibial nerve or one of its branches (medial calcaneal or lateral plantar nerve) in the tarsal tunnel just below the medial malleolus.
- More likely to occur in the overpronated athlete, where increased load on the flexor tendons results in swelling and increased pressure.
- May also be associated with anatomical variations such as ganglions and varicosities.
- Athletes feel pain and occasionally paraesthesia from the medial aspect of the heel and along the medial longitudinal arch.
- Symptoms can occur at night and may disturb sleep.
- Tinels sign may be positive over the entrapped nerve at the level of the flexor retinaculum.

Investigation
EMG and nerve conduction studies may be positive.

Treatment
- Orthoses to correct overpronation.
- Cortisone injection to the tarsal tunnel can provide temporary relief of symptoms.
- Surgical release of the entrapped nerve usually gives permanent cure and return to sport is possible approximately two months post-surgery.

Medial plantar nerve entrapment

(Also see p.267.)

History and examination

- Entrapment occurs in the midfoot, especially in athletes who overpronate or have a valgus heel alignment. May also be found secondary to chronic ankle instability.
- Athlete experiences pain in the medial longitudinal arch, radiating to the toes.
- Often aggravated by running uphill or around bends.
- May be accompanied by numbness affecting the medial border of the foot.
- Tenderness is found at the medial plantar aspect of the longitudinal arch.

Treatment

- Correct overpronation with orthotics.
- Surgery may be necessary in resistant cases.

Stress fractures of the calcaneus

History and examination

- Stress fractures of the calcaneus are relatively uncommon, having been described mostly in military populations.
- The history is of an insidious onset of heel pain on impact activities.
- On clinical examination there will be pain compressing the calcaneus from the sides.

Investigations

- X-rays usually show a sclerotic line parallel to the posterior margin of the calcaneus on the lateral view.
- Isotope and/or MRI scanning may be necessary to make the diagnosis.

Treatment

- Treatment is conservative with return to impact activities as the symptoms and signs permit (usually 6–8 weeks). There is no need to advise a period of non-weight-bearing.
- Fitness can be maintained through non-impact training—aqua jogging and cycling.
- On return to impact activities, footwear which provides adequate shock attenuation should be worn.

Stress fractures of the navicular

History and examination

- The exact cause of navicular stress fractures is unclear.
- They occur through the sagittal plane of the central third which is felt to be relatively avascular.
- Impingement and shearing of the navicular between the talus and first, second, and third rays is thought to occur in sprinting and jumping activities.
- Occur most commonly in sprinters and jumping athletes, but also in footballers.
- Usually present insidiously with midfoot pain and localized tenderness to palpation over the proximal, dorsal surface of the navicular (the so called 'N' spot).

Investigations

Plain X-rays are often negative and the diagnosis should be confirmed with isotope, CT, or MRI scanning.

Treatment

- These fractures are prone to non-union and require aggressive treatment—initially strictly non-weight-bearing in a cast for 6–8 weeks. Fitness can be maintained through cycling during this phase.
- Once the cast is removed the 'N' spot is palpated—if there is residual tenderness then a further 2 week period of immobilization is employed.
- If there is no localized tenderness at this stage then gradual weight-bearing activities can be resumed, with return to full training over the next 6–8 weeks.
- Non-union or delayed union is a major problem and surgery may be required for those fractures that fail to unite with conservative treatment.
- Recovery from these injuries is often prolonged. A gradual return to impact activities is required and footwear should be carefully checked to ensure that it is appropriate to the individual.
- Orthoses are indicated for those athletes who have an excessively overpronated gait.

Stress fractures of the metatarsals

History and examination

- These are very common—most often involving the second ('March fracture') and third metatarsal shafts.
- Stress fractures or the second metatarsal are especially common in ballet dancers.
- These fractures present with increasing pain on impact activities and localized tenderness over the affected bone.

Investigation

Plain X-rays may not be positive for 3 or 4 weeks and isotope scans are used to make an earlier diagnosis.

Treatment

- Conservative—strapping or use of a cast brace/walker with return to impact activities over a period of 6–8 weeks.
- Fitness can be maintained with low-or non-impact exercise such as aqua jogging.
- Return to full activity to be expected over eight to ten weeks.

Jones fracture

History and examination

- This is a stress fracture at the junction of the metaphysis and diaphysis of the proximal 5th metatarsal (although this fracture can also occur acutely as the result of an inversion/plantarflexion injury).
- These fractures represent a special group, as they are prone to non-union due to the relative avascularity of this area.

Investigation

In stress fracture, plain X-rays may not be positive for 3 or 4 weeks and isotope scans are used to make an earlier diagnosis in this situation.

Treatment

- These fractures should be immobilized in a short leg cast, non-weight bearing for 8 weeks—subsequent non-union is treated with intra-medullary screw fixation or bone grafting.
- Early surgical intervention should be considered in the professional or elite athlete.

Metatarsalgia

History and examination
- Forces while walking are normally transmitted through the first and fifth metatarsal heads.
- Loss of the transverse arch of the forefoot will result in excessive stress being placed on the other MTPJs causing synovitis and pain.
- The second and third MTPJs are commonly affected and there may be callous formation in this area reflecting the excessive stress.

Investigation
Diagnosis is based on clinical examination. There is pain compressing the metatarsal heads and manipulation of the affected joints.

Treatment
- Includes the use of a metatarsal pad (this must be placed on the plantar surface of the foot, proximal to the MTPJs to restore the normal transverse arch), and orthoses to correct any overpronation.
- Occasionally a cortisone injection into the affected MTPJ may give good relief.

Morton's (interdigital) neuroma

History and examination
- Swelling and scar tissue around the interdigital nerve due to compression between the metatarsal heads.
- Typically occurs between the third and fourth metatarsal heads and causes pain and interdigital numbness and paraesthesia.
- On clinical examination there will be pain compressing the metatarsal heads and a Mulders click may be felt between the MT heads, representing compression of the swollen nerve and scar tissue.

Investigation
Diagnosis is clinical but can be confirmed by MRI scan.

Treatment
- Treatment is the same as that for metatarsalgia and cortisone injections to the affected area may give temporary relief of symptoms.
- Metatarsal pads and orthotic correction of any abnormal gait pattern should be advised.
- Surgical excision is the definitive treatment.

Sesamoid injury

History and examination

- The medial and lateral sesamoid bones lie within the tendon of flexor hallucis brevis and injuries are frequent in sport. They act to increase the efficiency of the tendon and to stabilize the first MTP joint.
- The medial sesamoid is most commonly affected due to repetitive loading leading to the development of sesamoiditis/osteonecrosis or stress fracture. Athletes who overpronate are particularly vulnerable to these problems.
- On clinical examination there will be tenderness to direct palpation over the medial sesamoid and the patient may tend to walk on the lateral border of the foot in an attempt to unload the painful area.

Investigation

- Specific 'sesamoid views' on plain X-ray may show fragmentation or fracture of the involved bone—however, a bipartite sesamoid is a common finding and differentiation from a stress fracture may be difficult (the fibrous joint of a bipartite sesamoid is also prone to injury).
- Isotope or MRI scanning can be used to make the diagnosis.

Treatment

- These stress fractures are prone to non-union and initial treatment should be in a non-weight bearing cast for 6 weeks followed by gradual resumption of impact activities if bony tenderness is no longer present. Overpronation should be corrected with orthoses and padding may be used to unload the area on return to training.
- Sesamoiditis may occasionally respond to a cortisone injection.
- Generally excision of the sesamoid bones should be avoided as there can be significant problems following such procedures (although excision of a partial fragment can produce good results).

Cuboid syndrome

- Occasionally the lateral aspect of the cuboid may be subluxed dorsally due to excessive pull of the peroneus longus tendon. This results in lateral foot pain when weight bearing.
- Treatment is by manipulation of the subluxed cuboid and taping may be used post-reduction to hold the cuboid in place.
- Any biomechanical problems, such as overpronation, should be corrected.

Os naviculare syndrome

- An accessory ossicle at the tuberosity of the navicular occurs in approximately 10% of people and is generally asymptomatic.
- Pain may occasionally occur due to traction from the tibialis posterior tendon, especially in an individual with an overpronated gait.
- Treatment is aimed at reducing the traction with activity modification and orthoses to correct the abnormal gait pattern.
- A traction apophysitis may occur at this site in the adolescent athlete—treatment is along similar lines.

Sever's disease (traction apophysitis calcaneum)

History and examination

- 2nd commonest traction apophysitis after Osgood–Schlatter disease.
- Usually presents in children between 10 and 13 years.
- Unilateral or bilateral heel pain related to running and jumping activity.
- Pain may be associated with limping.
- Heel pain often worst on rising from bed.
- In severe cases, swelling develops over the posterior calcaneum.
- Hyperpronation and flat feet may be associated.
- Calf and hamstring flexibility usually poor.
- Focal tenderness at posterior border of the calcaneum at the insertion of the Achilles tendon.
- Ankle dorsiflexion may be reduced.
- Differential diagnosis includes a calcaneal stress fracture.

Investigations

- Rarely required.
- X-rays will demonstrate fragmentation of the calcaneal apophysis.

Treatment

- Limit running and jumping activities.
- Heel raise in shoe will ↓ pain.
- Ice heels after activity.
- Calf and hamstring stretching programme implemented.
- Calf strength programme.

Prognosis

- No long-term complications.
- Activity may need to be modified during vulnerable periods.

Iselin's disease (traction apophysitis affecting base of fifth metatarsal)

History and examination
- Presents with pain over lateral aspect of foot at site of insertion of peroneus brevis tendon into base of fifth metatarsal.
- Pain reproduced by passive foot inversion and resisted eversion.

Investigation
Not required.

Treatment
- Unloading tendon with standard ankle taping in eversion (as is done for the prevention of lateral ligament injuries).
- Exercise programme to stretch and strengthen the peroneal muscles.
- Prognosis is good.

Traction apophysitis navicular (insertion tibialis posterior tendon)

History and examination
- Presents with medial mid-foot pain.
- Pain reproduced by passive foot eversion and resisted inversion.
- Flat feet and hyperpronation commonly associated.
- No investigations are required.

Treatment
- Unload tibialis posterior tendon with orthotic device.
- Programme to stretch and strengthen tibialis posterior.
- Prognosis is good.

Tarsal coalition

- Congenital abnormality resulting in bony, cartilaginous or fibrous fusion of two tarsal bones.
- Causes abnormal mechanics around affected bones.
- Most common coalitions are calcaneo-navicular followed by talo-calcaneal and calcaneo-cuboid.
- In 40% of cases, tarsal coalition is bilateral and a family history of tarsal coalition is common.

History and examination

- Can present in several different ways depending on bones involved.
- Common presentations include recurrent ankle sprains, mid-foot pain, or a painless, rigid, asymmetric flat foot.
- May be asymptomatic in childhood and only present in adult life as a result of degenerative changes caused by altered foot mechanics.

Investigations

- X-rays useful when appropriate views are requested.
- A 'Harris–Beath' view will show bony coalition of middle subtalar facet in bony talocalcaneal coalitions.
- Lateral views useful for diagnosing talocalcaneal coalitions (continuous 'C' sign) and for identifying talonavicular spurring, which results from altered mechanics at the subtalar joint.
- Bony calcaneonavicular coalitions are often seen with an oblique foot X-ray.
- CT scanning will usually identify cartilaginous and fibrous unions, which cannot be detected on plain X-ray.

Treatment

- Depends on site of coalition and symptoms.
- Orthotics for symptom relief.
- Immobilization in neutral or inverted position in child with pronounced peroneal spasm.
- If symptoms severe and unresponsive to conservative measures or if indications of degenerative changes occurring in other joints, surgical excision of the bar may be required.

Prognosis

- Tarsal coalition is commonly missed in childhood and presents as severe arthritic change in the tarsal joints of adults.

Freiberg's disease (also called Freiberg's infraction or Freiberg's osteochondritis)

History and examination

- Freiberg's disease is an avascular necrosis of the metatarsal head, most commonly presenting between the ages of 12 and 18 years.
- Initial synovitis is followed by sclerosis, resorption, and collapse of the metatarsal head, leading to secondary degenerative changes.
- The second metatarsal head is most commonly affected, although the third can also be involved.
- Usually seen in running athletes and dancers, probably secondary to compressive forces at the metatarsal heads.
- This is the only ostechondrosis more common in females, perhaps due to preponderance of females in dancing.
- Gradual onset forefoot pain, worse with push-off and dancing en-pointe.
- Focal tenderness and ↓ROM over involved metatarsal head.
- Morton's foot (foot in which second metatarsal is longer than first) is commonly associated and increases the load on the second metatarsal head.

Investigations

- X-ray often normal initially.
- Later shows fragmentation of epiphysis, followed by flattening of metatarsal head.
- If the X-ray is normal, early in course of symptoms, a bone scan or MRI will confirm the diagnosis.

Treatment

- In the acute phase rest from all impact activity is necessary.
- Limit activity and modify footwear (use metatarsal bar to unload metatarsal head and avoid high-heeled shoes).
- In severe cases, immobilization may be required.
- Persistent pain may necessitate surgical intervention, but this should be delayed until after re-ossification has occurred.
- If symptoms do not resolve with conservative measures, excision of the metatarsal head is sometimes required.
- Freiberg's disease may cause long-term disability.

Kohler's disease

- Avascular necrosis of navicular.
- More common in boys than girls.
- Ischaemia and stress have been implicated as causative factors.

History and examination

- Presents earlier than other osteochondroses (around age 3–5).
- Presents with a painful limp and focal tenderness over the navicular.
- Passive eversion and resisted inversion often reproduce the pain.

Investigation

X-ray shows patchy sclerosis of the navicular, followed by compression and collapse.

Treatment

- Symptomatic.
- Analgesia.
- Rest from running activities.
- Medial arch-support orthotic improves pain by unloading the navicular.

Prognosis

- Excellent prognosis.
- Despite marked abnormalities on initial imaging, navicular returns to its normal shape before growth is complete.

Sub-ungal haematoma

- Painful condition. Should be drained by piercing the nail with a needle or heated paper clip to prevent loss of the nail, which would otherwise occur in 2 or 3 weeks. Dress to avoid infection.
- Black nails can also occur as the result of wearing poorly fitting shoes.

Ingrowing toenaills

- Usually affects the great toe and is caused by ill-fitting shoes or injudicious nail clipping.
- Can readily become infected and require antibiotic treatment.
- May require wedge resection of part of the nail and ablation of the nail bed with phenol to prevent re-growth.
- Prevention through proper and regular nail care is the best solution.

Callouses

- Skin thickens in response to pressure, forming callouses which can be painful.
- Common at heel and over the second metatarsal head.
- Hard skin can be pared back with a sharp scalpel.
- Attention should be paid to footwear to prevent recurrence.

Verrucae

- Verrucae (warts) are viral infections and can be spread, especially in shower areas or around pools.
- Can be self treated by paring back and applying a proprietary wart remover.
- May require to be burnt using podophyllin or frozen with liquid nitrogen.
- Recurrence is common.

Shoulder

Anatomy

Important areas of shoulder anatomy:
- Musculotendinous units of the rotator cuff and biceps.
- Bony landmarks of the humerus, scapula, and clavicle.
- Four joints of the shoulder.

Rotator cuff

The rotator cuff is comprised of the tendons of four muscles.
- The subscapularis is located anteriorly on the scapula.
- The supraspinatus, infraspinatus, and the teres minor are located posteriorly on the scapula.
- All are closely associated with the glenohumeral capsule, as is the biceps tendon.
- The primary function of the rotator cuff is to position the humeral head in the glenoid allowing larger muscles to provide necessary power.

Humerus

Important bony landmarks of the shoulder.
- Greater tuberosity of the humerus:
  - The insertion site of the supraspinatus, infraspinatus, and teres minor.
  - This prominence is often associated with impingement.
  - When testing for impingement on physical exam most tests attempt to force the greater tuberosity under and against the acromion and the coracoacromial ligament thus 'impinging' the subacromial structures.
- The bicipital groove is a palpable indentation immediately medial and anterior to the greater tuberosity of the humerus:
  - It houses the tendon of the long head of the biceps.
  - It is easily identified if the humerus is alternately internally and externally rotated while palpating this area.
- On the anterior and inferior border of this groove is the lesser tuberosity, the insertion site of the subscapularis.

Articulations

There are three true joints of the shoulder.
- The glenohumeral joint, acromioclavicular joint, and the sternoclavicular joint:
  - All three may have a fibrocartilagenous disc present within the articulation.
  - As with all true joints, they are susceptible to arthritides and trauma.

The fourth joint, the scapulothoracic joint, is a physiologic joint and may be associated with pain syndromes, bursitis, and neuropathies.

The clavicle and its attachments with the sternum, acromion, and coracoid processes are the only bony attachment of the shoulder to the thorax.
- These connections absorb a large portion of traumatic stresses to the upper extremity and are therefore more susceptible to injuries.

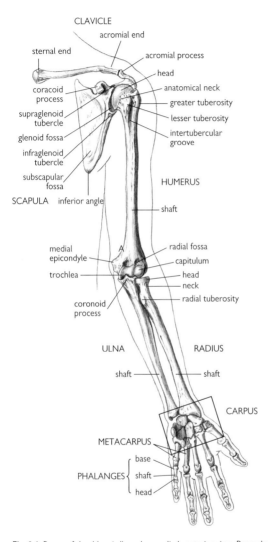

Fig. 9.1 Bones of shoulder girdle and upper limb; anterior view. Reproduced with permission from MacKinnon P and Morris J (2005). *Oxford Textbook of Functional Anatomy Vol 1*. Oxford University Press, Oxford. ©2005.

Glenohumeral joint
- The glenohumeral joint sacrifices the bony and ligamentous stability of other joints for increased range of motion.
- The primary stabilizers of the joint are the musculotendinous complex of the rotator cuff and the joint capsule.

Bursae

There are 4 important bursae in the shoulder
- The subacromial bursa.
  - Located immediately inferior to the acromioclavicular joint and superior to the glenohumeral joint .
  - It is often involved in impingement syndrome.
  - Injection into this bursa to eradicate symptoms is the basis of the impingement test.
- The subdeltoid bursa.
  - Located inferior to the deltoid tendon on the lateral shaft of the humerus.
- The subcapular bursa.
  - Located between the joint capsule and the tendon of the subscapularis muscle.
- The subcoracoid bursa.
  - Located between the joint capsule and the coracoid process of the scapula.

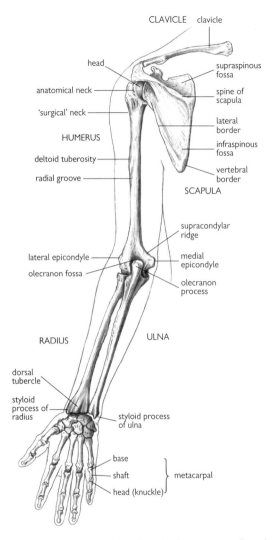

Fig. 9.2 Bones of shoulder girdle and upper limb; posterior view. Reproduced with permission from MacKinnon P and Morris J (2005). *Oxford Textbook of Functional Anatomy Vol 1*. Oxford University Press, Oxford. ©2005.

History

The key to developing an effective differential diagnosis for the patient with shoulder pain is a thorough history. Key questions in the evaluation are:
- What is the predominant symptom?
- Chief complaints may range from pain to instability to weakness.
  If pain is the predominant symptom, ask the patient to describe the quality of the pain, its location, and quantify the severity of the pain on a scale from 1 to 10. This helps you assess the results of treatment.
- How long have the symptoms been present? How did it develop or how has it changed? Have you had similar symptoms in the past? Was there a history of trauma?

These questions help to determine whether the problem is chronic or acute in onset. If trauma was involved, the exact mechanism may help to determine the diagnosis. A history of dislocation or recurrent subluxations may be a clue to instability. Chronic pain with overhead activities may be due to impingement.
- Where did the pain begin and has it changed in its location? Does the shoulder hurt at night? Are there certain positions or activities that bother it more than others?

These questions attempt to localize the problem. Night pain or pain with overhead activities may signify impingement, while pain with lifting, pushing open a car door, or carrying luggage may be due to instability.
- What is your job? What are your hobbies or sports activities?
- Injuries due to overuse are often seen in workers who have to work overhead often. They are especially susceptible to impingement syndrome, subacromial bursitis, and acromioclavicular problems. Certain sports have an increased incidence of shoulder injuries, especially volleyball, swimming, the overhead throwing sports, racquet sports, hockey, and wrestling.
- What has been done for treatment? Have there been any previous injuries to either of the shoulders?

These are important because they may alter the exam, or the comparison with the opposite shoulder.
- Do you have problems with neck pain? Is there pain that radiates into the shoulder or down the upper extremity? Is there associated abdominal pain, or chest pain? Is there a history of weight loss, fatigue, or fevers?

Determining whether pain is referred from the cervical spine, abdomen, or chest wall may prevent an expensive and inappropriate work-up. Constitutional signs of malignancy or a septic arthritis are rare, but may be helpful in the work-up.

Examination

Inspection

- Exposure (including shoulder blades).
  - Women may use bra and/or tie gown around neck with arms out.
- Muscle atrophy .
  - Biceps atrophy may be due to musculoskeletal nerve injury.
  - Scapular winging may be due to long thoracic nerve injury.
- Asymmetry.
  - A pronounced bicep may be due to biceps tendon rupture known as Popeye defect.
  - Prominence of the scapular spine may be due to palsy in young patients, or a long-standing rotator cuff tear in older patients.

Screen for referred pain

- Cervical spine.
- Cardiopulmonary.
- Abdominal.

Palpation

Localize the point of maximum tenderness only after the remainder of the exam is complete. Discomfort felt by the patient initially in the exam may cause guarding to the point of missing an important exam finding or making the exam significantly less useful.

Bony palpation

- Suprasternal notch
- Sternoclavicular joint
- Clavicle
- Coracoid process
- Acromioclavicular joint
- Acromion
- Greater tuberosity of the humerus
- Bicipital groove
- Spine of the scapula
- Medial border of the scapula

Palpation of the soft tissues

- Rotator cuff muscles
- Subacromial and subdeltoid bursa
- Axilla
- Major muscles of the shoulder

Active and passive movements

- There are nine movements described in the shoulder:
  - Abduction (normal 180°).
  - Adduction (normal 45°).
  - Flexion (normal 180°).
  - Extension (normal 45°).
  - Internal rotation (normal 70°).
  - External rotation (normal 75°).
  - Protraction, retraction, and elevation.

- Assess smoothness of the scapulohumeral and scapulothoracic movement, and test for a painful arc which may suggest impingement, rotator cuff problems, or labral tears.
  - Impingement pain is usually from 90–120° of abduction.
- Restricted or painful internal rotation at 90° of abduction may also signify shoulder impingement.
- Internal rotation is best observed with Apley's (behind the back) scratch test.
  - At least 55° of internal rotation is required to perform this manoeuvre, and you can quantitate the range of motion according to the level of the thoracic spine they can reach (T7 is at the inferior angle of the scapula) for comparison after treatment.

Special tests

The special manoeuvres for evaluation of the shoulder are presented below as described in the literature and organized according to the problem they evaluate. The reader may have been taught varying techniques for the tests presented here. Be cautious in modifying the test, as validity testing will no longer be applicable. A literature review of these manoeuvres is summarized in Table 9.1, but you should be aware that additional well-designed studies are needed in many cases.

Glenohumeral joint stability

Anterior apprehension test

With the scapula stabilized (or in the supine position), the arm is passively moved to 90° of abduction and gently externally rotated until there is apprehension and the patient resists further external rotation. Apprehension (the feeling that the joint is going to dislocate) constitutes a positive test. Pain alone does not necessarily signify instability. Caution should be exercised not to completely dislocate the joint with this manoeuvre.

Relocation test

The patient is supine and in the apprehension position as described above. With a positive test, a posterior force placed on the anterior humerus will relieve the apprehension. Further external rotation may then be possible. If the posterior force is removed, apprehension returns.

Augmentation test (fulcrum test)

To define an occult instability, placement of the examiner's hand under the humeral head posteriorly while the patient is supine and in the apprehension position may then elicit or 'augment' a positive apprehension test.

Load and shift test

While stabilizing the scapula, the humeral head is loaded medially against the glenoid while in the neutral position. A posterior and anterior stress is applied to the humeral head as if to shift it anteriorly and posteriorly. Translation of up to 50% of the width of the humeral head is considered normal.

Posterior apprehension

The shoulder is passively moved to 90° of abduction and gently internally rotated until the patient is apprehensive and resists further internal rotation. A posteriorly directed force placed upon the humeral shaft may intensify the feeling of instability.

Sulcus sign

The arm is passively at the side in the standing or sitting position. The humerus is distracted inferiorly. The sulcus sign is an indentation seen immediately inferior to the acromioclavicular joint and signifies an inferior instability. Normal is less than one centimetre.

Table 9.1 Shoulder (glenohumeral) joint: movements, principal muscles, and their innervation[1]

Movement	Principal muscles	Peripheral nerve	Spinal root origin
Flexion	Pectoralis major (clavicular part)	Pectoral nerve (medial and lateral)	C 5, 6
	Deltoid (clavicular part)	Axillary nerve	C 5, 6
Extension	Latissimus dorsi	Nerve to latissimus dorsi (thoracodorsal nerve)	C 6, 7, 8
Abduction	Supraspinatus (initial 20°)	Suprascapular nerve	C 5, 6
	Deltoid	Axillary nerve	C 5, 6
Adduction	Pectoralis major	Pectoral nerves (medial and lateral)	C 5, 6
	Latissimus dorsi	Nerve to latissimus dorsi	C 6, 7, 8
Medial (internal) rotation	Pectoralis major	Pectoral nerves (medial and lateral)	C 5, 6
	Latissimuss dorsi	Nerve to latissimuss dorsi	C 6, 7, 8
	Subscapularis	Subscapular nerves (upper and lower)	C 5, 6
	Teres major	Lower subscapular nerve	C 5, 6
Lateral (external) rotation	Infraspinatus	Suprascapular nerve	C 5, 6
	Teres minor	Axillary nerve	C 5, 6
	Deltoid (posterior fibers)	Axillary nerve	C 5, 6
Circumduction	Combinations of the above		

1 Reproduced with permission from MacKinnon P and Morris J (2005). *Oxford Textbook of Functional Anatomy Vol 1*. Oxford University Press, Oxford. ©2005.

Impingement syndrome

Neer's sign (impingement sign)
This test attempts to force the greater trochanter under the acromioclavicular joint to compress the bursa, rotator cuff, and biceps tendon. The arm is placed into maximum forward flexion and internal rotation while stabilizing the scapula (similar to a Nazi salute). The test is positive if pain is experienced.

Hawkin's sign
With the elbow flexed at 90° and the shoulder forward flexed at 90° the humerus is progressively internally rotated in order to grind the proximal humerus against the acromioclavicular joint. The test is positive if pain is experienced.

Impingement test
The impingement test involves the injection of 10cc of a 1% lidocaine solution into the subacromial space. Greater than 80% resolution of the pain with repeat testing for impingement signs is a positive test and suggests impingement syndrome.

Posterior impingement sign
Executed with the patient supine. The arm is placed in 90–110° of abduction and in slight extension (10–15°). The shoulder is rotated into maximum external rotation. Recreating symptoms marked by complaints of pain deep within the posterior aspect of the shoulder is indicative of a positive test for posterosuperior glenoid impingement.

Rotator cuff

Drop arm test
With the arm straight, shoulder abducted past 90°, and then forward flexed to 30° the patient is asked to slowly lower it to the side. With a supraspinatus tear they are unable to lower the arm slowly and the arm drops to the side.

Jobe's manoeuvre (empty can test)
With the arm straight, and the shoulder abducted to 90° and horizontally adducted to 30°, the humerus is internally rotated to 45° (as if emptying a beverage can). With a supraspinatus tear they are unable to maintain the position against resistance. The shoulder must be compared to the opposite side. In a recent study the position of supination (full can position) provided improved isolation of the supraspinatus. It is therefore recommended that both pronation and supination be utilized.

Gerber's lift off test (lift off test)
With the dorsum of the hand placed over the sacrum, the patient is asked to push away from the back against resistance. With subscapularis weakness or tear they are weaker on the affected side compared to the contralateral side.

External rotator test
With the elbows at their side and at 90° of flexion, and the humerus in 45° of internal rotation, the patient is asked to externally rotate the

humerus against resistance. With infraspinatus weakness they are weaker on the affected side as compared to the contralateral side.

External rotation lag sign

This tests infraspinatus and supraspinatus integrity. The patient is seated with their back to the examiner. The elbow is passively flexed to 90°, and the shoulder is held at 20° of abduction and near maximal external rotation (maximal external rotation minus 5° to avoid elastic recoil). The patient is then instructed to maintain this position as the examiner releases the arm supporting only the elbow. The sign is positive if a >10° lag or an angular drop is seen.

The drop sign

This tests mainly the infraspinatus integrity. The patient is seated with their back to the examiner. The affected arm is held at 90° of abduction and at almost full external rotation with the elbow flexed at 90°. They are then asked to maintain this position as the examiner releases the hand and supports only at the elbow. The sign is positive if a >10° lag occurs.

The internal rotation lag sign

This tests mainly the subscapularis integrity. The patient is seated with their back to the examiner. The affected arm is held behind the back. The elbow is flexed to 90° and the shoulder is held at 20° of abduction and 20° of extension. The patient's hand is then pulled away from the back until in almost maximal internal rotation. They are then asked to maintain this position as the examiner releases the hand and supports only at the elbow. The sign is positive if a >10° lag occurs.

Acromioclavicular joint

Crossover test

With the elbow extended the arm is brought across the chest stressing the acromioclavicular joint. Tenderness is felt in the lateral shoulder if the test is positive.

Biceps

Yergason's test

With the elbow at 90° and the wrist held in pronation the patient will experience pain if they attempt to supinate the wrist against resistance.

Speed's test

With the elbow flexed at 30°, shoulder at 60° of flexion and the wrist supinated, the patient will experience pain if they attempt to flex the arm against resistance.

Labral tears

Biceps load test II

With the patient in the supine position the examiner holds the patient's wrist and elbow with the shoulder in 120° of abduction and maximally externally rotated. The elbow is placed in 90° of flexion and the forearm supinated. The patient is asked to flex the elbow against the examiner's resistance. The test is considered positive for a labral lesion if there are increased complaints of pain with resisted elbow flexion.

Clunk test
While applying gentle axial pressure to the humerus with the elbow at 90°, rotate the humerus internally and externally while simultaneously abducting the arm. If the examiner's opposite hand is placed under the humeral head a clunk, pop, or snap may be felt if a labral tear is present.

Crank test
With the patient in the sitting or standing position the arm is elevated to 160° in the scapular plane. An axial load is applied to the humerus while simultaneously internally and externally rotating the humerus. Pain or reproduction of the patient's symptoms (usually pain or catching) is considered a positive test.

O'Brien test.
Performed with the patient in the sitting position the shoulder is abducted to 90° with the elbow in full extension. The forearm is then pronated with the thumb pointing down. A downward force is placed on the arm by the examiner. The force is repeated with the forearm in the supinated position with the thumb pointing upwards. Pain or clicking inside the shoulder joint is considered a positive test for a labral lesion. Pain over the acromioclavicular joint indicates pathology in the acromioclavicular joint.

Thoracic outlet syndrome

Adson's manoeuvre
While feeling the radial pulse the arm is passively abducted, extended, and externally rotated (abduction and external rotation of the arm compresses the brachial plexus against the scalene muscles). The head is extended and turned to the side of the lesion while the patient holds their breath. Loss of pulse is a positive test.

Wright's manoeuvre (hyperabduction manoeuvre)
Similar to Adson's manoeuvre but the arm is hyperabducted over the head while externally rotated and extended (this simulates compression of the neurovascular bundle beneath the pectoralis tendon). Loss of or a diminished radial pulse is a positive test.

Costoclavicular manoeuvre (military brace position)
The patient sits upright and thrusts the shoulders backward while the hands rest on the thighs. This narrows the space between the clavicle and the first rib. This may reproduce the symptoms if a 'backpacker's neuropathy' is present.

Roos test (overhead exercise test)
The arms are abducted to 90°, shoulders externally rotated, and the elbows flexed to 90°. The hands are opened and closed for 3 minutes to reproduce the symptoms. This may be positive in baseball pitchers with symptoms while in the cocking phase (though this mechanism may also represent an anterior instability).

Subscapular bursa
- Located between the scapula and the thoracic wall.
- May become inflamed with overuse.

Nerves

The brachial plexus is a complex array of roots, trunks, divisions, cords, and branches.

- Any of these areas may be injured with stretching of the brachial plexus.
- Because of the high incidence of anterior dislocations the most likely peripheral nerve to be damaged is the musculocutaneous nerve.
- Other peripheral nerves that are likely to be damaged include the axillary, suprascapular, and the long thoracic nerves.

Shoulder disorders

Epidemiology

- Shoulder pain is the second most common musculoskeletal complaint seen by practitioners: 1.2–2.5% of attendances in primary care.
- Rotator cuff lesions (65%).
- Pericapsular soft tissue pain (11%).
- Acromioclavicular joint pain (10%).

Factors related to early recovery:
- Mild trauma.
- Acute onset.
- Overuse problems.
- Early presentation.

Problems that are related to prolonged recovery are:
- Diabetes mellitus.
- Cervical spondylolysis.
- Radicular symptoms.
- Advancing age.
- Involvement of the dominant extremity.

Causes

Causes of increased susceptibility to injury include:
- An inherently less stable joint.
- The fact that we 'abuse' the joint with repetitive work activities and participate in sports that push the limits of the joint.

Differential diagnosis

Acute problems with rapid onset over days to a few weeks include:
- Trauma.
- Acute overuse.
- Cervical nerve root compression.

The age of the patient and the history may narrow the differential diagnosis.
- Patients below the age of 45 often have a biomechanical cause to their problem such as instability or tendonitis.
- Those older than 45 are more likely to have degenerative conditions such as osteoarthritis or rotator cuff tears.
- Evaluate the patient for adhesive capsulitis if there is a history of diabetes mellitus, progressive pain, and loss of motion.

Acute traumatic causes

Anterior glenohumeral instability

From grade I, with less than 50% subluxation of the humeral head beyond the glenoid fossa, to grade IV, which is a complete dislocation.

Anterior dislocation

- If a patient lands on the posterior aspect of the shoulder during a fall forcing the humeral head anteriorly on the glenoid or by forced external rotation while the upper extremity is abducted.
- The pressure of the anterior glenoid on the posterior humerus during dislocation may cause a small compression fracture or divot on the posterior humeral head known as a Hill Sach's lesion.
- While the humeral head is being forced anteriorly, the anterior capsule may tear the labral cartilage away form the underlying glenoid, termed a Bankart's lesion, worsening the anterior instability.

History and examination

- Patients usually present with pain in the anterior and lateral shoulder.
- They will often complain of an inability to move the shoulder without significant pain and in many cases 'know' it is dislocated.
- With an acute anterior dislocation, the acromioclavicular joint may be prominent on exam.
- Patients will hold the arm in a partially abducted and externally rotated position.
- If the shoulder has relocated they may have signs of instability on examination, or a positive Speed's test.

Investigation

- Diagnosis of dislocation is usually obvious on inspection.
- May be identified by X-ray evaluation, particularly the scapular Y view.
- A thorough neurovascular exam should be documented in all cases.

Treatment

- Immediate reduction preferably after evaluation by X-ray.
- Surgical intervention after the first dislocation is unusual but may be appropriate in:
  - High performance athlete at risk for repeated dislocations (football, hockey, or other collision sport).
  - Worsening symptoms of instability despite conservative treatment.
- Consider a rotator cuff tear in the first time dislocater older than 45 years of age.

Posterior glenohumeral dislocation

Posterior dislocations account for only 4% of dislocations. Posterior dislocations generally require great force and are often seen after motor vehicle accidents, seizure activity, repetitive weight lifting, or in football linemen. The mechanism is usually a force applied to the forward flexed upper extremity at 90°, forcing the humerus posteriorly. It may also occur after an anterior blow to the shoulder. A small avulsion of the posterior glenoid labrum may occur resulting in a reverse Bankart lesion.

History and examination

- Patients with posterior dislocations will present with the arm in internal rotation, and held close to the thorax.
- They are generally unable to abduct or externally rotate the shoulder.
- The coracoid may be prominent and the humeral head difficult to palpate.

Investigations

- Routine shoulder films may miss this injury.
  - Only axillary or scapular Y views demonstrate this well.

Treatment

Treatment is reduction.

Inferior glenohumeral dislocation

Inferior glenohumeral dislocations are unusual because of the protection given by the acromion. This may represent a generalized laxity and be associated with multidirectional instability. The mechanism is usually a forced abduction injury aided by caudal pressure on the proximal upper arm. The acromion acts as a fulcrum and forces the humeral head inferiorly.

History and examination

- With chronic instability there is pain while the arm is down by the side or overhead.
- These patients may also complain of easy fatigability while carrying loads.
- On inspection the acromion may be prominent.
- There may be a positive sulcus sign.
- Forced abduction may cause pain or apprehension.

Investigations

- Scapular Y views demonstrate this dislocation well.

Treatment

- Treatment is by immediate reduction with pre- and post-reduction films.
- Rehabilitation.
- Surgical stabilization may be possible even if multidirectional instability is present.

Conservative management of shoulder dislocation

For the elite athlete, or in cases of reoccurrence, a surgical stabilization may be the treatment of choice. For most athletes, however the first time dislocation will be managed conservatively. Estimated time to return to sport with conservative management: 3 months.

During all rehabilitation programmes following shoulder dislocation, it is important to ensure the appropriate balance and restoration of scapulo-thoracic stabilization, glenohumeral stabilization and humeral control, and the various neuromuscular mechanisms involved in their modulation.

Immobilization stage

Initially this will involve immobilization in a sling for 2–4 weeks. Longer periods of immobilization may be reserved for younger athletes.

Aims
- Minimize atrophy of the shoulder muscles.
- Maintain elbow mobility/strength.
- Maintain wrist mobility/strength.

Treatment
- Electrical muscle stimulation.
- Isometrics:
  - Elbow—flexion/extension.
- Grip strengthening.
- Active/assisted shoulder mobilizations within the limits of pain.

Early stage: weeks 1–3
Aims
- Begin to assess/manage underlying risk factors.
- Begin strengthening of the rotator cuff complex.
- Begin joint approximation/proprioceptive exercises.
- Gain full passive ROM.
- Enhance static and dynamic control of shoulder complex.
- Improve shoulder complex positional awareness.

Assess risk factors
Some athletes are predisposed to shoulder dislocation. Internal risk factors interact with an inciting event (e.g. fall on an outstretched arm) or in certain cases extrinsic risk factors (e.g. poor underfoot conditions), to cause the injury. Highlighting risk factors and implementing an appropriate rehabilitation programme can greatly decrease the chance of reoccurrence.

Note: adolescent athletes run a high risk of re-dislocating their shoulder, if they are managed conservatively. This should be clarified at the early stages of rehabilitation.

Common intrinsic risk factors include:
- Mechanical instability.
- Functional instability/decreased joint positional sense.
- Muscle weakness of:
  - The rotator cuff complex.
  - Lower trapezius.
  - Rhomboids.
  - Serratus anterior.
- Poor scapulo-humeral rhythm.
- Poor technique. e.g. tackling in contact sports.
- Inappropriate training drills.
- Poor general conditioning.
- Previous injury.
- Injury from inciting event e.g. Bankart lesion, Hills-Sachs lesion, acetabular labrum damage.

General exercises
Mobility
- Progress active assisted exercises up to full elevation through flexion.

Shoulder complex control
- Postural correction
  - Athlete focuses on finding/maintaining a neutral position of the shoulder complex.
  - Maintaining neutral shoulder adding active flexion/abduction through to 60°.
  - Increase the speed of the movements.
  - Add gentle oscillations of movement through the range.
- Strengthening: with all strengthening exercises, the athlete is encouraged to maintain a neutral shoulder position.
- Isometric strengthening of all muscle groups:
  - This should be performed in a neutral position with the flexed elbow resting on a table or similar surface.
  - The athlete adds resistance to the affected limb using the unaffected side (5s hold x 8reps x 3sets). Movements strengthened should include:
    —Flexion.
    —Extension.
    —Internal rotation.
    —External rotation.
    —Abduction.
    —Adduction.
  - After 2 weeks, the athlete should perform these exercises in various degrees of shoulder flexion and/or abduction ensuring at all times that neutral scapular position is maintained.
  - Lower traps/rhomboid exercises:
    —Shoulder blade squeezes: athlete is instructed to pull shoulder blades together and downwards.
    —Arms in neutral position.
    —Arms in 45° abduction.
  - Pillow squeezes:
    —Pillow in axilla, the athlete squeezes the pillow into his/her body.
  - Theraband exercises:
    —IR: from neutral to full IR.
    —ER: from full IR to neutral.
    —IR: from full ER to full IR.
    —ER: from full IR to full ER.
    —Flexion: neutral to 30°.
    —Abduction: neutral to 30°.
  - Serratus anterior strengthening:
    —Supine lying, straighten arm into end position for bench press.
    —Reach towards ceiling to protract scapula.
    —Ensure that shoulders do not roll forwards into slouched position.
    —15 reps x 3 sets.

- Joint approximation/positional sense training:
  —In a prone position with both forearms in contact with the ground, the athlete gently transfers weight over to the injured side. Note: both forearms remain in contact with the ground at all times. Athlete must aim to prevent shoulder blade protraction/winging.
  —In a supine position with arm in 90° flexion. Therapist applies manual approximation—athlete maintains a neutral position within shoulder complex.

Middle stage: weeks 4–10

Aims
- Progress strengthening.
- Increase joint approximation/joint positional sense.

Excercises
Joint approximation/positional sense/balance (throughout all exercises, the athlete is encouraged to maintain neutral shoulder position e.g. avoiding protraction/winging).
- Four point kneeling:
  - Keeping knees/hands in contact with the floor, gently transfer weight to all four corners of support.
  - Lift uninjured arm through elevation.
  - Lift uninjured arm through elevation, simultaneously extend the contralateral hip.
  - To progress:
    —Increase the speed of the movements.
    —Use dynamic surface e.g. Wobble board, balance pad.
    —Add manual perturbation.
- Gym ball: athlete standing, using both arms (at 90° shoulder flexion), presses a gym ball/football against a wall.
  - To progress:
    —Gradually increase the force/body weight transferred against the ball.
    —Single arm.
    —Add small oscillations—increase speed.
- Press ups:
  - Alternate hand position.
  - Dynamic surface.
  - Push ups plus.
    —In press-up end position, arms straight, protract shoulder.
    —Ensure movement happens in straight line and that shoulders do not round.
    —Keep head in neutral position.
    —Try to keep shoulder blades flat against back.
  - 3x15reps Step press ups:
    —Alternate leading arm.
    —Add reaction.

- Standing positional control exercises:
  - Stand in front of wall with shoulder in 90° flexion.
  - Slowly fall forwards against wall onto outstretched hand.
  - Push backwards off wall using protraction of shoulder—NOT elbow or wrist movement.
  - 3x15reps.
  - Progress by standing further away from wall.

Bodyblade exercises
- A bodyblade can be extremely useful in encouraging muscle activation, improving endurance, and enhancing positional sense.
- Oscillate the bodyblade as quickly as possible ensuring that movement occurs through rotation of the glenohumeral joint NOT wrist, elbow, or shoulder girdle movement.
- Perform in the following positions:
  - Neutral with elbow bent to 90°.
  - 45° abduction side with elbow bent to 90°.
  - 90° abduction side with elbow bent to 90°.
  - Arm above head.
  - Throwing position.
  - All fours with arm raised in front (as for superman exercise).

Strengthening
Once the athlete has gained a good baseline of shoulder control and strength in a neutral position, strengthening through range is essential and should focus on improving rotator cuff strength. The following exercises may be included:
- IR.
- ER.
- Rhythmic stabilizations.
- Scaption with internal rotation (empty can) using theraband or light dumbbell.
- Resisted assistive scaption using cable.
- Resisted assistive horizontal abduction using cable.
- Horizontal abduction using theraband or light dumbbell.
- Seated row using cable pulley or theraband.

Further progression should focus on combined movements through various planes.
- Add multi-directional PNF strengthening through shoulder diagonal patterns. Focus predominantly on the following movement patterns:
- ER/abduction/flexion.
- IR/adduction/ext (Sword draw).

End stage: weeks 10–12
Aims
- Progress JPS training/joint approximation exercises.
- Begin power/plyometric loading.
- Increase strength of gross shoulder movements.
- Begin sports-specific rehabilitation.

Joint approximation/positional sense/balance
- Wax on/wax off
- Press up to rotate:
  - In full elbow extension the athlete lifts the uninjured arm, and brings it into abduction, whilst maintaining single arm support and control with the weight bearing injured arm.
  - Gym ball walk outs—progress by multi-station step ups with hands. This can be further progressed by placing hands onto labile surfaces e.g. balance pad, medicine ball.
  - Add time constraints.
  - Mirroring.
  - Movement memory drills.
- Clap press ups:
  - Add dynamic surface.
    —Medicine ball.
    —Wobble cushion.
    —Gym ball.
- Pro-fitter exercises: Key element of pro-fitter exercises is to maintain shoulder position over the centre of the fitter whilst controlling upper limb movement. All movements should be smooth and controlled
  - Bilateral horizontal flexion/extension.
  - Bilateral flexion/extension.
  - Progress by performing exercise on affected side only.

Eccentric external rotator strength is essential for safe return to throwing activities. Eccentric external rotator strengthening should be carried out only when the athlete has adequate control and stability to do so. High load eccentric training should be introduced gradually at first to avoid significant muscle soreness and associated reduction in upper limb control.
- Eccentric external rotation can be trained using the following exercises:
  - Sit with arm in 90° abduction, use unaffected arm to position shoulder in external rotation. Theraband can be used in the early stages to provide resistance. Slowly and in controlled manner internally rotate the shoulder.
  - This can be progressed by using a cable pulley system or dumbbell.
  - Further progression is then introduced be removing any support for the elbow and moving further into a functional throwing position.
  - Gradually increase the speed of movement.
- Advanced eccentric external rotation training:
  - Use a modified dumbbell that has weight applied to only one end.
  - Athlete holds the other end and, with the shoulder in the correct position, forcefully internally rotates the shoulder as quickly as possible.
  - The external rotators must eccentrically contract to brake the movement.
  - Begin with 3 sets of 4 reps progressing to sets of 12 reps.

Strength and conditioning
Initially the athlete should carry out each activity using dumb bells, form and fatigue can be compared with the uninjured side.

A typical circuit might include:
- Bench press
- Shoulder press
- Chin ups
- Up right rows
- Bicep curls
- Tricep extensions.

On successful completion of a dumbbell strengthening programme, the athlete may progress back into Olympic lifting. Technical drills should be used initially before increasing weight and resistance.

Athletes returning to contact sports may have a higher risk of reoccurrence, therefore other higher demanding conditioning drills may be of benefit in the later stages of rehabilitation, and these include:
- Single arm cleans.
- Pec fly/alternate pec fly.
- Eccentric dumbbell catch.
  - High speed ER rotation, at 90° of abduction.
- Medicine ball throws
  - These should begin with two hands using:
    —Chest pass.
    —Overhead—forwards and back.
    —Lateral throw at waist height/shoulder height/in elevation.
  - Progressing to single arm:
    —Throwing forwards from 90° abduction.
    —These can be carried out lying on a gym ball or standing and throwing the ball against a wall.
- Overhead squat.
- Snatch progression through wide arm shoulder press, snatch balance.

Return to play
Prerequisites: prior to a safe return to play, the athlete must have achieved the following:
- Full painfree ROM.
- Negative apprehension test eg. couch based.
- Regained/improved static and dynamic control of the shoulder complex through all resisted movements/weight bearing movements.
- Strength equal to uninjured side—in particular through IR and ER.
  - An isokinetic measurement of IR and ER in 90° of abduction may be the most challenging and functional test of strength.
- Full participation in strength and conditioning.
- Negative apprehension/sound technique during higher risk sporting activity e.g. front- or side-on tackling in rugby football.

Example of final pitch-based rehabilitation

E.g. rugby football
The very nature of contact/collision sports increase the risk of injury, therefore prior to a full return to training, athletes must be strong enough and confident enough to perform every potential match scenario that may involve direct or indirect shoulder contact.

Note that in each of these drills, the athlete should be technically and tactically proficient; therefore the lead rehab therapist may require input and advice from coaching staff.

● Down and ups:
  • Front on.
  • R/L side.
● Down and ups to retrieve a ball.
● Contact drills:
  • Side contacts (athlete makes side on contact with a tackle pad/bag or player using the injured shoulder, with his/her arm remaining in minimal abduction).
  • Hit and spins.
  • Hand off:
    —As the arm is.
  • Taking tackles:
    —Ground contact: initially this can be performed at walking pace.
    —Falling to present ball/pop ball up.
  • Making tackles: note: initially the target (tackle bag/pad/player) should be static.
    —Front on tackle.
    —Side on tackle.
    —Recovery.
    —To progress:
      –Gradual increase of speed/strength of hit/intensity of the session.
      –The athlete should then progress to hitting a dynamic target.
      –Add tactical decision making.

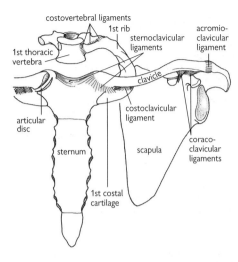

Fig. 9.3 Bones and ligaments of the shoulder girdle. Reproduced with permission from MacKinnon P and Morris J (2005). *Oxford Textbook of Functional Anatomy Vol 1.* Oxford University Press, Oxford. ©2005.

Acromioclavicular joint separations

Acute acromioclavicular sprains or separations are a common traumatic injury usually resulting from a fall onto the lateral shoulder.

- Type 1 is a mild sprain to the acromioclavicular ligaments. There is no separation of the acromioclavicular joint compared to the unaffected side.
- Type 2 involves rupture of the acromioclavicular ligament, but the coracoclavicular ligament is intact. There is less than one centimetre displacement of the acromion from the clavicle.
- Type 3 involves complete rupture of both acromioclavicular and coracoclavicular ligaments.
- Type 4, 5, and 6 injuries are also described and will usually require referral, but these are rare.

History and examination

- Patients will usually present with pain in the lateral shoulder. Sometimes over the distal trapezius with radiation to the proximal humerus..
- Motion is usually intact, but limited by pain.
- Palpation over the acromioclavicular joint may be tender.
- The patient may not feel pain if there is a grade 3 separation and may only sense instability.
- The crossover test may be positive.

Investigations

- The diagnosis is usually made on examination.
- Grading of sprains relies on radiologic examination with comparison to the opposite shoulder.
- Weighted films to overcome splinting due to pain has not been shown to be necessary.

Treatment

- Treatment is primarily symptomatic.
- The shoulder should be immobilized for a short period of time (1–2 days for a grade I, and 5–7 days for a grade III).
- Braces and long term slings are not recommended.
- Range of motion exercises should be started as soon as tolerated.
- Surgical stabilization is usually not necessary. Only indicated for chronic pain, instability, or for aesthetic reasons. In cases of aesthetics, the patient may only be 'trading a bump for a scar'.

Sternoclavicular joint separations

Sternoclavicular joint separations are much less common than acromioclavicular separations. Anterior subluxations are seen much more frequently than posterior subluxations. The injury involves disruption of both the sternoclavicular and costoclavicular ligaments. They are graded as first, second, or third degree injuries depending on the degree of associated capsular disruption. The most common mechanism is a fall onto the lateral or posterolateral shoulder often with a concurrent force applied to the opposite shoulder. This may be seen in a takedown in wrestling or a pile up in football or rugby. Less commonly, a posteriorly directed force directly over the sternoclavicular joint may occur which can result in a posterior dislocation.

History and examination
- While elevating the shoulder there may be a visually or palpably obvious subluxation accompanied by a pop or click.

Investigations
- The dislocation is more easily seen on the serendipity view during plain film examination.
- If suspicion is high but not obvious on plain film there may be a role for MRI in the diagnosis.

Treatment
- Treatment consists of rest, ice, and NSAIDs.
- Third degree injuries are rare but serious if present because of the possibility of superior mediastinal injury. These cases must be reduced immediately.

Glenoid labrum tears

Glenoid labrum tears are most often seen after a glenohumeral dislocation. These patients typically have fallen onto the outstretched arm or have an overuse injury such as in throwing athletes. During an anterior dislocation, the humeral head may tear the anterior and inferior labrum off the underlying glenoid. This may result in a Bankart lesion. If the lesion is present in the superior labrum extending anteriorly to posteriorly beneath the biceps tendon it is termed a SLAP lesion (Superior Labrum Anterior to Posterior). SLAP lesions are associated with marked anterior instability, Bankart's lesions, and rotator cuff tears. Labral lesions are graded as follows:

- Type 1—fraying of the superior labrum.
- Type 2—fraying plus separation from glenoid.
- Type 3—bucket-handle tear of the superior labrum.
- Type 4—bucket-handle tear extending into the biceps tendon.

Posterior impingement

Partial tear of the posterior superior glenoid labrum which may lead to impingement of the rotator cuff. Seen in throwing athletes. The tear itself may be due to traction of the biceps tendon on the superior labrum and posterior rotator cuff weakness. This leads to anterior and superior humeral translation and pinching of the posterior inferior structures during the cocking phase of throwing or in overhead activities.

History and examination

- Glenoid labrum tears are often seen in throwers with pain during the cocking, release, and/or follow-through phases of the throw.
- The pain is usually present in the posterior shoulder.
- Popping, clicking, and snapping are also common complaints.
- They may notice that they cannot throw as hard or as long as previously.
- On examination, patients with labral tears often have a positive Speed's test and often have positive labral tests.
- They may be tender to palpation around the anterior and posterior glenohumeral capsule.
- Signs of anterior instability may also be present.

Investigations

- Routine X-rays are usually normal unless a Bankart or Hill-Sachs lesion is seen.
- Diagnosis is usually based on MRI or CT evaluation. (Double contrast CT scans may elucidate labral pathology but not as well as MRI. An MRI arthrogram may delineate labral lesions best.)

Treatment

If a labral tear is suspected, referral is appropriate because of the chronic nature of the injury, instability, and impingement symptoms.

Biceps tendon rupture

Complete disruption of the tendinous fibres of the biceps occurs most often within the bicipital groove. Occasionally, it presents at the distal tendinous pole. Rupture occurs during a forceful flexion of the elbow, often during weight lifting or catching a heavy object.

History and examination

- The patient has immediate pain either in the shoulder and proximal biceps or in the distal biceps.
- Occasionally there is swelling and ecchymosis.
- They may feel a pop or snap during the initial injury.
- On exam they usually have an obvious bulging defect in the biceps, caused by the retraction of the muscle belly, and referred to as the 'Popeye defect'.
- They may have mild weakness to resisted flexion of the elbow and supination of the forearm if there is a proximal rupture. This may be quite pronounced if there is a distal rupture.

Investigations

- Plain films are usually normal.
- An MRI is only necessary if the diagnosis is uncertain.

Treatment

- Treatment of biceps ruptures is conservative with good results especially in the elderly. The defect generally remains.
- Surgery is indicated if there is a distal tendon rupture at the elbow or a complete tear of the tendons of both the short and long heads of the proximal biceps.
- With single proximal tendon tears, there may only be a surgical indication for heavy manual workers, certain athletes, or for cosmetic reasons.

Biceps tendon dislocation

Biceps tendon dislocation occurs because of retinacular incompetence allowing the long head of the biceps to separate from the bicipital groove of the humeral head. This is often seen in conjunction with a rotator cuff tear or in impingement syndrome.

History and examination
- The patient will present with pain in the anterior shoulder sometimes associated with a snapping or clicking sensation.
- These symptoms may be more pronounced with overhead activities, or with internal and external rotation.
- On exam they usually have a positive Speed's and Yergason's test.
- They may also have signs of a rotator cuff injury or impingement.

Investigations
- Diagnosis is by history and clinical exam.
- MRI is not usually indicated.

Treatment
- Conservative treatment if there is an isolated biceps tendon dislocation.
- If the patient fails conservative treatment, surgical stabilization may be attempted.
- Associated rotator cuff tears and impingement should be treated as indicated.

Fractures of the shoulder

Clavicle fractures

History and examination

- Clavicle fractures are very common and usually follow a fall or a direct blow to the clavicle.
- There is immediate pain and, if there is an associated pneumothorax, there may be shortness of breath or signs of a tension pneumothorax.
- With severe displacement, the brachial plexus may be damaged.
- Evaluate the patient for swelling and deformity of the clavicle, any subcutaneous crepitation, pneumothorax, or neurovascular deficits of the upper extremity.
- X-ray should include clavicular views and a chest film.

Treatment

- Even significantly displaced fractures of the middle third of the clavicle will heal well functionally.
- Management of uncomplicated clavicular fractures includes a sling or figure of eight brace until comfortable, followed by range of motion exercises.
- Referral is necessary with comminuted fractures.
- Treatment of very proximal and very distal fractures is controversial and referral may be appropriate.

Scapular fractures

- Fractures of the scapula are rare.
- Because of the severe trauma required to fracture the scapula, always assess for trauma to other areas.
- The treatment of most scapular fractures involves immobilization in a sling for two to three weeks accompanied by early range of motion exercises as tolerated.
- Significantly displaced scapular fractures or those that involve the glenoid, neck, acromion, or coracoid require orthopaedic referral.

Fractures of the proximal humerus

- Most proximal humeral fractures can be treated by immobilization in a sling for one to three weeks.
- The patient should start range of motion exercises as soon as tolerated.
- In about 20% of fractures there is displacement of the humeral head, the lesser or greater tuberosity, or the humeral shaft. Fractures of the anatomic neck, epiphyseal plate, greater tuberosity avulsion fractures, or fractures involving the humeral head also need to be referred.

Chronic overuse disorders

Instability of the glenohumeral joint

History and examination

- Some patients may present with pain but no history of trauma. This is often seen with repetitive throwing and overhead work which can cause small labral or capsule tears and place extra stress upon the rotator cuff muscles. Recurrent microtrauma may lead to impingement syndrome or osteoarthritis.
- Those with anterior instability typically have a positive apprehension sign, relocation test, and possibly an anterior load and shift test.
- In posterior instability there may be a positive posterior apprehension sign, and perhaps a positive posterior load and shift test.
- Having the patient do a pushup against the wall may reproduce symptoms.
- Inferior instability may show up on exam as a positive sulcus sign.
- Carrying weights or suitcases may reproduce symptoms.
- Multidirectional instability may have signs of anterior, posterior, and/ or inferior instability. These patients may have generalized joint laxity (assess the knees and elbows for hyperextensibility, the ability to abduct the thumb to the forearm when the wrist is flexed, or extension of the metacarpophalangeal joints past 90°).

Investigation

- Routine X-rays may show signs of chronic subluxation such as erosion of the glenoid rim, Hill-Sachs lesions, and lesser tuberosity fractures. X-ray can also show a Bankart lesion.
- An MRI may be useful in diagnosing small labral tears and demonstrate a rotator cuff tear, if suspected.

Treatment

- 80–90% of non-traumatic instabilities respond well to physical therapy but do poorly with surgical intervention.
- If the initial dislocation occurred before the age of thirty, only about one third need operative treatment.
- If a Hill-Sach's lesion, attenuated ligaments, or a torn labrum are present, recurrent dislocations occur after rehabilitation or if the patient plateaus at an unacceptable level, physical therapy will not likely resolve the problem and the patient may benefit from a stabilizing procedure.

Impingement syndrome and rotator cuff tendonitis

Impingement syndrome is an overuse injury with impingement of the rotator cuff between the greater tuberosity of the humerus and the acromion, coracoid, and/or coracoacromial ligament. The rotator cuff, biceps tendon, and the subacromial bursa may all be affected. It occurs with overuse of the shoulder or in chronic instability. The supraspinatus and biceps tendons are at particular risk because of their position under the coracoacromial arch. If the humeral head is allowed to move superiorly due to the laxity, instability may accentuate impingement. Increased mechanical irritation on the bursa and rotator cuff over time

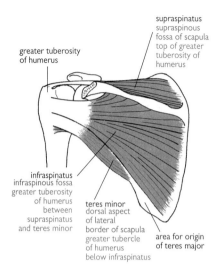

Fig. 9.4 Supraspinatus, infraspinatus, teres minor; acromion removed. Reproduced with permission from MacKinnon P and Morris J (2005). *Oxford Textbook of Functional Anatomy Vol 1*. Oxford University Press, Oxford. ©2005.

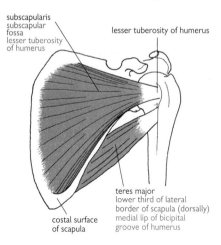

Fig. 9.5 Suscapularis and teres major. Reproduced with permission from MacKinnon P and Morris J (2005). *Oxford Textbook of Functional Anatomy Vol 1*. Oxford University Press, Oxford. ©2005.

leads to increased fibrosis and partial thickness rotator cuff tears and/or partial thickness biceps tendon tears. Eventually this may lead to full thickness rotator cuff and biceps tendon tears. The combination of laxity and impingement is often seen in swimmers and overhead throwers. Impingement syndrome may also result from direct trauma (such as a fall onto an elbow or an outstretched hand), muscular imbalances, posterior capsule tightness, or anatomical overgrowth of the acromion process. Impingement is rarely seen in patients less than 40 years of age, unless there is trauma involved or they are a pitcher. Sports at particular risk are pitching, swimming, tennis, weight lifting, and golf, especially if the patient is overtraining or has poor technique.

History and examination
- The onset of pain is usually gradual and may be present for weeks or months. It is usually located in the lateral deltoid just distal to the tip of the acromion. It may also present with pain in the biceps radiating down to the elbow.
- Pain is usually worsened with overhead activities and when lying on the involved side and may be worse at night.
- The patient may complain of popping, snapping, or grinding.
- On examination, there may be pain between 90–120° of abduction (painful arc).
- There may be tenderness with internal and external rotation while the shoulder is at 90° of abduction.
- Hawkin's, and Neer's tests may be positive.
- The impingement test is usually positive.
- There may be signs of rotator cuff and biceps tendon irritation as well as frank weakness due to pain. This must be re-evaluated after treatment to rule out a complete or partial tear of these tendons.

Investigation
- Radiographic evaluation is usually normal unless there is acromial overgrowth or degenerative joint disease.
- Radiologic evidence of calcification suggests calcific tendonitis (see calcific tendinopathy, p.196).

Treatment
- Treatment is with rest, range of motion exercises, and strengthening exercises of the scapula and thorax.
- Injection of steroids across (but not into) the superior aspect of the rotator cuff may be of benefit to some patients.
- If conservative measures fail after 6 weeks or if partial or complete tears are present surgical intervention should be obtained.
- Prevention is by avoidance of improper techniques used in overhead sport activities and minimizing offending activities.

Rotator cuff tears

Rotator cuff tears occur when there is a complete separation of the tendinous fibres. Most cases are seen in patients over 40 years of age and most have longstanding impingement symptoms. This may be due to age, vascular changes, trauma, attrition, or impingement. If acute trauma is involved, it is usually due to a fall onto an abducted arm or a direct blow to the lateral shoulder. The most likely tendon to be affected is the supraspinatus. The tear may then extend to the infraspinatus, and in severe cases, it may involve the teres minor and biceps tendon. The subscapularis is rarely involved.

History and examination

- The patient usually presents with weakness and poorly localized pain that may radiate to the humerus.
- Pain is worsened with overhead activities.
- Approximately 50% associate their pain with a specific trauma.
- Inspection may demonstrate wasting of the supraspinatus and infraspinatus if the problem has been longstanding.
- The rotator cuff may be tender to palpation or there may be crepitus in the subacromial bursa.
- Direct testing of the muscles of the rotator cuff will find weakness when compared with the unaffected side (Jobe's test and Gerber's manoeuvre).
- The strength of the external rotators may be affected in extensive tears due to the involvement of the infraspinatus.
- Patients usually have less tenderness with passive than active range of motion.
- Most patients will have one or more of the lag signs present, and possibly a positive drop arm test.
- Tests for impingement are often positive including the Hawkin's, Neer's, and the impingement test.

Investigation

- Plain films may only show acromial overgrowth.
- The gold standard had been the arthrogram but it is less reliable in diagnosing partial thickness tears and unreliable in determining the size and extent of tears.
- MRI is now used more often as a non-invasive replacement which can differentiate complete and partial tears and even visualize other shoulder conditions such as articular cartilage damage or tears of the glenoid labrum.
- Unless a complete rotator cuff tear is suspected, an MRI or CT need not be obtained unless the patient has failed 6–8 weeks of conservative therapy. An arthrogram or MRI adds little information unless planning intervention. Ultrasound is less expensive, and may be less sensitive and specific but specificity and sensitivity are highly reliant on technician expertise.

Treatment

- Treatment is usually with rest, and protection and avoidance of all overhead activities.
- Physical therapy.
- Subacromial injections are recommended by some experts but the evidence from randomized controlled trials is equivocal and there is some suggestion that they may impede tendon repair. Use in patients over 40 with caution.

- If symptoms persist for more than 6–8 weeks, or if there are high demands by the patient, they should be referred to orthopaedic assessment for debridement of partial thickness tears or repair of full thickness tears.

Proximal humeral epiphysiolitis (Little Leaguer's shoulder)

- Stress injury to proximal humeral physis 2° shear forces associated with throwing and pitching.
- May be the first stage of a continuum to a physeal stress fracture.

History and examination

- Usually presents in adolescence with shoulder pain on throwing.
- No history of specific injury.
- Usually full ROM.
- Swelling uncommon.

Investigation

AP X-ray in external rotation demonstrates widening of proximal humeral physis. May need to compare with other side.

Treatment

- Rest from throwing (usually >2 months required).
- Graduated return to throwing when asymptomatic.
- Adhere to age guidelines regarding pitching limits and correct throwing technique (if needed) to prevent recurrence.

Prognosis

- Usually good.
- Small risk of premature growth plate closure and subsequent humeral length discrepancy.

Biceps tendonitis

Biceps tendonitis is characterized by pain and inflammation of the long head of the biceps tendon within the bicipital groove. These patients are usually young or middle aged. This condition is often due to repetitive elbow flexion or supination, and in particular activities that require reaching, and overhead lifting; recreational activities such as tennis, swimming, golf, or throwing sports. It is often associated with impingement syndrome and/or rotator cuff tears.

History and examination

- The patient will present with diffuse pain in the anterior shoulder.
- The pain is usually worse during and directly after activity and improves with rest.
- There is usually no pain at night.
- Symptoms may be present for a variable length of time.
- On examination there is tenderness with resisted flexion of the elbow and supination of the wrist.
- There may be tenderness to palpation within the bicipital groove and along the long head of the biceps tendon.
- There may also be limitation of the extremes of abduction, internal rotation, and external rotation.
- Speed's and Yergason's test are typically positive for pain.
- There may be biceps weakness secondary to pain.

Investigations
- X-rays are usually normal.
- MRI is usually not warranted unless a repairable biceps or rotator cuff tear is suspected.

Treatment
- Rest, ice, local heat, and protection.
- Gentle stretching and exercise.
- The patient may benefit from a formal physical therapy programme if a quick return to activities is important.
- Oral anti-inflammatories may be of benefit.
- While injection of the tendon with corticosteroids directly is not recommended, subacromial injection may be of benefit.

Calcific tendonitis

With degeneration of the collagen fibers of the rotator cuff tendons, calcium salts may infiltrate the substance of the tendon and cause inflammation. This may be associated with acute or chronic symptoms and may secondarily involve the bursa. The most common site is the supraspinatus tendon, but it may also involve the biceps tendon, infraspinatus, or subscapularis.

History and examination
- There may be severe pain affecting sleep.
- If calcification is chronic, the patient may have symptoms more like an impingement syndrome.
- On examination, the patient may hold the arm splinted against the body and be in such pain that examination is not possible.
- Any palpation over the affected area produces significant tenderness.
- The tenderness may affect range of motion.
- A globally tender shoulder that he is unwilling to move.

Investigations
- X-ray examination of the shoulder may show calcifications.
- AP views in external rotation and internal rotation will show the rotator cuff best.
- Bicipital groove views show biceps tendon calcifications.

Treatment
- Treatment by injection of a lidocaine and steroid preparation may be effective and provide dramatic relief. Protect biceps movement for two weeks after such an injection.
- Oral anti-inflammatories rarely provide as significant an improvement.
- Physical therapy.
- Surgical intervention is rarely required.

Acromioclavicular degenerative joint disease

Degenerative joint disease of the acromioclavicular joint is common and develops much earlier than that of the glenohumeral or sternoclavicular joint.

History and examination
- The patient usually complains of intermittent pain, gradual in onset, but may present after trauma.
- There may be intermittent swelling, popping, clicking, or grinding.
- On examination the patient is usually tender over the superior and anterior aspect of the acromioclavicular joint.
- There may be a prominence to the acromioclavicular joint on inspection.
- The crossover test is usually positive.

Investigations
- X-ray.
- Diagnosis can be verified by injection of lidocaine into the joint and resolution of the pain supports the diagnosis.

Treatment
- Treatment is usually symptomatic.
- Injection with a steroid may be of benefit.
- Surgical intervention consists of resection of the distal clavicle and removal of the intra-articular disc, if present, but is unusual.

Adhesive capsulitis (frozen shoulder)

Adhesive capsulitis may be due to prolonged immobilization or disuse due to pain, reflex sympathetic dystrophy, or idiopathic. The pathophysiology is unclear. Patients with diabetes mellitus are more at risk. The patient is often female with involvement of the nondominant arm.

History and examination
- The pain is usually gradual in onset and located over the insertion of the deltoids.
- Patients may report difficulty sleeping on the affected side.
- On examination, active and passive range of motion to abduction, internal rotation, and external rotation, are limited by adhesions in the capsule.
- There is no specific point tenderness but often a diffuse tenderness exists especially with movement.

Treatment
- Treatment is by intensive physical therapy.
- It may take years to completely resolve.
- Surgical manipulation under anesthesia may be required.

Osteolysis of the distal clavicle

Often caused by chronic overuse, but may also be initiated by an acute traumatic injury. Weight lifters appear to be more prone. Osteolysis of the distal clavicle usually presents with chronic pain in the lateral superior shoulder lasting longer than four months.

History and examination

Pain is usually a dull ache over the acromioclavicular joint. There may be weakness and pain with flexion and adduction.

Investigation

Diagnosis is usually by plain X-ray which may show osteopenia with tapering of the distal clavicle, and associated osteophytes, subchondral erosions, and cysts.

Treatment

Treatment is usually by surgical resection if the pain is unacceptable.

Atraumatic causes

Thoracic outlet syndrome

There are four areas of potential compression:

1 Compression of the subclavian vein between the anterior scalene, clavicle, and first rib.
2 Compression of the brachial plexus and subclavian artery between the anterior scalene, middle scalene, and first rib.
3 Compression of the neurovascular bundle between the clavicle and the first rib.
4 Compression of the neurovascular bundle as it passes under the tendinous portion of the pectoralis minor.

Cervical ribs are the most common bony anomaly seen with thoracic outlet syndrome. 10% of these however are asymptomatic. Trauma, as a precipitating factor, is not uncommon.

History and examination

- Patients may complain of neurologic, vascular, or combined symptoms.
- Neurologic symptoms consist of pain, often sharp but sometimes aching, that radiates from the neck or shoulder into the forearm or hand, often following an ulnar nerve distribution.
- Paresthesias and hyperaesthesias may also be present.
- Symptoms may be exacerbated by overhead activity.
- Vascular symptoms that originate from the subclavian artery may cause pain over the supraclavicular space.
- There may be associated pale, cold, or numb fingers.
- Activities that involve elevation or abduction of the arm may worsen such symptoms.
- Compression of the subclavian vein may cause pain over the supraclavicular space or the feeling of pressure in the extremity.
- On examination, the extremity may appear dusky, swollen, mottled, or blue, or it may appear entirely normal.
- The patient may have a positive Wright's manoeuvre, Roos manoeuvre, and/or Adson's test.

Investigations

- X-ray evaluation of the cervical spine and chest.
- If vascular compromise, Doppler studies will usually define the area of concern. Angiograms are usually necessary if there are abnormalities seen on Doppler.
- Electrodiagnostic studies may be needed if neurologic compromise is suspected.

Treatment

- Shoulder strengthening exercises concentrating on posterior scapular stabilization, if the patient's symptoms are not disabling or consistent with vascular compromise.
- If there is vascular compromise, or conservative treatment fails, surgical intervention usually consists of resection of the first rib.

Reflex sympathetic dystrophy (shoulder-hand syndrome)

History and examination

- Shoulder involvement is common in reflex sympathetic dystrophy.
- Clinically it presents as pain and limitation of motion with dystrophic skin changes of the ipsilateral hand and arm.
- There may be pain and swelling in the distal extremity.
- It is bilateral in 25–30% of cases.
- Risk factors include cardiovascular disease, recent myocardial infarction, cervical disc disease, and shoulder, arm, or neck trauma.
- No obvious inciting event is present in at least 25% of the patients.

Investigations

- Abnormal resting sweat output (RSO) studies in combination with quantitative sudomotor axon reflex tests (QSART) are thought to correlate strongly with the diagnosis of reflex sympathetic dystrophy.
- Technetium pyrophosphate bone scan is a sensitive tool and demonstrates increased blood flow to the involved extremity and mild synovitis.
- X-rays may show periarticular osteoporosis, and erosions.

Treatment

- Treatment with a short course of steroids and active, assisted range of motion of the hand, elbow, and shoulder provides adequate treatment in most patients.
- Sympathetic blockade or surgical sympathectomy may be needed for patients with persistent symptoms.

Septic arthritis

Septic arthritis of the shoulder is rare. It is most frequently seen in infants and children two years of age or younger, but may be seen at any age. It represents a surgical emergency. If left untreated it could lead to septic shock, arthritis, or a fused joint. There is an increased incidence in those patients with diabetes mellitus, cancer, hypogammaglobulinemia, or chronic liver disease and in those receiving corticosteroid or immunosuppressive drugs. The more common organisms to infect the joint are *S. aureus* (most common in adults), *N. gonorrhoeae*, *Strep. pneumoniae*, *Strep. pyogenese*, *H. influenza* (most common in neonates), and gram negative bacilli.

History and examination

- The patient usually presents with pain, swelling, and loss of range of motion of the joint with no apparent portal of entry.
- Occasionally they may present following an aspiration or injection procedure of the joint.

Investigations and treatment

- Diagnosis is by aspiration of joint fluid.
- If frank pus is present, immediate incision and drainage should be performed and the patient started on intravenous antibiotics.
- If the clinical suspicion is high and the joint fluid appears normal or equivocal the patient should be started on intravenous antibiotics until the cultures return.

Osteonecrosis (ischaemic necrosis, avascular necrosis)

- Ischemia of the humeral head is typically referred to as avascular necrosis (AVN) of the humeral head.
- It is associated with hemoglobinopathies, pancreatitis, alcoholism, and connective tissue disease. It has also been documented in gout, osteoarthritis, burns, Goucher's disease, prolonged immobilization, pregnancy, hyperparathyroidism and cytotoxic treatments.
- The patient will usually present with chronic shoulder pain and limited range of motion.
- X-ray changes are not seen until several months after the onset of pain.
- Technetium pyrophosphate bone scanning is useful in detecting early ischemic necrosis as is MRI.
- Treatment is limited to supportive care, but in cases of severe pain total joint arthroplasty may be necessary.

Cervical radiculopathy

- Always consider the cervical spine in any evaluation of shoulder pain
- Cervical radiculopathy causes deep burning pain that radiates from the shoulder to the fingertips and may be associated with paresthesias.
- It is often relieved by forward shoulder elevation or repositioning of the neck.
- Range of motion of the cervical spine should be tested.
- Spurling's manoeuvre and an atlanto-occipital axial compression test should be performed.
- Motor function should be evaluated in the upper extremity, arm, and hand. Fine movements of the hand should be evaluated.
- Deep tendon reflexes should be tested in the upper extremity as well as a sensory exam.
- An appropriate cervical work-up should precede a shoulder work-up if any abnormalities are found.

Tumours of the shoulder

- The most common malignant bony tumors of the humerus are Ewing's sarcoma and osteosarcoma. These tend to occur in adolescence.
- Chondrosarcomas, though rare, tend to occur during the third to seventh decade. Most cases in adults, however, represent metastatic lesions (especially hypernephroma) or multiple myeloma.
- Other lesions seen include osteochondromas, chondroblastomas, giant cell tumors, aneurysmal bone cysts, and Pancoast tumors.
- Tumors may present with pain that is worse at night and in some cases may be significantly improved with NSAIDs.
- Plain radiographs may identify the lesions but MRI is usually needed for clarification.

Referred pain from the chest and abdomen

- The phrenic nerve arises from the fourth cervical nerve but also receives branches from the third and fifth nerves. It begins at the posterior scalene muscle, descends the chest in the lateral part of the pericardium and ends at the diaphragm. Branches of this nerve provide sensory innervation to the mediastinal and diaphragmatic pleura, diaphragmatic peritoneum, and probably the liver, gallbladder, and inferior vena cava. Irritation of the diaphragm or the innervated areas of the pleura or peritoneum will stimulate the phrenic nerve.

- Since these nerves also innervate the skin of the neck, supraclavicular area, and shoulder, pain may be referred to these areas.
- Pneumonia, pulmonary infarction, empyema, neoplasm, hepatobiliary disease, subphrenic abscess, splenic injury, or a pseudocyst of the pancreas can all produce shoulder pain.

Elbow and forearm

History

- Onset, mechanisms, previous injuries.
- Symptoms including pain site(s) and radiation, provocative factors/movements, swelling, locking, tingling, numbness, clicking.
- Are there neck, forearm, or hand symptoms?

Examination

Inspection

- Look at soft tissue contour for evidence of wasting or asymmetry of muscle bulk, muscle fasciculation, scars, deformities, and alignment. Over-development of the dominant arm is common.
- Look for swelling and soft tissue masses in the antecubital fossa.
- Estimate the carrying angle with the arm extended.
- Inspect posteriorly for dislocation, olecranon bursa, effusion, and triceps tendon tear (excessively bony prominence, with a gap just above).
- Inspect laterally for synovitis or effusion which may be evident in the triangular space between the lateral epicondyle, the head of the radius, and the tip of the olecranon.

Palpation

- Examine the bony landmarks with the arm flexed at 90°.
- Tenderness in the area of the MCL indicates injury.
- Palpate the radial head for tenderness (fracture, synovitis, osteoarthritis, dislocation).
- Check the biceps tendon and brachial pulse in the cubital fossa.
- Palpate the lateral collateral ligament and the lateral epicondyle.
- Palpate the ulnar nerve posterior to the medial epicondyle for thickening and/or irritability. Anterior subluxation of the ulnar nerve is often evident with flexion and reduced with extension.
- The flexor-pronator muscle group may be tender at its origin with medial epicondylitis.

Movements

- Assess passive and active range of motion and movement against resistance (for specific muscle groups) and compare sides.

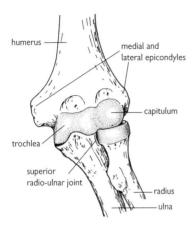

Fig. 10.1 Articular surfaces of elbow joint (anterior aspect). Reproduced with permission from MacKinnon P and Morris J (2005). *Oxford Textbook of Functional Anatomy Vol 1*. Oxford University Press, Oxford. ©2005.

Special tests

Assess MCL and LCL with elbow in 30° of flexion looking for pain and laxity.

Lateral epicondylitis

- Resisted wrist extension is tested with the forearm pronated/supinated and the elbow in two positions: firstly extended then flexed to 90° (extensor carpi radialis brevis).
- Patient extends elbow, pronates the forearm and extends the fingers. The examiner applies downward force to the middle finger (extensor digitorum communis).

Medial epicondylitis

- Resisted wrist flexion with the elbow flexed and forearm supinated.
- Resisted forearm pronation with the forearm extended and in neutral rotation.

Neurovascular status

- Tests of ulnar nerve entrapment: Tinel's test—elbow flexion test (similar to Phalen's test at the wrist).
- Ulnar nerve instability: repeated flexion/extension of the elbow reproduces ulnar nerve symptoms and nerve subluxation.

Medial collateral ligament injury

History and examination

Acute or chronic MCL injury in adults is due to repetitive valgus extension overload which occurs usually in throwers but can occur with direct trauma. MCL instability and a wedging effect of the olecranon into the olecranon fossa may cause a posterior osteophyte which can irritate the ulnar nerve. A sudden onset of pain during throwing, with an associated 'pop' or 'snap' may indicate an acute injury. In chronic cases there is progressive medial elbow pain that is functionally limiting and worse during the acceleration phase of throwing.

On examination there is swelling, local MCL tenderness and instability. Flexion contractures and cubitus valgus deformities are common in throwers. Posteromedial osteophytes may be palpable. Olecranon tenderness is worsened by bringing the arm into valgus and extension.

Investigations

Plain X-rays may be normal. In chronic cases there may be ectopic bone formation in the MCL, posteromedial osteophyte formation at the olecranon and conoid tubercle and loose bodies. Stress films may confirm medial instability. MRI allows assessment of the MCL.

Treatment

Aim to settle the acute symptoms where present and to restore normal range of motion with relative rest, ice, analgesics, and NSAIDs. Commence passive and active range of motion exercises early, with a strengthening regime. Throwing activities are resumed when there is full range of motion. Surgery is considered with chronic instability and impairment. Excision of osteophytes and local debridement or a straight osteotomy, 1cm proximal to the tip of the olecranon may be considered in those with impingement. For instability, reconstruction using a tendon graft; repair may be performed in the acute rupture.

Prevention of the condition is important through adequate conditioning, warm-up, stretching, and appropriate technique.

Medial collateral ligament instability in children

History and examination

This usually occurs in relation to throwing or racket sports. Medial apophysitis is a true epicondylitis due to traction and inflammation of the growth plate at the medial epicondyle. 'Little Leaguer's elbow' is due to a variable combination of a medial apophysitis, MCL injury, and instability, compressive changes at the radiocapitellar joint and osteochondrosis. There is usually gradual onset of an aching pain at the medial elbow and there may be weakness of grip and paraesthesiae in the distribution of the ulnar nerve. An acute avulsion injury at the apophysis can also occur. In the acute avulsion there is a 'pop', followed by medial swelling and weakness.

On examination, there may be swelling and tenderness at the medial epicondyle, and perhaps bruising and flexion contracture. Pain is exacerbated by passive extension of the elbow and wrist. With an avulsion injury, a fragment may be palpable. Stress testing may show medial instability. Lateral elbow tenderness, pain on movement and on compression of the joint indicates lateral compressive changes.

Investigations

Plain X-rays may be normal or may show widening of the physis, fragmentation or avulsion of the apophysis, in comparison to the other side. Gravity valgus stress views may be necessary.

Treatment

Relative rest, analgesics, ice, stretching. Healing can be prolonged. When avulsion has occurred, treat according to degree of displacement. Immobilize for 2 weeks with mild displacement followed by progressive rehabilitation. With large or rotated fragments, consider open reduction and fixation.

Traction apophysitis medial humeral epicondyle ('Little Leaguer's elbow')

This condition is commonly seen in the young, throwing athlete. The valgus force imparted to the elbow when throwing causes compression of lateral elbow structures and stretching of medial elbow structures. This results in traction of the wrist flexors on the apophysis of the medial epicondyle.

History and examination
- Insidious onset of pain over the medial epicondyle (common flexor origin), exacerbated by pitching, bowling, and throwing long distances.
- May have difficulty fully extending the elbow.
- Focal tenderness ± swelling over the common flexor origin.
- Pain is reproduced by passive dorsiflexion of the wrist with the elbow in the extended position and with resisted wrist flexion.

Investigation
- Diagnosis is usually based on clinical findings.
- If onset of pain is acute, X-ray may be warranted to exclude an avulsion fracture of the medial epicondyle.

Treatment
- Rest from throwing activities until pain resolves.
- Stretching programme for wrist flexors.
- As pain improves, a strengthening program should be instituted to avoid further injury on resumption of throwing.
- Full recovery can be expected.

Lateral epicondylitis

History and examination

This is a tendinopathy of the common extensor—supinator tendon rather than epicondylitis. Degenerative microtears (due to repetitive mechanical overload) are found in the common extensor—supinator tendon, with the origin of ECRB most commonly affected.

There is often a history of overuse, involving repetitive flexion-extension or pronation-supination activity. There is acute or chronic lateral epicondylar pain and tenderness worse with gripping. Among tennis players, the backhand stroke is commonly implicated and less skilled players with a faulty technique are most likely to be injured. Equipment factors may play a role; the tennis racquet that may be too heavy or too light, a grip that is too big, string tension that is too tight, and the use of heavy or wet tennis balls. 13% of elite players and up to 50% of non-elite tennis players have symptoms suggestive of lateral epicondylitis and approximately half of these have symptoms for an average duration of 2½ years. It may occur in other sports (e.g. golf—where it is more common than 'golfers elbow'). It particularly affects those aged 40–60 years.

On examination there is tenderness over the ECRB origin at the lateral epicondyle. The tenderness may be diffuse, over the origins of EDC and/or ECRL. One or more provocation tests may be positive. Look for other possible causes of lateral elbow pain including the neck. Examine the equipment and assess technique.

Investigations

Imaging studies are not routinely performed. A 'gun-sight' oblique plain radiograph of the lateral epicondyle may show irregularity punctate calcification in the region of the lateral epicondyle in chronic cases. Ultrasound shows decreased echogenicity, inhomogeneity, and thickening of the tendon, and a local fluid collection may be seen. In chronic cases there is often local calcification at the tendon insertion and irregularity of the bone surface. On MRI there may be increased signal intensity of the extensor tendons close to their insertion on the lateral epicondyle.

Treatment

Relative rest, ice (10–20 minutes every 2 hours in the acute stages), analgesia, and NSAIDs (topical NSAIDs are preferable). In chronic cases, transverse friction massage helps to breakdown scar tissue at the site. Compression straps or counterforce braces applied distal to the bulk of the extensor mass may help. The brace is tightened to a comfortable degree of tension with the forearm muscles relaxed, so that a maximum contraction is limited. Constant use of the brace not advised.

Corticosteroid injections may provide short-term pain relief, but there is no evidence of benefit over placebo in the longer term. The patient must be warned of the significant risk of subcutaneous atrophy, tendon rupture, and other standard risks and informed consent must be obtained.

Stretching of the forearm extensors and range of motion exercises at the elbow and wrist should start early. Progressive rehabilitation for strength and endurance of the forearm extensor-supinator group as soon as pain allows, progressing according to symptoms. Use ice after early rehabilitation sessions to limit an excessive inflammatory response.

The cause. In tennis players, technique and equipment factors must be addressed. Proper racket handle size can be estimated by distance from mid-palmar crease to the ring finger. Evaluation of technique with the help of a coach may prove beneficial. Improvements may be noted by avoidance of the leading elbow during backhand, ensuring that the forearm is only partially pronated, the forward shoulder is lowered, and the trunk is leaning forward. The patient should also consider reducing string tension to 2–3 pounds less than the manufacturers' recommendations (i.e. 50–55 pounds), using slower, lighter tennis balls, and playing on slower courts.

Surgery is reserved for those patients with disabling symptoms who fail to respond to all the above measures over the course of 1 year. Options include repair of the extensor origin after excision of the torn tendon, granulation tissue and local drilling of the subchondral bone of the lateral epicondyle, with an aim to increasing blood supply. The elbow is placed in a posterior plaster splint for a week, then in a lighter splint for 2 weeks, with the elbow in 90° flexion and in neutral rotation. Range of motion exercises are commenced thereafter, with a progressive strengthening regime. Light activities can be recommenced at 3 months, but the patient can expect to wear a counterforce brace initially.

Other surgical options include reduction of the tension on the common extensor origin by fasciotomy, direct release of the extensor origin or lengthening of the ECRB tendon distally. Fasciotomy and complete extensor tendon release can result in loss of strength, and lengthening of ECRB distally appears to be effective only in the minority of cases. Whilst intra-articular procedures such as synovectomy and division of the orbicular ligament have been suggested, these seem inappropriate for an extra-articular condition. Some surgeons advocate decompression of the radial or posterior interosseous nerves on the basis that PIN entrapment is contributing to—or is the primary cause of—chronic symptoms.

Medial epicondylitis

History and examination

This is not a true epicondylitis but an overuse injury of the common tendinous origin of the flexor-pronator muscle group. It commonly occurs with repetitive flexion and pronation, less commonly with valgus stresses, and is seen in throwing and racket sports and in golfers ('golfer's elbow').

It causes an acute/chronic aching pain at the medial elbow and proximal flexor musculature of the forearm. There may be weakness of grip. Some patients have paraesthesiae in the ring and little fingers suggestive of an ulnar neuropathy.

On examination there is tenderness at the medial epicondyle and there may be reduced range of motion at the elbow, due to pain on stretching of the flexor-pronator group with full extension. Other causes of medial elbow pain should be considered including radiation from the neck. One or more of the provocation tests may be positive.

Investigations

Ultrasound shows decreased echogenicity, inhomogeneity and thickening of the tendon and more rarely a local fluid collection. Local calcification within the tendon may occur in chronic cases.

Treatment

Relative rest, ice, analgesics, NSAIDs, and a reverse counterforce brace. Deep transverse friction massage may be used in chronic cases, to breakdown scar tissue. Aim to commence rehabilitation, including early stretching of the wrist and elbow and a progressive strengthening regime of the wrist flexors and forearm pronators. Return to activities when there is full pain free range of movement and strength of grip, forearm pronation and wrist flexion has returned to at least 80% of normal. Corticosteroid injections are rarely necessary and care must be taken because of the proximity of the ulnar nerve.

Prevention includes adequate conditioning of the forearm, attention to technique, and adequate warm-up, stretching, and cool down. Reduce the causes through proper sporting technique and equipment.

Surgery is rarely required. Standard approaches include release of the tendinous origin of pronator teres, and usually a portion of FCR, debridement, and decompression of the ulnar nerve distal to the medial epicondyle. Post-operative rehabilitation is continued for 6 months before a return to full activities. Complications of surgery include loss of full elbow extension (up to 5°) in 1% of cases, superficial infection (in less than 1%), and damage to the ulnar nerve and MCL.

Osteochondritis dissecans and osteochondrosis

History and examination

Osteochondritis dissicans (OCD) is a spontaneous necrosis of the capitallum.

Osteochondrosis (Panner's disease) is necrosis, fragmentation, and regeneration of the capitellar growth plate. These may occur with repetitive stresses and usually in 10–15 year olds involved in gymnastics, racket, and throwing sports. The main symptoms are of pain in the lateral elbow with progressive restriction.

- Focal area of avascular necrosis affecting the subchondral bone of the capitellum, or less commonly, the radial head.
- It is thought to result from compression of lateral elbow structures, leading to vascular compromise and softening of the articular cartilage, followed by fragmentation of the subchondral bone and, later, loose body formation.
- Pain exacerbated by throwing or upper-limb weight bearing.
- May have difficulty fully straightening their elbow.
- May describe locking sensation secondary to loose body formation.
- Elbow effusion and loss of full extension.
- Tenderness localized to the capitellum or radial head.

Investigations

In OCD, X-ray may show fragmentation of an island of subchondral bone. In osteochondrosis there is fragmentation and irregularity of the whole capitellar ossifyc nucleus. X-rays may be normal and, if suspected, further imaging, usually using CT scan is necessary.

- X-rays may show flattening of the capitellum ± fragmentation and loose body formation.
- In early stages it may be necessary to X-ray other side for comparison to detect subtle changes.
- CT scanning is useful for detecting loose bodies, which may be difficult to visualise on X-ray.

Treatment

Osteochondrosis is a self-limiting condition so no intervention is necessary other than relative rest during the acute phase. In OCD, relative rest is important for a minimum of 6 weeks where pain and/or contracture has occurred. Arthroscopic assessment and removal/reattachment of fragment may be required.

- Early recognition is important.
- Rest from aggravating activities.
- Local physiotherapy to reduce swelling and restore range of movement.
- Exercise programme to improve forearm strength should follow.
- If loose bodies present, a surgical opinion should be sought.
- Return to sport when there is resolution of symptoms and effusion and restoration of a full pain-free range of motion.

Prevention

Guidelines regarding pitching should not be exceeded and activity should stop if symptoms recur.

Prognosis

- Early diagnosis will improve prognosis.
- With disruption of the joint surfaces and loose body formation, long-term disability and osteoarthritis can result.

Acute injuries

Rupture of the biceps

History and examination

This may occur with trauma, usually with the elbow in 90° flexion. There is a sudden tearing pain in the antecubital fossa followed by a deep aching discomfort, with bruising and weakness of supination and flexion and grip strength. It is more common with anabolic steroid use.

On examination, there is a palpable gap, a bulbous swelling in the arm, and weakness. A partial rupture of the tendon produces pain and local crepitus on supination and pronation.

Investigation

MRI or ultrasound.

Treatment

Management is early surgical repair.

Triceps rupture

History and examination

Triceps rupture is usually an avulsion injury at the tendo-osseous junction. Patients may describe a sudden tear or pop, pain, swelling, and weakness of elbow extension. Partial ruptures, usually in the central third of the tendon, can also occur. Other injuries may occur simultaneously, including fracture of the radial head. The injury usually occurs after a fall onto the outstretched hand, but can occur after a direct blow. If there is spontaneous rupture, consider anabolic steroid use. On examination there is swelling, a palpable gap, and weakness of elbow extension.

Investigations

In most cases a lateral plain X-ray will show flecks of avulsed bone proximal to the olecranon. It is also important to exclude a fracture of the head of the radius. Ultrasound will confirm tendon rupture.

Treatment

Tendon reattachment is usually recommended with acute rupture. Reconstruction may be considered if there is delay or if there is underlying tendon disease.

Elbow dislocation

History and examination

These may be complicated (with fracture) or simple (without). Displacement is usually posterior or posterolateral and there is considerable soft tissue injury. They usually occur after a fall onto the outstretched hand with the elbow in extension. On examination there is pain, swelling, deformity, and possible neurovascular symptoms. It is important to assess neurovascular status.

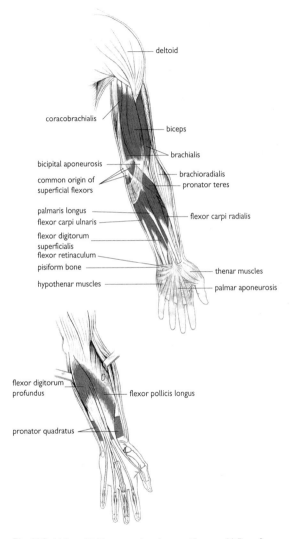

Fig. 10.2 (a) Superficial flexor muscles of arm and forearm. (b) Deep flexor muscles of the forearm. Reproduced with permission from MacKinnon P and Morris J (2005). *Oxford Textbook of Functional Anatomy Vol 1*. Oxford University Press, Oxford. ©2005.

Investigation

X-ray confirmation looking closely for fractures, especially of the radial head and olecranon process.

Treatment

Analgesia and relaxants. Closed reduction is preferably performed under general anaesthetic. Apply longitudinal traction with one hand and with the other apply pressure to relocate the olecranon back onto the trochlea. Assess neurovascular status and elbow stability (extent of soft tissue damage) afterwards.

Supracondylar fractures

History and examination

These usually occur in children and often with a fall onto outstretched hand with elbow pushed into extension. On examination there is pain, swelling, and S-deformity of elbow. Most are displaced so it is essential to check neurovascular status (15% have a neurological injury).

Investigation

X-ray to confirm.

Treatment

With an undisplaced, place in a collar and cuff for 3 weeks and monitor serially to assess for displacement. Displaced fractures and most adults require a closed reduction and, if necessary, fixation.

Lateral condylar fractures

History and examination

Separation can occur at growth plate especially aged 4–10 years and this may cause long-term growth plate damage. Patients describe lateral elbow pain, swelling, dysfunction.

Investigation

Confirm on X-ray.

Treatment

Splint an undisplaced separation in a backslab at 90°. If displaced, reduction and fixation is necessary.

Radial head and neck fractures

History and examination

Radial head fractures usually occur in adults and radial neck injuries in children. They occur after a fall onto an outstretched hand, with the elbow pushed into valgus. On examination there is tenderness, swelling, and there may be limitation in supination/pronation.

Investigation

X-ray.

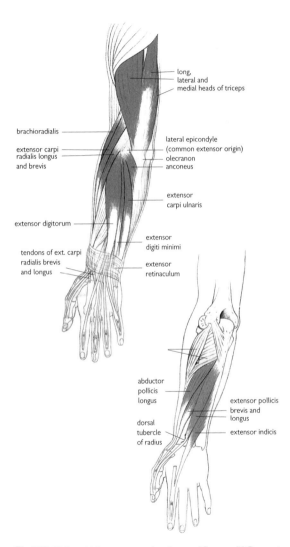

Fig 10.3 (a) Superficial extensor muscles of arm and forearm. (b) Deep extensor muscles of the forearm. Reproduced with permission from MacKinnon P and Morris J (2005). *Oxford Textbook of Functional Anatomy Vol 1.* Oxford University Press, Oxford. ©2005.

Treatment

An undisplaced fracture of the radial head in adults is treated in a back-slab. A displaced fracture requires open reduction and fixation or if comminuted, excision may be necessary. In children, where the fracture is of the radial neck, closed or open, reduction is needed if there is angulation beyond 20° of radial tilt.

Monteggia fractures (ulna fracture with radial head dislocation, in children)

History and examination

This usually occurs after a fall onto an outstretched hand. There is diffuse elbow pain, swelling, and there may be global limitation.

Investigation

On X-ray, the line through the middle of the radial shaft should bisect the radial head in all views. This fracture can be missed.

Treatment

Closed reduction and immobilization. Monitor for displacement on X-ray.

Chronic elbow injuries

Distal biceps tendinopathy

Tendinosis of the distal end of biceps brachii can occur with repetitive supination and pronation activities. Pain is felt in the antecubital fossa and local swelling and tenderness may be noted. Pain is worse with resisted supination. Treatment includes relative rest, ice, NSAIDs, and modification of activities. Failing to address the problem can result in rupture.

Ulnar neuropathy

History and examination

The ulnar nerve is vulnerable along its path through the cubital tunnel posterior to the medial epicondyle and particularly if there is a shallow ulnar groove within the tunnel, hypermobility, or laxity of the soft tissue constraints of the nerve in the tunnel. Those who perform repetitive throwing or flexion activities are particularly vulnerable to dislocation or subluxation of the nerve. Recurrent dislocation of the ulnar nerve occurs in 16% of the normal population. The nerve is at risk of direct trauma. The nerve can also be compressed by hypertrophied forearm musculature, by the aponeurosis of flexor carpi ulnaris, a ganglion situated in the cubital tunnel, local bony anomalies, or by adhesions within the cubital tunnel. The ulnar nerve may be injured with fractures or dislocations, in progressive valgus deformity after UCL injury, or lateral epicondylar fracture. There may be entrapment between the two heads of FCU, distal to the medial epicondyle. At the wrist injury may occur through compression, OA, pressure against bicycle handlebars, tumours, haemorrhage, and the usual causes of mononeuritis (diabetes, vasculitides, sarcoid, amyloid, RA, SLE, malignancy).

There may be a sharp deep aching pain at medial elbow and proximal forearm, which may radiate proximally or distally and may be noted only during flexion and valgus stresses. Neurological disturbances including paraesthesia, dysaesthesia and anaesthesia in the ulnar one and a half digits are noted early in the condition. Whilst clumsiness is frequently reported, true motor weakness is rare. Recurrent dislocation or subluxation of the nerve can cause a 'popping' or 'snapping' sensation with elbow flexion and extension.

On examination, look for valgus deformity of the elbow, a mild flexion contracture and MCL instability, soft tissue swelling at the ulnar groove, with tenderness and thickening of the nerve. There may be wasting of the small muscles of the hand and hypothenar eminence but sensory changes occur late. Elbow flexion and Tinels tests are insensitive. Those with ulnar nerve subluxation may be able to demonstrate the phenomenon and it may be possible to dislocate the nerve from the groove. A Martin Gruber anastamosis, where there is communication between the median and ulnar nerves in the forearm, occurs in 15% of people and may confuse clinical findings. Examine the cervical spine and look for hypermobility syndrome.

Investigations

Nerve conduction studies may show reduced conduction velocity by more than 33% across the site of compression compared to the unaffected arm. An X-ray will show bony abnormalities (in particular, osteophytes).

Treatment

Relative rest and protection; splinting the elbow at 30° of flexion may provide symptomatic relief. Ice, NSAIDs, and simple analgesics are often unhelpful. Gentle range of motion exercises are commenced as soon as tolerated. Return to normal activities can commence after full strength is regained with a progressive strengthening regime of forearm musculature and correction of faulty technique/instability where appropriate.

Surgical decompression, transposition and correction of instability/other pathology may be necessary. All potential sources of compression of the nerve should be explored, even when a specific site of compression has been indicated by electrodiagnostic studies, since more than one site of compression can exist.

The pronator syndrome

History and examination

Median nerve compression at the elbow and proximal forearm is known as the pronator syndrome. It causes a vague aching pain at the proximal, volar surface of the forearm. There is often a history of repetitive strenuous use of the forearm. There may be dysaesthesias in the distribution of the median nerve in the hand. If compression occurs at the ligament of Struthers (a band between the medial epicondyle and the supracondylar process), symptoms are worse with flexion of the elbow against resistance between 120° and 135° flexion. Compression at the bicipital aponeurosis can cause indentation of the pronator muscle mass below the medial epicondyle and symptoms are increased by active and passive forearm pronation. Compression can also occur within the pronator teres due to hypertrophy or tightness of the muscle, when symptoms are worse with resisted pronation of forearm with the wrist in flexion (to relax FDS) or at FDS, when the symptoms are aggravated by resisted flexion of FDS of the middle finger, and with passive stretching of finger and wrist flexors. If there is weakness of pinch grip, the condition should be differentiated from anterior interosseous syndrome.

Investigation

Electrodiagnostic studies help to confirm median nerve latency but may not localize the lesion to the forearm.

Treatment

Passive stretching of the forearm musculature, NSAIDs, and elbow splinting in neutral rotation. Symptoms may take 2–3 months to improve. Surgical intervention involves exploration of the nerve from 5cm proximal to the elbow and in the forearm, at potential sites of compression.

Anterior interosseous syndrome

History and examination

This occurs with lifting heavy weights and where there is cumulative trauma. Compression of the anterior interosseous nerve results in a pure motor paralysis of FPL and the index flexor digitorum profundus. There may be weakness of pronator quadratus. Those patients with a Martin Gruber anastamosis may experience weakness of the ulnar intrinsic muscles and/or weakness of flexor profundus to other fingers. Patients may describe a short episode of pain, which subsides to leave motor weakness. On examination there is weakness of pinch grip.

Investigation

After 2–3 weeks, EMG studies will show signs of denervation of affected muscles.

Treatment

NSAIDs and relative rest for 8–12 weeks. Those who remain symptomatic are considered for surgery, which involves a similar approach to pronator syndrome.

Radial nerve lesions

History and examination

Depending upon which portion of the nerve is affected, symptoms may be motor (posterior interosseous nerve, PIN), sensory (superficial radial nerve), or both. Posterior interosseous nerve entrapment occurs at 5 sites, but most commonly at the arcade of Frohse at the proximal edge of supinator, deep to extensor carpi radialis longus. Nerve compression can also occur due to synovitis at the radiocapitellar joint, fractures, ganglia tumours, vascular anomalies, or other local masses. The superficial radial nerve can be entrapped alone or in combination with the posterior interosseous branch. The radial nerve can also be entrapped above the level of the elbow, due to a lateral intermuscular septum, although this is rare.

The injury occurs with repetitive rotary movements e.g. discus throwing and racquet sports. There is aching pain in the belly of the extensor muscles, of insidious onset, worse with forearm pronation and wrist flexion. Pain may be more diffuse over the extensor forearm; there may be exacerbation after exertion and pain at night. Patient may have been diagnosed with 'resistant tennis elbow'. On examination there is tenderness to palpation over the course of the PIN, deep to the extensor muscle belly and just distal to the radial head. Pain may be reproduced with resisted extension of the middle finger with the elbow extended, and on resisted supination of the extended forearm.

Investigation

Neurophysiology studies are frequently normal. There may be a decrease in motor conduction velocity in the radial nerve across the entrapment site, and changes in the muscles innervated distal to the entrapment site.

Treatment

Stretching and activity modification. In resistant cases, exploration of the nerve is necessary. Surgical procedures used in the treatment of lateral epicondylitis may be followed.

Forearm compartment syndrome

History and examination

This may occur acutely after trauma or may present with chronic symptoms. It is less common than in the lower legs and is associated with lifting heavy weights and, in particular, activities that involve elbow and wrist flexion. Aanabolic steroid use can be a factor. It causes exertional forearm pain and there may be paraesthesiae in the forearm and hand. The symptoms gradually resolve with cessation of activity. On examination, there may be little to find at rest, although the forearm is usually muscular.

Investigation

The diagnosis may be confirmed by intracompartmental pressure monitoring before and after exercise (normal range 0–8mmHg), although diagnostic levels for forearm compartment syndrome have not been set.

Treatment

Fasciotomy.

Radial head bursitis can occur with repetitive pronation/supination and may be confused with distal biceps tendinitis. There is local pain and tenderness in the antecubital fossa and there may be fullness or swelling in this area. Pain is worse with pronation. Treatment is symptomatic with modification of activities, ice, and NSAIDs.

Other causes of lateral elbow pain include articular disorders: arthropathies, osteochondritis dissecans and osteochondrosis of the humeral capitellum, synovitis of the radiohumeral head, and fractures.

Olecrannon bursitis

History and examination

Bursitis usually occurs as a result of trauma; a direct blow or repetitive friction. It may be acute or chronic, septic or aseptic and caused by trauma, sepsis, crystals, inflammatory arthritis, uraemia, or calcific deposits. Septic bursitis (most commonly *Staphylococcus aureus*) can arise due to direct inoculation through local skin. Steroid injections precede infections in up to 10% of cases.

On examination there is discrete swelling at the posterior elbow, representing thickened bursa and/or bursal fluid. In sepsis or crystal induced bursitis the patient may be systemically unwell with a fever, cellulitis, and local lymphadenopathy.

Investigation

Inflammatory markers (ESR, CRP) and white cell count may be elevated in systemic sepsis and crystal induced bursitis. If sepsis is suspected, blood cultures and sterile aspiration of the bursal fluid, plus analysis by Gram stain and culture and crystals is essential. X-rays are not performed routinely; calcification and olecranon spurs may also be evident but may be coincidental.

Treatment

Most uncomplicated cases are managed symptomatically with regular ice, NSAIDs, and local protection by an elbow pad or dressing. Aspiration without injection can help to relieve pain and allows bursal fluid to be obtained for examination. Injection of hydrocortisone 10mg is rarely necessary but may benefit persisting bursitis especially with an inflammatory arthritis/crystals. Relative rest for 5 days after aspiration is recommended.

In the acute post-traumatic bursitis, repeat sterile aspiration of blood provides symptomatic relief and should be followed by a compressive dressing, regular icing, and NSAIDs. Steroid injections have no role. Return to contact activities is permitted once the patient is asymptomatic but a protective elbow pad should be worn initially.

Where sepsis is confirmed in those who are systemically well and with little cellulitis, aspiration of the bursa is followed by oral broad spectrum antibiotics. Progress should be monitored and intravenous antibiotics commenced in those who fail to respond, and early in those with systemic symptoms. Open drainage and lavage may be necessary.

Table 10.1 Radio-ulnar and wrist joints: movements, principal muscles, and their innervation[1]

Movement	Principal muscles	Peripheral nerve	Spinal root origin	
Supination	Biceps	Musculocutaneous nerve	C 5, 6	
	Supinator	Radial nerve (deep branch)	C	6, 7
Pronation	Pronator teres	Median nerve	C	6, 7
	Pronator quadratus	Median nerve	C	7, 8
Flexion	*Common flexor origin muscles*			
	flexor carpi radialis	Median nerve	C	6, 7
	flexor carpi ulnaris	Ulnar nerve	C	7, 8
	(palmaris longus)	Median nerve	C	6, 7
	Long digital flexors	Median and ulnar nerves	C	6, 7
Extension	*Common extensor origin muscles*			
	extensor carpi radialis	Radial nerve (trunk and deep branch*)	C	6, 7
	longus and brevis			
	extensor carpi ulnaris	Radial nerve (deep branch*)	C	7, 8
	Long digital extensors			
Abduction	Flexor carpi radialis	Median nerve	C	6, 7
	Extensor carpi radialis longus and brevis	Radial nerve	C	6, 7
	Abductor pollicis longus and brevis	Radial nerve (deep branch*)	C	7, 8
Adduction	Flexor carpi ulnaris	Ulnar nerve	C	7, 8
	Extensor carpi ulnaris	Radial nerve (deep branch*)	C	7, 8

* The deep branch of the radial nerve is also called the posterior interosseous nerve from its position in the extensor compartment posterior to the interosseous membrane.
[1] Reproduced with permission from MacKinnon P and Morris J (2005). *Oxford Textbook of Functional Anatomy Vol 1*. Oxford University Press, Oxford. ©2005.

Wrist and hand

Epidemiology

- Overall, wrist and hand injuries account for between 3–9% of all sports injuries.
- Incidence varies between sports, with up to 87% of gymnasts reported to experience wrist pain during their career, due to the wrist being a weight bearing joint in many of the activities of this sport.
- Hand injuries account for 44% of all injuries in rock climbing.
- Injuries to the hand and wrist are common in tennis and golf (especially the left hand in right-handed golfers).
- The majority of injuries are soft tissue, but a diagnosis of 'wrist sprain' should only be made by exclusion of other more serious injuries.
- Hand and wrist injuries are more common in children, and may involve the epiphyseal plates with the potential for growth disturbance.

Wrist biomechanics

- Normal daily activities require 30° of extension, 5° flexion, 10° radial deviation, and 15° of ulnar deviation.
- Throwing requires a similar degree of extension and radio-ulnar deviation, but flexion is increased to 80–90° at the end of the acceleration phase prior to ball release.
- Studies of the golf swing have shown a flexion-extension arc of 103° in the right wrist compared with 71° in the left wrist for right handed players (advanced players show less movement at the left wrist but more at the right).
- With an intact TFCC, the radius bears 82% and the ulna 18% of the force during axial loading of the wrist.
- This pattern of force transmission can be altered in sports such as gymnastics, where a significant load can be applied to the ulnar side of the wrist.
- Excision of the TFCC increases the load on the radius to 94%.
- Ulnar shortening (negative ulnar variance) of 2.5mm reduces the ulnar load bearing to 4%, while lengthening by 2.5mm increases it to 42%.

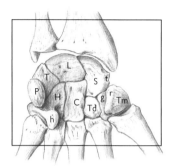

Fig. 11.1 Carpal bones; anterior view. Reproduced with permission from MacKinnon P and Morris J (2005). *Oxford Textbook of Functional Anatomy Vol 1.* Oxford University Press, Oxford. ©2005.

Fracture of the distal radius/ulna (Colles' fracture)

History and examination

- Common in the elderly athlete (approximately 7% of all Colles' fractures occur during sport) and are caused by a fall on the outstretched hand.
- Dorsal angulation and impaction leads to the classic 'dinner fork' deformity.
- May involve the epiphyseal plate in children (especially distal radius) and careful follow up is required to ensure that premature growth arrest does not occur (see also 'gymnasts wrist').

Investigation

Diagnosis confirmed by X-ray.

Treatment

- Accurate closed reduction and cast immobilization for 6–8 weeks with regular review to ensure that a satisfactory position is being maintained.
- Any intra–articular involvement in the young athlete should be treated by open reduction and internal fixation to restore joint congruity.

Fracture of the scaphoid

History and examination

- Caused by a fall onto the outstretched hand and therefore common in football, basketball, hockey, and rugby. These injuries may also occur in boxing.
- Clinical findings include tenderness in the anatomical snuff box (always compare with the uninjured side) and over the palmar scaphoid.
- There will be pain when an axial load is applied to the first metacarpal.
- Common in sport and are important not to miss, as they have the potential for delayed or non-union, with subsequent avascular necrosis and long-term disability.

Investigations

- Plain X-rays may initially be normal and therefore if suspected, initial treatment should be immobilization in a scaphoid POP followed by repeat X-ray in ten days.
- MRI scan, if available, is very useful in making an early diagnosis of scaphoid fracture.

Treatment

- Fractures with a good potential to heal include incomplete, undisplaced fractures, and those involving the distal scaphoid.
- Treatment is immobilization in a scaphoid cast for a period of 8–12 weeks (average time to union $9^1/_2$ weeks).
- Those requiring surgery include displaced or proximal pole fractures and those with greater than 15° of angulation.
- Non-union occurs in approximately 10–15% of cases—this complication is preventable by early recognition and appropriate treatment as detailed above.
- A diagnosis of a 'sprained wrist' can only be made by exclusion, and it is much better to err on the side of caution and immobilize all cases of suspected scaphoid fracture, even if the initial X-rays are negative.

Fracture of the hamate

History and examination

- These fractures occur in racquet sports and golf, caused by the butt of the racquet or golf club forcibly impacting on the hypothenar eminence and hamate hook. In golf may be due to the club being gripped too close to the butt.
- Fractures of the hook of the hamate comprise 2–4% of all carpal fractures.
- Injury to the ulnar nerve may occur in this area and cause the patient to present with numbness and paraesthesia or weakness of the ulnar innervated muscles, as well as pain and tenderness to direct palpation.

Investigation

Diagnosis is confirmed on CT scan—fractures of the hamate are difficult to see on plain X-rays.

Treatment

Non-displaced fractures are treated conservatively with cast immobilization for 4–6 weeks, whilst displaced fractures require open reduction and internal fixation, or excision of the fractured hook.

Fracture of the pisiform

History and examination

The pisiform may occasionally be fractured by a direct blow.

Treatment

Treatment is excision with preservation of the flexor carpi ulnaris tendon.

Fracture of the metacarpal bones

History and examination

Fractures of the neck of the 5th metacarpal are common in combat sports (hence the term 'boxer's fracture').

Investigations

- X-ray. Fractures of the metacarpal bones may be transverse, oblique, or comminuted.
- It is important to check for malrotation (best observed by asking the patient to make a clenched fist).

Treatment

- Non-displaced fractures should be treated conservatively with cast immobilization—any displacement should be managed surgically.
- Return to sport depends on the need for hand function, but can be expected after approximately 2 weeks in stable, non-displaced fractures.
- Angulation is common, but if greater than 60° then the fracture should be reduced and immobilized in a metacarpal splint.
- Shortening may occur and percutaneous pinning should be considered in the competitive boxer.

Bennett's fracture

- A fracture/dislocation of the base of the first metacarpal.
- The pull of abductor pollicis longus causes displacement of the metacarpal shaft.
- Treatment is by closed or open reduction and pinning, followed by 4–6 weeks cast immobilization.
- A further period of splinting is necessary on return to sport.

Phalangeal fractures

- It is very important to check for malrotation (most common in spiral fractures of the proximal phalynx)—ask the patient to make a clenched fist and any rotational deformity should become obvious.
- Also assess for any tendon or volar plate injury.
- Stable fractures can be managed conservatively by 'neighbour' splinting for 3–4 weeks, but careful follow up of all injuries is advised to ensure return of full function.

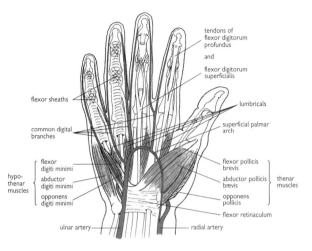

Fig. 11.2 Superficial aspect of palm. Reproduced with permission from MacKinnon P and Morris J (2005). *Oxford Textbook of Functional Anatomy Vol 1.* Oxford University Press, Oxford. ©2005.

Dislocation of the carpal bones

History and examination

- Acute dislocations of the lunate may occur following a fall.
- The lunate dislocates anteriorly and may cause compression of the median nerve.
- More common than an acute dislocation is the development of scapholunate dissociation following a tear of the scapholunate ligament.
- There is tenderness over the radial side of the lunate and Watson's test will be positive (pressure over the scaphoid tuberosity as the wrist is moved from ulnar to radial deviation will result in the scaphoid being felt to sublux dorsally).

Investigation

A clenched fist PA X-ray will demonstrate a gap between the scaphoid and the lunate in cases of scapholunate dissociation (the 'Terry Thomas' sign).

Treatment

- Treatment of lunate dislocation is by open reduction and repair of the torn ligaments followed by eight weeks cast immobilization.
- Treatment of dissociation following a tear is surgical with ORIF and repair of the damaged ligament.

Dislocation of the 1st metacarpophalangeal joint

History and examination

Rarely the 1st MCP joint can be dislocated dorsally.

Investigation

X-ray.

Treatment

- This requires open reduction as the metacarpal head becomes button holed between the lumbrical and long flexor tendons.
- Following reduction a splint should be worn to prevent the terminal 30° of extension at the MCP joint for 6 weeks.

Dislocation of the interphalangeal joints

History and examination

- Dislocations of the DIP joints are often caused by a ball hitting the tip of the finger e.g. in cricket.
- Dislocations of the PIP joints are extremely common in sport and may be reduced on the field of play.

Investigations

- X-rays should be performed to exclude a volar plate injury—the more serious of which will require ORIF.
- It is important not to undertreat these injuries as residual deformity and disability can result.

Treatment

Following successful reduction the PIP joint should be splinted for 3–4 weeks in slight flexion with a block of approximately 30° to full extension.

Mallet finger

History and examination

- Rupture of the long extensor tendon at or near its attachment to the terminal phalanx results in an inability to actively extend the tip of the finger.
- They commonly occur when the point of the finger is struck by a ball, e.g. in attempting to catch a cricket ball or football.

Investigation

X-ray.

Treatment

- Occasionally a small avulsion fracture may be evident on X-ray and should be treated by surgical fixation to achieve the best results.
- Otherwise treatment is with a splint which holds the distal IP joint in extension for a period of 8 weeks.
- It is very important that the splint is worn continuously, even in bed at night. If removed e.g. for washing, then care should be taken to ensure that the terminal phalanx is held in full extension at all times.
- Splinting is effective even in injuries up to 3 months old.

Jersey finger

History and examination

- Avulsion of the flexor digitorum profundus tendon at its attachment to the flexor aspect of the distal phalanx results in an inability to actively flex the tip of the finger.
- As the name suggests, it is usually caused when a player tries to grab the jersey of an opponent and the finger is forcibly extended.
- The ring finger is most often involved.
- When examining for this injury, the PIP joint should be fixed in extension and the patient asked to actively flex the DIP joint.

Investigation

X-ray.

Treatment

Treatment is by early surgical intervention to reattach the avulsed fragment followed by a period of immobilization in a splint.

Ulnar collateral ligament injuries (skier's thumb)

History and examination

- Injury to the ulnar collateral ligament of the thumb is common in skiers and results from a fall on the outstretched hand forcing the thumb into abduction and extension against the ski-pole.
- It may also occur on dry slopes when the thumb is caught between the spaces in the carpet.
- On examination there will be tenderness to palpation at the ulnar side of the thumb at the level of the 1st MCP joint.
- There will be excessive (more than 30° compared to uninjured side in a complete tear) laxity when the thumb is stressed into abduction.

Investigation

X-ray to exclude an avulsion fracture.

Treatment

- Partial tears of the UCL (10–20° of laxity with a definite end point) can be treated conservatively with splint immobilization for a period of 6 weeks.
- Complete tears should be repaired surgically as there is a significant chance of the torn ligament becoming interposed between the adductor aponeurosis (the so-called Stener lesion) and its distal attachment, preventing healing of the ligament and resulting in chronic instability and disability.
- Following surgery the thumb is immobilized for 6 weeks and should be protected with strapping for another 8 weeks on return to sport.
- The term 'gamekeepers thumb' is used to describe a chronic injury of the UCL—due to the gradual attenuation of the ligament over years caused by breaking rabbits' necks.
- Injuries to the Radial Collateral Ligament of the thumb may also occur. These can generally be treated conservatively with cast immobilization as the risk of soft tissue interposition is less and good results can be expected.
- Tears of the collateral ligaments of the PIP joint can occur at any of the fingers, e.g. when attempting to catch a ball or falling onto the finger.
- Stable injuries (where the joint surfaces are exactly parallel) can be managed conservatively by neighbour strapping—unstable injuries require surgical intervention.
- Collateral ligament sprains can result in many months of discomfort and swelling.

Carpal tunnel syndrome

History and examination

- Due to compression of the median nerve within the carpal tunnel at the wrist joint. May occur in athletes secondary to flexor tenosynovitis.
- More common in pregnant patients and those with diabetes and hypothyroidism, it can occur with repetitive overuse.
- The patient presents with pain or tingling in the distribution of the median nerve in the hand (thumb, index, middle, and radial half of the ring finger).
- Symptoms are often worse at night and in chronic cases can lead to muscle wasting of the thenar eminence.
- Tinel's sign may be positive over the median nerve at the wrist.
- Phalen's test is positive if numbness is elicited by holding the wrist in hyperflexion for 30 seconds.
- The differential diagnosis includes cervical radiculopathy and a thorough examination of the cervical spine should be performed.

Investigation

The clinical diagnosis may be confirmed by nerve conduction studies although this is generally not necessary unless surgical treatment is being considered.

Treatment

- Milder cases can be treated by corticosteroid injection, while more severe cases will require surgical decompression.
- Splinting of the wrist and NSAIDs may be helpful.

Ulnar nerve compression

History and examination

- Compression of the ulnar nerve at the wrist can occur as the nerve passes through the Canal of Guyon between the pisiform and the hamate.
- This is common in cyclists and is due to pressure of the hands against the handlebars.
- Symptoms can be motor (weakness of finger abduction), sensory (numbness or tingling in the ulnar 1 and 1/2 digits), or mixed, depending on the branch of the nerve affected.

Investigation

The clinical diagnosis may be confirmed by nerve conduction studies.

Treatment

Treatment includes the use of cycle gloves or handlebar padding and changes to the position of the hands when cycling, anti-inflammatory medication or, in severe or chronic cases, surgical decompression.

Other nerve injury syndromes

- Direct compression of the *posterior interosseous nerve* (radial tunnel syndrome) can occur in gymnasts due to hyperextension of the wrist and in athletes who repetitively supinate and pronate their forearms (racquet sports, golf).
- It can mimic lateral epicondylopathy of the elbow, although the site of tenderness is distal to the common extensor origin.
- Can cause aching pain in the wrist and paraesthesia in the hand.
- Repetitive traction of the superficial branch of the radial nerve can occur and cause pain and numbness over the radial aspect of the dorsum of the hand and thumb.
- Treatment is activity modification and splinting the wrist in a dorsiflexed position.

De Quervain's tenosynovitis

History and examination

- Inflammation of the tendons of *extensor pollicis brevis* and *abductor pollicis longus* can occur as they pass through a tight fibrous tunnel at the level of the radial styloid.
- Common in racquet sports and rowers as well as in certain occupations, for example carpenters.
- In the acute stage there will be swelling, tenderness, and occasionally palpable crepitus at the base of the thumb with pain on resisted testing.
- Finkelstein's test is performed by adducting the thumb across the palm of the hand and then placing the wrist into ulnar deviation—this manoeuvre will cause pain in affected individuals.

Investigation

None required—this is a clinical diagnosis.

Treatment

- Treatment may include avoidance of aggravating activities, a short period of immobilisation in a splint and corticosteroid injection to the tendon sheath.
- Response to corticosteroid injection is variable, with one third of patients requiring more than one injection.
- In chronic cases the tendon sheath may become thickened and stenosed requiring surgical decompression.
- Pain may arise more proximally, at the site where the tendons of APL and EPB cross over the wrist extensors.
- This condition is known as Intersection syndrome and occurs approximately 6–8 cm from Lister's tubercle.
- Treatment is similar that used for De Quervain's tenosynovitis.
- Surgery is occasionally necessary.

Other tendinopathies

- All tendons which cross the wrist are subject to overuse and can become painful—extensor (ECU) and flexor carpi ulnaris and radialis are particularly prone to developing problems.
- ECU tendinopathy is associated with the double handed backhand technique in tennis.
- Ulltrasound scanning of the affected area is useful to assess the injured tendon and to differentiate tenosynovitis from tendinopathy or intratendinous tear.
- Acute subluxation of ECU can occur in sports such as tennis, golf, and weightlifting. Dynamic ultrasonography can be used to demonstrate this.
- If identified acutely, immobilization in pronation and radial deviation is generally successful.
- Surgical stabilization is necessary in recurrent or chronic cases.
- Patients with tendinopathy/tenosynovitis should be referred to a physiotherapist for treatment with local electrotherapeutic modalities and a programme of eccentric strengthening exercises.
- Stenosing tenosynovitis can affect any of the flexor tendons of the hand at the level of the MCP joint, causing a triggering effect (*trigger finger*).
- A tender thickening or nodule is felt at this level.
- A single steroid injection to the affected tendon sheath is usually curative.
- Surgery is only very rarely necessary.

Ganglion

History and examination
- A ganglion is a degenerative cyst of either a joint capsule or tendon sheath.
- They are very common at the wrist, especially at the scapho-lunate joint.

Treatment
- Often asymptomatic, larger ganglions may be treated by aspiration and cortisone injection.
- However, recurrence is very common—the only definitive treatment is complete surgical excision.

Impaction syndromes

History and examination
- Several impingement or impaction syndromes can occur at the wrist joint—these are especially common in gymnasts.
- Entities described include the ulnar-triquetral, scaphoid, and triquetro-lunate impaction syndrome.
- Soft tissue impingement (capsulitis) may also occur (diagnosed by excluding other causes of dorsal wrist pain, e.g. ganglion).

Investigations
- MRI scan may be helpful in showing bone stress and in excluding other causes of wrist pain.
- These conditions require rest from the impact activities which cause pain until symptoms resolve.

Radial epiphysitis (gymnast's wrist)

- Stress reaction at the distal radial epiphysis.
- Occurs secondary to overloading.

History and examination

- Most commonly seen in gymnasts secondary to upper limb weight bearing.
- Insidious onset of unilateral or bilateral dorsal wrist pain with or without swelling.
- Pain is exacerbated by upper limb weight bearing, e.g. hand stands, bench presses, or use of parallel or uneven bars.
- Limitation of wrist dorsiflexion often present.
- Focal tenderness over the distal radial epiphysis.
- Forced extension of the wrist reproduces the pain.

Investigations

- Affected epiphysis appears widened, sclerotic, and irregular on X-ray.
- Imaging of the asymptomatic side may be required to detect subtle changes.

Treatment

- As with other stress reactions, management involves unloading the injured area (i.e. avoiding upper limb weight bearing) until the pain resolves.
- Physiotherapy is aimed at restoring full range of movement and strengthening the wrist flexors.
- If the distal radial epiphysis appears to be closing prematurely, specialist referral is warranted.

Prognosis

- If untreated, radial epiphysitis can cause premature closure of the distal radial epiphysis.
- Radial epiphysitis may be associated with positive ulnar variance (a relative overgrowth of the ulna) which is a common finding in gymnasts.

Triangular fibrocartilage complex (TFCC)

Tears

- The triangular fibro-cartilage complex is composed of triangular fibro-cartilage and ligaments on the ulnar side of the wrist between the ulna and the carpus.
- This is a cartilage disc which covers the ulnar head and blends with the dorsal and palmer radio-ulnar ligaments.
- It contributes to the stability of the ulnar side of the wrist joint.
- The TFCC can be injured as the result of a fall or tears may occur with repetitive overuse (e.g. in gymnasts) or degeneration.

History and examination

- Can be torn with activities involving wrist extension and ulnar deviation. e.g. gymnastics and tennis.
- Ulnar wrist pain and swelling exacerbated by wrist dorsiflexion and ulnar deviation.
- May be tender to palpation in this region.
- Compression and ulnar deviation of the wrist may elicit pain.
- A clicking sensation may be present.
- Grip strength is commonly reduced.
- May be a previous history of radial epiphysitis.
- The 'piano key' sign is elicited by getting the patient to lean onto a desk with the palms facing down—if the TFCC is torn then the ulna will sublux dorsally.

Investigations

- Plain X-rays are generally unhelpful, although positive ulnar variance may be seen.
- X-ray may reveal positive ulnar variance but MRI is diagnostic.
- When MRI is not available, arthrography can be used to determine the presence of a tear.

Treatment

- Conservative treatment involves rest from provocative activities and splinting or taping to prevent excessive dorsiflexion and ulnar deviation.
- Local physiotherapy can reduce pain and swelling.
- If symptoms do not settle with conservative treatment, orthopaedic referral is required for wrist arthroscopy, removal of the torn cartilage and sometimes an ulnar osteotomy to correct positive ulnar variance.
- Surgical treatment may include debridement or repair of the injured tissue (peripheral tears are within the vascular zone and may be repaired).
- Symptoms are likely to recur when associated with positive ulnar variance and when provocative activities are continued.

Kienbock's disease

- This is an avascular necrosis affecting the lunate of unknown aetiology, affecting mostly young males aged between 15–25 years.
- Often associated with repeated minor wrist trauma.

History and examination

- Commonly presents in adolescence or later with a restricted range of movement in the wrist and loss of grip strength.
- Dorsal wrist pain is exacerbated by loading the wrist in dorsiflexion.
- Often a history of recurrent loading of the wrist, e.g. gymnasttics, racquet sports, repetitive falls.
- This condition is often associated with a short ulna—normally 80% of forces are directed through the scapho-lunate/distal radius articulation. If the ulna is shortened (negative variance) then more force is transmitted through the lunate.

Investigations

- X-ray may be normal in the early phases but later demonstrates sclerosis and flattening of the lunate.
- May be associated with negative ulnar variance.
- Bone scan and MRI will be positive in the early stages.

Treatment

- Treatment depends on the staging of the process, with stages 1 and 2 responding to rest and radial shortening/osteotomy if a short ulna is present.
- If diagnosed in the early stages before significant X-ray changes have occurred, rest from exacerbating activities and bracing or cast immobilization may prevent compression.
- If compression of the lunate has occurred, orthopaedic referral is required.
- In cases of chronic pain where conservative treatment has failed, wrist arthrodesis may be required.
- Long-term disability is common after compressive changes have occurred.

Head and face

Sports concussion

- Impairment of brain function caused by trauma. May be direct blow or impulsive (whiplash) force.
- Transient neurological symptoms that may or may not involve loss of consciousness.
- Normal neuroimaging studies.
- Incidence 0.25–5/1000 player hours of exposure for most sports.
- Professional jumps jockeys have the highest concussion rate of any sport.
- The pathophysiology is unknown. Speculated to affect the permeability and function of cell membranes within specific parts of brain or brainstem, which results in transient functional disruption.

Subtypes

Proposed by Prague consensus group (2005) but remain unvalidated

Simple concussion

The injury progressively resolves without complication over 7 days.

Complex concussion

Where athletes suffer persistent (>7 days) symptoms either at rest or with exertion.

Diagnosis is based on the presence of acute signs, symptoms, and cognitive impairment.

Symptoms

Symptoms	Signs	Cognitive
• Headache	• Loss of consciousness	• Disorientation
• Dizziness	• Poor balance	• Confusion
• Nausea	• Concussive convulsion	• Amnesia
• Unsteadiness	• Vomiting	• Easily distracted
• 'Foggy' or 'dazed'	• Slurred speech	• Poor concentration
• Ringing in the ears	• Personality changes	• Slow to answer
• Double vision	• Inappropriate playing behaviour	questions

History and examination

Key features on history include: time and place of injury, mechanism of injury (eyewitness or video), presence or duration of LOC, post-injury behaviour, presence of convulsions post-injury, past medical history, medication use, drug and alcohol history.

Physical exam centres on the exclusion of intracranial pathology (e.g. haemorrhage) by neurological examination. A baseline GCS should be recorded. There are no specific physical findings in uncomplicated concussion.

Key symptoms to flag

These signs and symptoms may indicate an intra-cerebral injury requiring urgent medical assessment. Err on the side of caution—'If in doubt, check it out'

- A deterioration in the level of consciousness following injury.
- Skull fracture.
- Penetrating skull trauma.
- Focal neurological symptoms or signs.
- Loss of consciousness >5 minutes.
- Persistent vomiting or headache after injury.
- Difficulty in assessing the patient due to alcohol, drugs, epilepsy, etc.
- Other high-risk medical conditions (e.g. haemophilia).
- The lack of a responsible adult to supervise the athlete post-injury.
- More than one concussion in a match or training session.
- Head injuries in children.

Diagnostic tests

Brain CT (or where available MR brain scan) contributes little to concussion evaluation but should be employed if you suspect an intra-cerebral structural lesion.

Genetic testing

ApoE4 is a risk factor for adverse outcome following all levels of brain injury. The significance of *ApoE4* in the risk of sports concussion or injury outcome is unclear.

Pre-participation physical examination

A detailed concussion and head injury (e.g. facial fractures) history is of value but many athletes will not recognize or remember all concussions suffered in the past.

Convulsive and motor phenomena

A variety of acute motor phenomena (e.g. tonic posturing) or convulsive movements may accompany a concussion. Although dramatic, these clinical features are generally benign and require no specific management beyond the standard treatment for the underlying concussive injury. Because of the unusual and infrequent nature of this complication, it is recommended that they be managed as for a 'complex' concussion.

Second impact syndrome

Diffuse cerebral swelling is a rare but well recognized complication of mild traumatic brain injury that occurs predominantly in children and teenagers. Although repeated concussive injuries are proposed as the basis for this syndrome, a single impact of any severity may cause this rare complication.

Prevention of head injury

There is no clinical evidence that currently available protective equipment will prevent concussion. Protective equipment may prevent other forms of head injury which may be important for those sports. But, remember the concept of *risk compensation*. This is where protective equipment results in behavioural change, including more dangerous playing techniques, with a paradoxical increase in injury rate.

Education

Athletes and their health care providers must be aware how to detect concussion, its clinical features, assessment techniques, and principles of safe return to play.

Management of sports concussion

Acute concussion management

When a player shows ANY symptoms or signs of a concussion:

1. The player should not be allowed to return to play in the current game or practice.
2. The player should not be left alone; and regular monitoring for deterioration is essential over the initial few hours following injury.
3. The player should be medically evaluated following the injury.
4. Return to play must follow a medically supervised stepwise process.

A player should never return to play while symptomatic. 'When in doubt, sit them out!'

Sideline evaluation

Sideline evaluation of cognitive function is an essential component in the assessment of this injury. Brief neuropsychological test batteries such as the Maddocks questions, Standardized Concussion Assessment Tool (SCAT) or the Standardized Assessment of Concussion (SAC) have been validated in this setting. Standard orientation questions (e.g. time, place, person) are unreliable in the sporting situation compared to memory assessment.

Maddocks questions

- Which ground are we at?
- Which team are we playing today?
- Who is your opponent at present?
- Which quarter is it?
- How far into the quarter is it?
- Which side scored the last goal?
- Which team did we play last week?
- Did we win last week?

Sideline assessment of cervical spine injury

Think cervical spine injury, always! If an alert patient complains of neck pain, has evidence of neck tenderness or deformity, or has neurological signs suggestive of a spinal injury, then neck bracing and transport on a suitable spinal frame is essential. If the patient is unconscious, then a cervical injury should be assumed until proven otherwise. Airway protection takes precedence over any potential spinal injury. In this situation, the removal of helmets or other head protectors should only be performed by individuals trained in this aspect of trauma management.

Concussion injury severity grading

International expert consensus has abandoned anecdotal grading scales in favour of combined measures (clinical symptoms, cognitive assessment) of recovery in order to determine injury severity and hence guide return to play decisions. There is limited published evidence that concussion injury severity correlates with the number and duration of acute concussion signs and symptoms and/or degree of impairment on neuropsychological testing.

Neuropsychological assessment post-concussion

Neuropsychological testing in concussion is of value and continues to contribute significant information in concussion evaluation. Neuropsychological assessment should not, however, be the sole influence on the decision to return to play, but is an aid to clinical decision making. Neuropsychological test batteries are most useful with baseline pre-injury testing and serial follow-up post-injury.

Post-concussion balance assessment

Balance testing, either with computerized platforms or clinical assessment, may offer additional information, and may be useful as part of the overall concussion management strategy.

Return to play protocol

Most injuries are simple concussions which recover spontaneously over several days and an athlete usually proceeds rapidly through the stepwise return to play strategy. During the first few days following an injury, it is important to emphasize to the athlete that physical AND cognitive rest is required. Activities that require concentration and attention may exacerbate the symptoms and as a result delay recovery.

Return to play follows a stepwise process:
1. No activity, complete rest. Once asymptomatic, proceed to level (2).
2. Light aerobic exercise such as walking or stationary cycling, no resistance training.
3. Sport-specific training (e.g. skating in hockey, running in soccer), progressive addition of resistance training at steps 3 or 4.
4. Non-contact training drills.
5. Full contact training after medical clearance.
6. Game play.

If any post-concussion symptoms occur, the patient should drop back to the previous asymptomatic level and try to progress again after 24 hours. In cases of complex concussion, the rehabilitation will be more prolonged and return to play advice will be more circumspect. Complex cases should be managed by physicians with specific expertise.

Concussed athletes should not only be symptom free but should not be taking any pharmacological agents/medications that may affect or modify the symptoms of concussion.

The SCAT (Standardised Concussion Assessment Tool) card cognitive screen in concussion

The Standardised Concussion Assessment Tool (SCAT) is a sideline assessment card that may be used in the initial assessment of cognitive function in concussed athletes. It is an alternative to the Maddocks questions and the Standardised Assessment of Concussion (SAC). The SCAT was derived from the outcome statement of the Prague Expert Consensus conference held in 2005.

Cognitive assessment
Memory (step 1)

5 word recall			Immediate	Delayed
		(Examples)	(after concentration tasks)	
Word 1	_____	cat	—	—
Word 2	_____	pen	—	—
Word 3	_____	shoe	—	—
Word 4	_____	book	—	—
Word 5	_____	car	—	—

Concentration/attention

Months in reverse order
Dec–Nov–Oct–Sep–Aug–Jul–Jun–May–Apr–Mar–Feb–Jan (circle incorrect)

Or

Digits backwards (check correct)

4–9–3	6–2–9	_____
3–8–1–4	3–2–7–9	_____
8–4–3–7–1	1–5–2–8–6	_____
7–1–8–4–6–2	5–3–9–1–4–8	_____

Memory (step 2)

Ask delayed 5-word recall now
Footnotes for administration of SCAT assessment

Memory

Select any 5 words (an example is given). Avoid choosing related words such as 'dark' and 'moon' which can be recalled by means of word association. Read each word at a rate of one word per second. The athlete should not be informed of the delayed testing of memory (to be done after the reverse months and/or digits). Choose a different set of words each time you perform a follow-up exam with the same candidate.

Concentration/attention

Depending upon the age of the person being assessed it may be more appropriate to initially ask the months of the year in order and if they can achieve this task without difficulty then ask the child to recite the months of the year in reverse order, starting with a random month. Circle any months not recited in the correct sequence.

For digits backwards, if correct, go to the next string length. If incorrect, read trial 2. Stop after incorrect on both trials.

Glasgow Coma Scale (GCS)

The most widely used traumatic brain injury severity scale throughout the world is the Glasgow Coma Scale (GCS). It is useful in categorizing the acute injury, mild, moderate, and severe injuries, and performed serially to monitor progress over time. Deterioration in the GCS score may herald intracranial complications requiring neurosurgical or neurointensive care intervention.

Category	Response	Score
Eye opening response (E)	Spontaneous	4
	To speech	3
	To pain	2
	No response	1
Verbal response (V)	Oriented	5
	Confused, disorientated	4
	Inappropriate words	3
	Incomprehensible sounds	2
	No response	1
Motor response (M)	Obeys commands	6
	Localizes	5
	Withdraws (flexion)	4
	Abnormal flexion (posturing)	3
	Extension (posturing)	2
	No response	1

Fig. 12.1 Glasgow Coma Scale

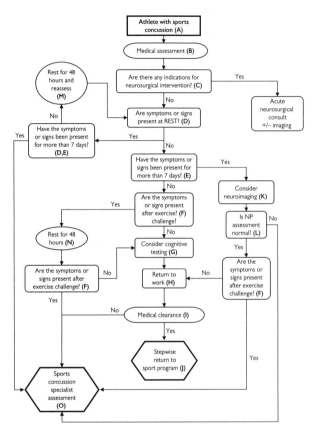

Fig. 12.2 Sports concussion algorithm

Footnotes for flow chart (Fig. 12.2)

The flowchart is a conceptual management approach to provide advice regarding return to work and sport. At least 7 days should have passed in order to detect resolution of symptoms. In the first 7 days there are currently no prognostic means of separating simple and complex concussive injury. There is still, therefore, an important role for physician discretion in neuroimaging and/or neuropsychological assessment in this early period. This management algorithm provides general guidance only. The letters in parentheses correspond to the flowchart.

(A) This refers to athletes with no evidence of previous concussion and no history of behavioral, neurological, psychological problems or learning disorder. Any return to sport also presumes that the athlete is free of any drugs, alcohol, or medication that may mask symptoms or interfere with cognitive performance.

(B) Initial medical assessment involves history, neurological exam, physical exam including examination of face, skull, and cervical spine and SCAT card assessment.

(C) Indications for neurosurgical intervention are detailed elsewhere.

(D) Symptoms and signs of concussion are presented in the box on p.442.

(E) The Prague guidelines allow 7–10 days for symptoms and signs of simple concussion to resolve. Until this timeframe is formally validated in athletes, we recommend 7 days, although recognize that physician discretion should apply.

(F) An exercise challenge requires the athlete to exercise until heart rate is greater than 60% of MPHR (maximum predicted heart rate). MPHR = 220–age in years. As a simple 'rule of thumb' this corresponds to a heart rate of >120 beats per minute.

(G) Formal neuropsychological testing is not required for simple concussion. However, the athlete must be able to score normally on the SCAT card mental status assessment. If this assessment is abnormal then more formal neuropsychological assessment may be warranted.

(H) Return to work or school is dependent upon complete resolution of symptoms, signs, and cognitive function both at rest and after exercise. Athletes should be medically reassessed after return to work or school to ensure functional recovery before proceeding to the stepwise return to play guideline. When considering return to school, it would be prudent for the teachers and parents to be aware of potential problems that may arise at this stage.

(I) Medical clearance involves an assessment of symptom recurrence after return to school and documentation that the athlete has completed all steps appropriately in the management plan and in particular, is asymptomatic at rest and following exercise challenge.

(J) Stepwise return to sport program under the return to play recommendations. All 6 steps must be completed, as described in the text and we would emphasise the important role of physician clearance at this stage.

(K) Athletes with symptoms/signs lasting ≥7 days may require brain CT or MRI.

(L) Neuropsychological (NP) assessment is recommended in all athletes with complex concussion.

(M) At 48 hours the athlete should be reassessed. Obviously, if there are any persistent symptoms or signs, the rest period will be greater than 48 hours. Once 7 days is reached and the patient is still symptomatic then the athlete would follow the complex concussion protocol and be assessed by a concussion specialist.

(N) At this stage in the flowchart, the athlete is asymptomatic at rest, but symptomatic after exercise. Therefore, the athlete must return to complete rest for another 48 hours before repeating the exercise challenge.

(O) A 'sports concussion specialist' is a neurologist, neurosurgeon, or sports medicine physician, with specific expertise in managing sport-related concussion and who has access to specialized formal neuro-psychological assessment and generally works in a multi-disciplinary management setting.

Traumatic brain injury (TBI)

Traumatic brain injury is an injury to the brain or central nervous system and incorporates injuries to other structures of the head (skull bones, soft tissues, and vascular structures of the head and neck).

The crude incidence for all traumatic brain injuries varies between countries and is approximately 300/100,000 per year with 80% of those injuries being mild. Males are more than twice as likely to suffer a traumatic brain injury than females. Sporting injuries contribute approximately 10% of all cases of TBI.

General management

The major priorities at this early stage are the basic principles of first aid. The simple mnemonic DR ABC may be a useful aide-memoire.

Initial on-field assessment of concussion

D	Danger immediate environmental	Ensuring that there are no dangers which may potentially injure the patient or treatment team. This may involve stopping play in a football match or marshalling cars on a motor racetrack.
R	Response	Is the patient conscious? Can he/she talk?
A	Airway	Ensuring a clear and unobstructed airway. Removing any mouthguard or dental device which may be present.
B	Breathing	Ensure the patient is breathing adequately
C	Circulation	Ensure an adequate circulation

Once these basic aspects of care have been achieved and the patient stabilized, only then consider moving the patient from the field to an appropriate facility. Before moving the patient, carefully assess for a cervical spine or other injury.

When in doubt, refer

Indications for urgent referral to hospital

Any player who has or develops the following:
- Fractured skull.
- Penetrating skull trauma.
- Deterioration in conscious state following injury.
- Focal neurological signs.
- Confusion or impairment of consciousness >30 minutes.
- Loss of consciousness >5 minutes.
- Persistent vomiting or increasing headache post-injury.

- Any convulsive movements.
- More than one episode of concussive injury in a session.
- Where there is assessment difficulty (e.g. an intoxicated patient).
- Children with head injuries.
- High risk patients (e.g.: haemophilia, anticoagulant use).
- Inadequate post-injury supervision.
- High risk injury mechanism (e.g. high velocity impact).

The management of traumatic brain injury

Acute management of sporting TBI

- An eyewitness account or, in the case of professional sport, videotape analysis may be available.
- Vital signs must be recorded following an injury. Abnormalities may reflect brain stem dysfunction.
- An acute rise in intracranial pressure with central herniation usually manifests rising blood pressure and falling pulse rate (the Cushing response).
- Hypotension is rarely due to brain injury, except as a terminal event, and alternate sources for the drop in blood pressure should be aggressively sought and treated. (Cerebral hypotension and hypoxia are the main determinants of outcome following brain injury and are treatable).

A neurological exam should be performed including measurement of the GCS. It serves as a reference to which other repeated neurological examinations may be compared. Record your findings. Skull palpation should be a quick and simple component of every physical exam in head trauma. It is important to check for any evidence of CSF leakage through the nose and/or ears.

When time permits, a more thorough physical exam should be performed to exclude co-existent injuries and/or to detect signs of skull injury (e.g. Battle sign). Restlessness is a frequent accompaniment of brain injury or cerebral hypoxia and may be confused with a belligerent patient who is presumably intoxicated. If the patient is unconscious but restless, attention should be given to the possibility of increased cerebral hypoxia, a distended bladder, painful wounds, or tight casts. Only when one is certain that these have been ruled out, drug therapy may be considered in consultation with a neurotrauma expert.

Investigations in head trauma

Indications for emergent cranial CT imaging in the initial evaluation of the head-injured patient include the following:

Indications for emergent neuroimaging

- History of loss of consciousness.
- Depressed level of consciousness.
- Focal neurologic deficit.
- Deteriorating neurologic status.
- Skull fracture.
- Progressive/severe headache.
- Persistent nausea/vomiting.
- Post-traumatic seizure.
- Mechanism of injury suggesting high risk of intracranial haemorrhage.
- Examination obscured by alcohol, drugs, metabolic derangement, or postictal state.
- Patient inaccessibility for serial neurologic examinations.
- Coagulopathy and other high-risk medical conditions.

CT evaluation as soon as the patient is haemodynamically stable and immediately life-threatening injuries have been addressed. Any deterioration in the neurologic examination warrants prompt evaluation by CT, even if a previous study was normal.

Compared to CT, MR is time-consuming, expensive, and less sensitive to acute brain haemorrhage. Moreover, access to critically ill patients is restricted during lengthy periods of image acquisition, and the strong magnetic fields generated by the scanner necessitate the use of non-ferromagnetic resuscitative equipment. Presently, MR imaging is best suited for electively defining associated parenchymal injuries following the acute event.

Plain skull radiographs are inexpensive and easily obtained, and often demonstrate fractures in patients with extradural haemorrhage. However, the predictive value of such films is poor. Other, more traditional, diagnostic tools have largely been supplanted by cranial CT in the initial assessment of the head-injured patient.

Management of post-traumatic seizures

Impact seizures or concussive convulsions are a well-recognised sequelae of head impact. These are not epileptic and require no specific management beyond the treatment of the underlying concussive injury.

Post-traumatic epilepsy may also occur and is more common with increasing severity of brain injury. A convulsing patient is at increased risk of hypoxia with resultant exacerbation of the underlying brain injury. Maintenance of cerebral oxygenation and perfusion pressure (blood pressure) is critical in the management of such patients.

Because convulsions may cause a dramatic increase in intracranial pressure, they should be prevented during the recovery phase of acute head injury. Phenytoin (or fosphenytoin) is usually the drug of choice because a loading dose can be administered intravenously to rapidly achieve therapeutic concentrations and because phenytoin does not impair consciousness. Benzodiazepines (e.g. lorazepam, clonazepam, diazepam) can be used for the acute treatment of post-traumatic seizures but they produce at least transient impairment of consciousness. Neither phenytoin, any of the benzodiazepines, nor any other anti-epileptic drug has been shown to be effective for preventing the development of post-traumatic epilepsy.

Post-traumatic epilepsy should then be managed in the same manner as symptomatic partial-onset epilepsy. Carbamazepine, phenytoin, and valproate are the drugs of choice for the initial management of secondarily generalized convulsions. Carbamazepine and phenytoin are drugs of choice for complex partial seizures, but valproate is also effective. New agents, such as gabapentin, lamotrigine, and topiramate, are also effective in the management of partial-onset seizures and generalized convulsions. Treatments do change and it is important to keep up to date.

Non-brain head injury

Various soft tissue, bony, ocular, and other injuries may occur to the head. Scalp wounds, although dramatic in appearance, usually heal well with good wound management. Blood loss from scalp wounds may be extensive, particularly in children, but rarely causes shock. Use the usual precautions against blood-borne infections such as hepatitis B and C and HIV infection. If large vessels are severed (for example, superficial temporal artery), the arterial bleeder should be located, clamped, and ligated. One should always inspect the wound carefully and palpate using a sterile glove inside the laceration for signs of skull fracture. A depressed skull fracture can be palpated, although a subgaleal hematoma may confuse the findings. All open fractures or depressed skull fractures should have neurosurgical consultation. Inspection of the wound will also detect CSF leaks.

The wound should be irrigated with copious amounts of saline before closing and any debris, including hair, must be removed from the wound. Bony fragments should not be removed until surgery. Primary repair should be accomplished using a sterile technique and the area immediately around the laceration should be well shaved. The galea should be closed first using interrupted sutures and then the superficial layer of the scalp is sutured.

Traumatic intracerebral hematomas/contusion

Subtypes/aetiology

Traumatic intracerebral hematomas are divided into acute or delayed types. Delayed traumatic intracerebral haemorrhages, which are more common, may occur from as early as 6 hours after injury to as long as several weeks.

Presentation

Clinical signs and symptoms depend on the size and location of the intracerebral haematoma as well as the rapidity of its development. In most cases, there is a brief period of confusion or loss of consciousness. Only one third of the patients remain lucid throughout their course. Impaired alertness is found frequently on initial examination.

The prime aim is to reduce post-traumatic oedema and ischaemia. Treatment includes adequate circulation and ventilation, aggressive monitoring and control of intracranial hypertension to ensure adequate cerebral perfusion pressures, close intensive care monitoring, correction of any coagulopathies or electrolyte abnormalities, and seizure prophylaxis. Interventions to control elevated intracranial pressure include mechanical hyperventilation, osmotic diuresis, and emergency ventriculostomies.

Head-injured patients should be monitored for coagulopathy for at least 24–48 hours after injury.

Prognosis

The overall cognitive impairment and the speed and quality of recovery are strongly related to the associated diffuse axonal injury. When occurring in isolation and when the volume is less than 30cc, an intracerebral haematoma is compatible with a favourable recovery. Brainstem compression and loss of consciousness significantly worsen prognosis regardless of treatment. Overall, mortality rates are in the range of 25–30%.

Subdural haematoma

Subdural haematomas can be the result of either non-penetrating or penetrating trauma to the head. There is bleeding into the subdural space due to stretching, and subsequent rupture of bridging cerebral veins. These injuries are typically seen following falls on hard surfaces or assaults with non-deformable objects rather than low velocity injuries. In most cases there is a brief period of confusion or loss of consciousness.

There is frequently impaired cognitive function and/or attention on initial examination. Soft tissue injuries are seen at the site of impact. Other signs of significant head trauma, which can result in subdural haematomas, include peri-orbital and post-auricular echymoses, haemotympanum, CSF otorrhea/rhinorrhea, and facial fractures. The focal neurologic deficits depend on the location and size of the lesion. Enlargement of the haematoma or an increase in oedema surrounding the haematoma produces additional mass effect, with further depression of the patient's level of consciousness, increases in motor or speech deficit, and eventually ipsilateral compression of the third nerve and midbrain.

The impact that produces acute subdural haematoma frequently causes severe injury to the cerebral parenchyma. This co-existing severe brain injury explains, in large part, the better outcome in extradural haematomas compared with acute subdural haematomas. Indeed, in most cases of acute subdural haematoma, it is likely that the extra-axial collection is less important in determining outcome than the parenchymal injury sustained at the time of impact.

Extradural haematoma

A direct blow to the head is essential for extradural haematoma formation. As the skull is deformed by the impact and the adherent dura forcefully detached, haemorrhage may occur into the pre-formed extradural space. This injury is most commonly seen in children due to flexibility of the skull. The source of bleeding may be arterial, venous, or both. In the supratentorial compartment, haemorrhage from the middle meningeal artery contributes to at least 50% of extradural hematomas; bleeding from the middle meningeal veins accounts for an additional 33%. Haemorrhage from a fracture line may also accumulate to create a mass lesion in the extradural space.

Presentation

There is remarkable clinical variability with extradural haemorrhage. Extradural haematomas may, rarely, be asymptomatic. Most, however, present with non-specific signs and symptoms referable to an intracranial mass lesion. The mode of presentation may be correlated with the size and site of the haematoma, the rate of expansion, and the presence of associated intradural pathology. Extradural hematomas involving the temporal lobe may cause a more precipitous decline than those at other sites, due to their proximity to the brainstem.

Alteration in consciousness can be quite variable in extent and duration. The so-called 'lucid interval' occurs in less than one third of patients, and thus is not a sensitive diagnostic discriminant.

Treatment

If a large traumatic extradural hematoma is unrecognized and/or untreated, there is progressive neurologic dysfunction due to the expanding mass lesion, ultimately resulting in transtentorial or uncal herniation, brainstem compression and ischaemia, and death. Rapid diagnosis and prompt surgical evacuation offer the best chance of a good outcome. If treatment is instituted prior to obtundation, pupillary dysfunction, and/or vegetative motor posturing, the probability of full functional recovery is high.

Prognosis

The expanding extradural lesion only partially accounts for the neurologic morbidity observed with extradural hematomas. Coincident intradural pathology is encountered in up to 50% of cases and is associated with lower admission Glasgow Coma Score, more substantial and prolonged intracranial pressure elevation, and higher mortality. In general, it is the sequelae of these lesions that dictate the degree of residual functional impairment in patients who survive extradural haematoma.

Traumatic subarachnoid haemorrhage

Traumatic subarachnoid haemorrhage is usually classified according to the site of arterial rupture and bleeding. It is usually due to vertebral artery injury—either a tear or dissection, although it may also be due to tearing of meningeal vessels. Sub-arachnoid bleeding typically presents with florid meningeal symptoms such as headache, neck stiffness, and photophobia.

The most common initial symptoms are neck pain and occipital headache that may precede the onset of neurological symptoms from seconds to weeks. Clinical symptoms and signs often develop with a 'stuttering' onset over days or weeks following the original injury.

Headache symptoms in most cases are ipsilateral to the vascular injury and the pain usually radiates to the temporal region, frontal area, eye, or ear. None of the reported cases of vertebral arterial rupture had cervical tenderness or objective restriction of neck movement, although a subjective exacerbation of pain did occur with neck movement.

Treatment

Medical management of SAH is the same as for intracerebral haematomas with intracerebral monitoring and control of ICP. Vasoactive substances released by the haematoma may promote further ischaemia, and the calcium channel blocker, Nimodipine is used to prevent vasospasm. Operative treatment is directed toward control of IP or treatment of hydrocephalus. The prognosis is variable and many cases result in fatal outcome.

Diffuse cerebral swelling

DCS or second impact syndrome?

Diffuse cerebral swelling is a rare but well-recognized complication of mild traumatic brain injury in sport that occurs predominantly in children and teenagers. It is likely that a single impact of any severity may result in this rare complication, however, participation in sport often draws attention to concussive injuries in this setting.

Pathophysiology

The injured brain swells within the cranial cavity. This increase in brain volume will eventually increase intracranial pressure (ICP). In the first few hours and days following severe head injury, ICP is often raised due to increased cerebral blood flow. Later brain swelling is due to an increase in brain tissue water content. Anecdotal evidence suggests massive traumatic cerebral oedema, documented on CT scanning, occurs within 20 minutes of cerebral injury.

Post-injury DCS can occur within minutes or be delayed for days or even weeks. Because of this theoretical risk, no athlete with a concussive injury should be allowed to return to playing or training until ALL clinical symptoms have fully resolved and cognitive function has returned to normal.

Downward displacement of the cerebrum due to increased intracranial pressure results in compression of the diencephalon and midbrain through the tentorial notch. During this process, the ipsilateral third cranial nerve and the posterior cerebral artery are compressed by the uncus and edge of the tentorium. Herniation can also compress the posterior cerebral artery to cause occipital lobe ischaemia.

Prognosis

In cases of cerebral herniation complicated by ischaemia, patients may suffer permanent neurologic sequelae if coma duration is 6 hours in duration or longer. Most patients with a maximum intracranial pressure increase of less than 30mmHg experience good recovery.

Head injury advice card

All patients, whether athletes or not, should be given a head injury card following their discharge from medical care. An example is shown below.

> **Head injury advice**
>
> This patient has received an injury to the head. A careful medical examination has been carried out and no sign of any serious complications has been found.
>
> It is expected that recovery will be rapid, but in such cases it is not possible to be quite certain.
>
> If you notice any change in behaviour, vomiting, dizziness, headache, double vision, or excessive drowsiness, please telephone
>
> ....
>
> or the nearest hospital emergency department immediately.
>
> Other important points:
> No alcohol
> No analgesics or pain killers
> No driving
> Patient's name
>
> ....
>
> Date & time of injury
>
> ....
>
> Date of medical review
>
> ....
>
> Treating physician
>
> ....
>
> CLINIC PHONE NUMBER
>
> ....

Mouthguards

There is no published evidence that mouthguards will prevent concussion but mouthguards should be mandatory to prevent oro-facial injuries.

Types of mouthguard

- 'Stock' mouthguards that may be purchased from sporting goods stores.
- 'Mouth-formed' or 'boil and bite' guards which are heated and immediately worn by the athlete allowing some adaptation to the dentition to occur.
- 'Custom-made' guards, which come in several types but all require an impression cast of the patients' dentition as the initial step and the guard is made on this cast.

A custom fitted design is necessary to ensure retention of the mouthguard in collision or contact sports and minimize the risk of oro-facial injury. These need to be made and fitted by a dentist or dental technician. The simper designs (e.g. boil and bite) do not afford much protection, tend to fit poorly, often interfere with breathing and speech, and may obstruct the airway in an unconscious patient. They are, however, cheap, available, and used widely.

There are no acceptable international standards for mouthguards, which makes the comparison difficult, but intuitively one would expect a laminated custom fitted guard to offer more protection, at least to the teeth.

The evidence that correctly fitting mouthguards reduce the rate of cerebral injuries is largely theoretical and no protective effect against concussion has been seen in randomized controlled trials.

Helmets and head protectors

Helmets theoretically reduce the risk of brain injury. There is published evidence for the effectiveness of sport-specific helmets in reducing head injuries in sports with high speed collisions, missile injuries (e.g. baseball) and falls onto hard surfaces (e.g. gridiron, ice hockey).

No sport-specific helmets have been shown to be of proven benefit in reducing head injury in sports such as soccer, Australian football, and rugby. Most commercially available soft helmets fail to meet impact-testing criteria that would be typical of sport-related concussion and randomized controlled trials in various football codes have failed to show a protective effect against concussion.

Other means of preventing sports concussion

Rule changes may be appropriate where there is a clear-cut mechanism of injury in a particular sport. Rule changes, such as banning spear tackles in American football, reduce the incidence of catastrophic head and neck injury.

Neck muscle conditioning may be of value in reducing impact forces transmitted to the brain. In theory, the energy from an impacting object is dispersed over the greater mass of an athlete if the head is held rigidly, but there is no scientific evidence that this can be effective

On-field recognition of concussive injury is a priority and application of appropriate validated guidelines in returning athletes to sport.

Epilepsy and sport

	Timing of event	Type of seizure	Likely aetiology
Immediate	Seconds to hours post-injury	Generalized/ myoclonic	Non epileptic
Early	Hours to 7 days post-injury	Focal	Epileptic
Late	>7 days post-injury	Generalized	Epileptic

Specific syndromes

Concussive convulsions

Defined as a convulsive episode that begins within two seconds of impact associated with concussive brain injury. Following impact, there is typically a phase of brief tonic stiffening followed by myoclonic jerking. The convulsive movements may be transient but can last up to 3 minutes in some cases. These episodes are not associated with structural or permanent brain injury and are a non-epileptic phenomenon.

Post-traumatic epilepsy

Seizures are common after severe head injury and account for 2% of the total cases of epilepsy. Post-traumatic epilepsy is categorized into immediate (within 24 hours of injury), early (within one week), and late (after one week) subtypes. Risk factors are prolonged unconsciousness, skull fracture, intracerebral haematomas, haemorrhagic cerebral contusion, and focal neurological signs. In addition, children have almost three times the risk of early post-traumatic epilepsy than adults for the same severity of brain injury.

Idiopathic epilepsy

One of the peaks of incidence of epilepsy is in the late teens and early twenties, the time when many sportsmen and women are actively involved in athletic pursuits. Exercise does not increase seizure frequency, affect anti-epileptic drug levels or induce epileptiform EEG changes. There is no evidence that epileptics are more prone to seizures after head injury, or that epileptics are more prone to injury than other athletes.

Other less common causes of convulsions in sport

Syncope

Patients who faint often have convulsive movements of the extremities which are thought to be due to a brainstem reflex phenomenon.

Cardiac rhythm disturbances

An anoxic convulsion may occur with a transient arrhythmia.

Movement disorders

Episodic involuntary movement disorders may be precipitated by movement or exercise.

Metabolic disturbances

Convulsive activity, dystonia, and syncope may occur secondary to hypoglycaemia, hyponatraemia, hypocalcaemia, and hypomagnesaemia, all conditions recognized in sports—particularly endurance running and ultra marathons.

Illicit drug use/alcohol

Pseudoseizures

Post-traumatic headache

Post-traumatic headache generally has a good prognosis for recovery although some patients may remain affected for considerable periods of time.

Paradoxically, headaches may occur more often and be of longer duration in patients with concussive injury than in patients with more severe traumatic brain injury.

Classification of post-traumatic headache (International Headache Society (IHS) criteria)

1. *Post-traumatic (or trauma-triggered) migraine*—in sports such as soccer, where repetitive heading of the ball gives rise to the term 'footballer's migraine'. Even mild head trauma may induce migraine.
2. *Extracranial 'vascular' headache*—periodic headaches at the site of head or scalp trauma.
3. *Dysautonomic cephalgia*—an unusual consequence of trauma to the anterior part of the neck, triggering autonomic symptoms from local injury to the sympathetic trunk and adjacent ganglia. This entity may be successfully treated with propranolol.
4. *Headache overlap syndrome*—persistent low grade occipital headache.

Diagnostic workup

The rate of significant neuropathological injury is between 1–3% in patients with headache, and the typical headaches found, even in life-threatening conditions, were non-specific in nature.

Post-traumatic headaches are generally treated in the same fashion as primary headache syndromes. Analgesic-rebound headache can complicate a post-traumatic headache disorder.

For post-traumatic migraine, aspirin and NSAIDs can be used with mild episodes and ergot preparations, and sumatriptan can be used to treat severe attacks.

Chronic post-traumatic migraine or recurrent episodes requiring prophylactic agents may be treated with amitriptyline or propranolol if no contraindications exist. Alternative agents include nadolol, timolol, amitriptyline, nortriptyline, doxepin, verapamil, nonsteroidal anti-inflammatory drugs, valproic acid, methergine, methysergide, fluoxetine, or phenelzine.

Prognosis

Acute post-traumatic headache has a good prognosis and, in most cases, symptoms resolve within 1–3 months. Education and support can help patients deal with transient cognitive difficulties associated with headaches. The chronic post-traumatic syndrome with prolonged disability is difficult to treat and generally requires specialist intervention.

Headaches and sport

Classification of exercise-related headache

The International Headache Society (IHS) in conjunction with the World Health Organization (WHO).

Clinical approach to headache

1. Exclude possible intracranial causes on history and physical exam. If intracranial pathology is suspected then an urgent workup is required which may include neuroimaging studies and laboratory investigations.
2. Exclude headaches associated with viral or other infective illness.
3. Exclude a drug-induced headache (see below) or headache related to alcohol and/or substance abuse.
4. Consider an exercise (or sex-related) headache syndrome.
5. Differentiate between vascular, tension, cervicogenic, or other cause of headache.

Many commonly used drugs can provoke headaches. Some of these drugs such as NSAIDs are in widespread use by athletes. If not recognized, this may be the reason for treatment failure.

Drugs commonly causing headache
- Alcohol
- Anabolic steroids
- Analgesics
- Antibiotics
- Anti-hypertensives
- Caffeine
- Corticosteroids
- Dipyridamole
- Nicotine
- Nitrazepam
- NSAIDs
- Oral contraceptives
- Sympathomimetics
- Theophylline
- Vasodilator agents.

Clinical
- Age of onset of the headaches
- Frequency and duration
- Time of onset of headache
- Mode of onset
- Site of pain & radiation
- Headache quality
- Associated symptoms
- Precipitating factors
- Aggravating & relieving factors
- Previous treatments
- General health
- Past medical history
- Family history

- Social & occupational history
- Drug & medication use.

A full neurological and general physical examination is required with particular attention to the cervical spine as a potential source of headache: general appearance (including skin lesions such as rashes), vital signs (pulse, blood pressure, and temperature), mental status and speech, gait, balance and coordination, cranial nerve and long tract examination, visual fields, acuity and ophthalmoscopic fundus exam, and skull palpation.

Key symptoms to flag

Certain symptoms may indicate the presence of more serious pathology, such as a mass lesion or infective process, and require urgent neurological assessment. These are set out below:

- Sudden onset of severe headache.
- Headache increasing over a few days.
- New or unaccustomed headache.
- Persistently unilateral headaches.
- Chronic headache with localized pain.
- Stiff neck or other signs of meningism.
- Focal neurological symptoms or signs.
- Atypical headache/change in the usual pattern of headache.
- Headaches that wake the patient during the night or early morning.
- Local extracranial symptoms (e.g. sinus, ear, or eye disease).
- Systemic symptoms (e.g. weight loss, fever, and malaise).

Specific common headache syndromes

Migraine

Migraine is an episodic headache that is usually accompanied by nausea and photophobia and may be preceded by focal neurological symptoms with a prevalence of 12–18% in community populations.

In elite athletes, there are specific management considerations related to the use of 'banned' drugs. Many conventional headache medications (such as beta-blockers, caffeine, codeine-containing preparations, dextro-propoxyphene, narcotics and opioids etc) are banned agents and their use, if detected, may result in severe penalties for the athlete concerned.

Tension-type headache

Tension-type headache results in a constant tight or pressing sensation that may initially be episodic and related to stress but can recur almost daily in its chronic form without regard to any obvious psychological factors.

Cervicogenic headache

Abnormalities of the neck including synovial joints, the intervertebral disks, ligaments, muscles, nerve roots, and the vertebral artery. Cervicogenic headache shares many of the clinical features of chronic tension-type headache. It is usually occipital in onset and may radiate to the anterior aspect of the skull and face. The headache is usually constant in nature, lasts for days to weeks and has a definite association with movement or manipulation of cervical structures.

Benign exertional headache

The formal criteria for BEH include:

(a) The headache is specifically brought on by physical exercise.

(b) The headache is bilateral, throbbing in nature at onset, and may develop migrainous features in those patients susceptible to migraine.

(c) Lasts from 5 minutes to 24 hours.

(d) Is prevented by avoiding excessive exertion.

(e) Is not associated with any systemic or intracranial disorder.

The major differential diagnosis is a subarachnoid haemorrhage. Exertional headache may be due to dilatation of pain-sensitive venous sinuses at the base of the brain as a result of increased cerebral arterial pressure. A similar type of vascular headache is described in relation to sexual activity and has been termed benign sex headache or orgasmic cephalgia.

Treatment strategies include NSAIDs such as indomethacin at a dose of 25mg three times per day. Other pharmacological strategies that have anecdotal support include the prophylactic use of ergotamine tartrate, methysergide or propranolol pre-exercise. These headaches tend to recur over weeks to months and then slowly resolve, although some cases may be lifelong. In the recovery period, a graduated symptom-limited weightlifting programme is appropriate.

Effort headache

Effort headaches differ from the exertional headaches in that they are not necessarily associated with a power or straining type exercise and occur in a variety of sports. The clinical features include:

(a) Onset of mild to severe headache with aerobic type exercise.

(b) More frequent in hot weather.

(c) Vascular type headache (i.e. throbbing).

(d) Short duration of headache (4–6 hours).

(e) Provoking exercise may be maximal or submaximal.

(f) Patient may have prodromal 'migrainous' symptoms.

(g) Headache tends to recur in individuals with exercise.

(h) Athlete may have a past history of migraine.

(i) Normal neurological exam and investigations.

Boxing and head injury

Boxing-related neurological injury

In amateur boxing, the rate of acute head injury (in contested bouts) varies between 0.14–0.4 injuries per 1000 exposures whereas in professional boxing the rate is up to 40 per 1000 exposures. The risk of such events is relatively low when compared to other sports. No studies have been reported to suggest that female boxers are at increased risk.

Few prospective studies enable a true estimate of the incidence or prevalence of chronic boxing-related neurological injury in either amateur or professional boxing.

The 'punch drunk' syndrome

In 1928, Harrison Martland anecdotally described a syndrome in prize-fighters that was known in lay boxing circles as the '*punch drunk*' or '*slug nutty*' state, although he did not actually examine any boxer with this condition. It was later labelled dementia pugilistica, traumatic encephalopathy, or chronic traumatic encephalopathy of boxers.

In the early stages, the clinical syndrome is mixed due to lesions affecting the pyramidal, cerebellar and extra-pyramidal systems. In the latter stages, cognitive impairment becomes the major neurological feature. Throughout the course of the condition, various neuropsychiatric and behavioural symptoms may occur. Compared to professionals, amateur boxers show milder neurophysiological and neuroimaging evidence of chronic traumatic encephalopathy. There are many differing symptoms with variable degrees of severity. Neuroradiological imaging techniques have not shown any systematic evidence of brain injury in boxers.

Neurophysiological studies show variable results. EEG abnormalities may occur in one third to one half of punch drunk professional boxers, and consist of diffuse slowing or flat, low-voltage records.

There is indirect evidence of compromise of the blood-brain barrier as revealed by increases in creatine kinase isoenzyme BB from astrocytes during the first 9 minutes after a boxing match, and as suggested by increased CSF protein. Similar changes are noted with creatine kinase and neuron-specific enolase with elevations following a single bout of amateur boxing. Surprisingly few detailed reports of neuropathological changes in ex-boxers have been performed.

Risk factors for chronic boxing-related neurological injury

The putative risk factors fall into two broad areas—exposure and genotype. Chronic boxing-related neurological injury is described in boxers who began fighting at a young age, had had several hundred professional fights and a long (>10 year) career. In addition, the *ApoE4* phenotype has been associated with an increased risk of chronic boxing-related neurological injury in boxers. The concept that punch-drunk boxers were mostly nonscientific 'sluggers' known for taking a punch has passed into medical folklore despite the lack of scientific support.

Prevention

There are no scientifically validated means by which chronic boxing-related neurological injury may be prevented and neuroradiological studies are not useful as a sole screening tool.

1. Monitoring of bout frequency—high exposure (>20 bouts) correlates with risk of chronic boxing-related neurological injury. A boxing 'passport is recommended.
2. Regular, preferably annual, neuropsychological and neurobehavioral assessment.
3. Regular, preferably annual, neurological examinations are recommended focusing on the cerebellar, pyramidal, extra-pyramidal systems, and gait rather than simply being a generic neurological exam.
4. An initial MR scan at first registration to exclude boxers with pre existing CNS abnormalities and to serve as a baseline for future comparison.
5. Ideally a boxer's apolipoprotein E genotype should be performed at the outset of his or her career with genetic counselling to discuss the implications of a positive finding.

A boxer's career should be terminated by the development of neurological signs.

Ideally, apolipoprotein E genotype should be performed at the outset of his or her career with genetic counseling to discuss the implications of a positive finding.

A 'high risk' notification system is to be encouraged:
- Boxers who have had >20 fights (including amateur fights).
- Boxers who have had >6 losses/knockdowns.
- Active boxers >35 years.
- Boxers who have an *ApoE4* genotype.
- Active boxing career >10 years.
- Boxers experiencing neurological symptoms post-bout.

Screening alone will not lead to injury reduction. Injury prevention, appropriate medical advice and remedial programmes, where indicated, must be implemented. Unless boxers, medical staff, trainers, and boxing officials act on the deficits discovered during the screening process, pre-participation screening will act solely as a predictor of injury, rather than as a preventive measure.

The post-concussion syndrome

The post-concussive syndrome (PCS) remains as controversial today as when it was first proposed in the 19th century. Symptoms may include headache, vertigo, dizziness, nausea, memory complaints, blurred vision, noise and light sensitivity, difficulty concentrating, fatigue, depression, sleep disturbance, loss of appetite, anxiety, loss of coordination, and hallucinations. These symptoms are not the same as the acute symptoms of concussion that typically resolve over several days. The investigation of PCS is in the exclusion of other causes of ongoing symptoms. No specific treatment is available for this condition beyond general advice and reassurance.

Fractures

Skull fracture

Athletes with a cranial fracture usually have a headache and may or may not have symptoms of an underlying brain injury. Local soft tissue swelling may also indicate an underlying fracture, and palpation of the skull should be a mandatory part of the clinical assessment of all head injuries. Percussion of the skull may result in a characteristic 'cracked pot' sound. Rhinorrhea and otorrhea are classic signs of skull fracture with torn dural membranes. If a glucose stick test of nasal or ear fluid leak is positive, the fluid is cerebrospinal fluid.

In all cases of skull fracture, especially if a CSF leak is present, an urgent neurosurgical consultation is required. When a skull fracture is suspected, the patient should always be hospitalized for observation and neurosurgical evaluation. The physician should cover the injured area of an open cranial fracture with a sterile dressing.

Nasal fractures

Nasal fractures are diagnosed radiographically, using lateral images.
The patient should be referred to a facio-maxillary or ear, nose, and throat specialist. Septum haematoma must be evacuated. Closed nasal bone reposition is the most common treatment. This should be done either immediately after the injury or 3–7 days later, when the swelling is reduced. The patient should wear a protective splint or face mask for 4 weeks when participating in training or competition.

Mandibular fractures

Mandibular fractures are the second most common group (13–45%) of sport-related facial injuries and are usually caused by a blow to the lower jaw, such as may occur in combat and team sports, or in a fall where the lower jaw or the chin hits a hard surface. Symptoms include swelling and haematoma, problems with occlusion, mucous membrane tears, differences in the level of the tooth row, mobility in the area of the fracture, and hypoesthesia with nerve damage in the mental nerve area. The standard radiographic examination is an orthopantomogram.

Most lower jaw fractures should be treated by a specialist. If proper occlusion is achieved after the operation, the prognosis is good.

Zygomatic fracture

Typical cheekbone fractures involve the zygomatico-maxillary complex: the infra-orbital rim, the orbital floor, and the lateral orbital rim. Cheekbone fractures are the third most common sport injury to the face. The clinical presentation is a flattening of the prominence of the cheekbone. If the cheekbone is pressed inward, it may be difficult for the patient to open the mouth wide. Double vision and nerve injury corresponding to the infra-orbital nerve are symptoms of a fracture in the orbital floor. A CT scan with axial and coronal views provides the best imaging.

Eye injuries

Contusion of the eyeball

Contusion of the eyeball may be caused by direct blows to the eye (boxing), a ball in the eye (squash), crashing into a hard object, and falling accidents. Tearing, light sensitivity, and blepharospasm (cramps of the eyelid) are signs and symptoms of contusion of the eyeball. Look out for swelling and bleeding in the eyelid, subconjunctival bleeding, corneal oedema, corneal damage, bleeding in the anterior chamber (hyphema), separation of the iris (iridodialysis), traumatic paresis of the pupil (mydriasis, oval pupil), accommodation paresis, lens damage or dislocation, bleeding in the vitreous, retinal damage (bleeding or oedema), or damage to the optic nerve. Visual acuity MUST be assessed in every eye injury and threshold for referral to an ophthalmologist should be low.

Perforation of the eyeball

Ski poles in the eye, bow and arrow shooting accidents, and accidents with other sharp objects frequently cause eye perforation. Ruptures of the eye may also be caused by powerful blunt contusion trauma. In that case, the eye ruptures at the weak points (along the limbus and the optic nerve). Visual acuity MUST be assessed in every eye injury. If perforation is suspected, the patient should be sent to the nearest ophthalmology department urgently.

Spine

History

Question the athlete and witnesses of injury. Study the videotape if available in acute injury.

Understand the demands of sport, exercise, and occupation.

Pain
- Character.
- Location and radiation.
- Relationship to exercise or activity.
- Alleviating or relieving factors.

Neurological symptoms
- Numbness, pins and needles.
- Weakness.

Past history
- Spinal problems.
- Orthopaedic problems.

Family history
- Spinal problems.

Notes: medical (insidious and persistent, worse in morning), mechanical (intermittent and associated with activity), disc herniation and nerve impingement (radiates to lower leg or foot), tumour (night pain), relief from aspirin (osteoid osteoma).

Problems which show familial predisposition—disc disease, ankylolising spondylitis, Reiter's syndrome, other spondylolarthropathies.

Red flags in history of patient with back pain[*]
- Less than 10 years of age.
- First episode of back pain and over 60 years old.
- Unexplained weight loss.
- Chronic cough.
- Night pain.
- Intermenstrual bleeding.
- Altered bowel function.
- Altered bladder control.
- Visual disturbance, balance problems, upper limb dysaesthesias.
- Past history of cancer or corticosteroid use.
- Bilateral weakness of lower extremities.

---

[*] Require consideration of pathology that might be life threatening or require urgent intervention.

Examination

Inspection

With patient standing.
- From behind—check level of shoulders, lateral curvature/scoliosis, normal alignment, lengths of lower limbs (level of posterior superior iliac spines), or hair tufts over spine.
- From side—check increased kyphosis, decreased lordosis.

Note: scoliosis may be due to unilateral muscle spasm, or nerve root irritation due to disc herniation.

Palpation

Palpate each spinous process, sacroiliac joints, facet joints for tenderness and muscle spasm and consider the anatomy.

Active and passive movement

Restriction of spinal movement may be due to muscle spasm as a result of pathology in one or more functional unit. Note pain during any of the movements tested.
- Lumbar flexion (normal 40° to 60°) occurs by reversing the lordosis (see lumbar spine becomes straight). During re-extension the lumbar lordosis is regained in the final 45°.
  Note: toe touching with straight legs is influenced by hip mobility, hamstring tightness—so not useful. However, this may be confirmed by measuring the increased distance between marked points over the spinous processes with flexion (Shrober's test).
- Lumbar extension (normal 20° to 30°) is painful with facet joint or pars interarticularis pathology—called 'posterior element pain'. This can be due to posterior disc pathology or closing of the foramen of nerve roots.
- Lumbar lateral flexion (normal 20°) is painful with ipsilateral facet joint pathology or lateral disc protrusion (radicular pain), but is often a non-specific sign.
- Lumbar rotation occurs with thoracic rotation (normal 90°) and is assessed with pelvis and hips fixed (held by examiner or sitting).

Neurological examination

- Sensory—light touch over back and abdomen, legs, perianal sensation.
- Lower limb reflexes (L4 knee, S1 ankle), superficial anal reflex—touching perianal skin causes contraction of sphincter and external anal muscles (S2, S3, and S4).
- Motor—squat and return to standing, walk on heels (weak ankle dorsiflexors exposed—L4) and then toes (weak triceps sura exposed—L5). Muscle strength testing for nerve root assessment (L1—hip flexion, L2—hip flexion, L3—knee extension, L4—foot dorsiflexion, L5—hallus extension, foot eversion, S1—knee flexion & foot plantar flexion). Sphincter tone and contractility.

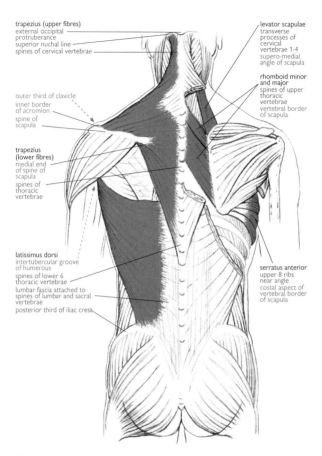

trapezius (upper fibres)
external occipital protruberance
superior nuchal line
spines of cervical vertebrae

levator scapulae
transverse processes of cervical vertebrae 1-4
supero-medial angle of scapula

rhomboid minor and major
spines of upper thoracic vertebrae
vertebral border of scapula

outer third of clavicle
inner border of acromion
spine of scapula

trapezius (lower fibres)
medial end of spine of scapula
spines of thoracic vertebrae

latissimus dorsi
intertubercular groove of humerous
spines of lower 6 thoracic vertebrae
lumbar fascia attached to spines of lumbar and sacral vertebrae
posterior third of iliac crest

serratus anterior
upper 8 ribs near angle
costal aspect of vertebral border of scapula

Fig. 13.1 Superficial muscles of the shoulder girdle and back. Reproduced with permission from MacKinnon P and Morris J (2005). *Oxford Textbook of Functional Anatomy Vol 1*. Oxford University Press, Oxford. ©2005.

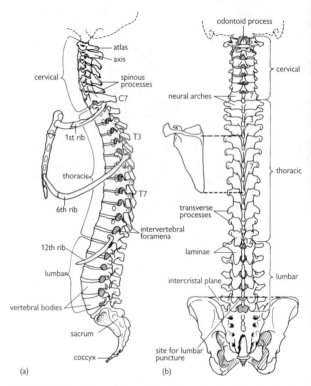

Fig. 13.2 Vertebral column: (a) lateral view; (b) posterior view. Reproduced with permission from MacKinnon P and Morris J (2005). *Oxford Textbook of Functional Anatomy Vol 1.* Oxford University Press, Oxford. ©2005.

Special tests

Sciatic and femoral nerve tension tests

Principle—stretching the dura and nerve root to produce leg pain. Positive will produce the patient's radicular symptoms.

Sciatic nerve tests

- Straight leg raise.
- Laseque test—patient supine with hips flexed to 90°. Knee slowly extended.
- Bowstring sign—examiner presses in popliteal fossa and causes increased pain in leg.
- Slump test—patient sits 'slumped'. Progressive increase in tension by flexing neck, extending knee, and dorsiflexing foot.

Notes: ankle dorsiflexion and neck flexion should aggravate radicular pain or decrease angle of straight leg raise.

False positive—pain with less than 30° of SLR, production of back pain with no leg pain.

Femoral nerve test

Prone—knee flexed to 90° and hip extended—a positive test is recorded if there is pain in the thigh with hip extension.

One-legged hyperextension and Fitch test

In those with posterior element pathology (see 'spondylolysis'), pain is reproduced in the back when the patient hyperextends while standing on one leg. The Fitch test includes rotation as well as one-legged hyperextension and may be more sensitive.

Investigation

Guided by history and examination.

General problem—degenerative changes appear in asymptomatic from early age.

X-rays

Routine AP and lateral, specialized oblique.
- Advantages cheap, low radiation dose, define bones.
- Disadvantage do not define soft tissues.

AP—check spinous process, 2 transverse processes, 2 pedicles, 2 laminae and 2 facet joints (vertical in lumbar spine) at each level, assess alignment.

Lateral—see bodies of vertebrae, disc spacing increasing from L1–L4, lumbar intervertebral foraminae alignment will give smooth curve of posterior aspects of the bodies forming the lumbar lordosis.

Oblique—for facets joints and pars interarticularis
See 'Scottie Dog'—neck is pars, nose is transverse process, eye is pedicle, ear is superior articular process, front legs are inferior articular process. Collar = spondylolysis.

Bone scan

Technetium labelled injection is taken up in areas of increased osteoblastic activity demonstrating increased metabolic activity in bone. Detected by gamma camera. Reveals stress fractures (i.e. spondylolysis), but also epiphyses and metaphyseal bone plates of young.
- Advantage—high sensitivity.
- Disadvantage—low specificity, radiation dose.

SPECT (single photon emission computer tomography)

Gives more precise anatomical localization of 'hot spot' than bone scan. Use to locate spondylolysis.

CT (computer tomography)

Allows visualization of bony configuration and good visualization of paraspinal soft tissues.
- Advantage—good to detect fractures and impingement of spinal canal, evaluate spinal tumours.
- Disadvantages—radiation dose, slices may miss pathology.

Myelography

An injection of radio-opaque dye into the spinal canal reveals an outline of the spinal cord and nerve roots on subsequent plain X-rays. This can reveal nerve root compression, though not its cause (i.e. prolapsed disc, osteophyte or tumour).

CT myelography

Myelography is combined with CT technology for even greater detail.

MRI (magnetic resonance imaging)

Provides excellent visualization of soft tissues—including discs. Can assess impingement of nerve roots. May see haemorrhage from ligamentous injury. Can detect atrophy in paraspinal muscles. Detects changes in the spinal cord, such as syringomyelia.

- Advantage—no radiation.
- Disadvantage—cost.

Discography

Injection of radiopaque dye into the disc space under pressure—pain response assessed.

Acute spinal injury

History and examination

Consider forces involved and take history from the patient and witnesses. Review video if available.

Clinical examination, carefully, to exclude injuries that could produce instability (threaten neurological structures). Inadequate immobilization in transporting player from pitch could worsen clinical picture!

When to immobilize?
- Pain in spine secondary to high velocity injury.
- Any neurological signs.
- Severe spinal pain (for comfort).

Transportation should be on a spinal board by trained personnel to ensure immobilization in position athlete was found. In general, equipment such as helmets should not be removed.

Cervical spine injury and potential instability should be presumed in anyone who is unconscious after head injury. The cervical spine will need assessment by cervical spine X-ray and CT of entire neck.

Acute injuries of the back in sport

- Muscular strains.
- Ligamentous sprains.
- Contusions.
- Fractures—transverse processes, ribs*, posterior elements—generally stable and not associated with neurological damage.
- Compression fractures of the vertebral bodies—unless trauma was extreme, are usually pathological (i.e. often osteoporosis in elderly athletes).
- Fracture dislocations—high-energy injuries (e.g. diving, car racing) with high risk of spinal cord injury.
- Thoracic disc herniation occurs occasionally in athletes, as in the general population (1.6 per 1000), but is not associated with athletic activities—lateral herniation presents with chest wall pain in dermatomal pattern and central herniation with lower extremity spasticity and paraparesis.
- Lumbar disc disease.

* Beware renal injury with injury at costovertebral angle—assess abdominal tenderness and haematuria and consider intravenous pyelogram or renal ultrasound.

Management of musculoligamentous injuries of the back

Sprains and strains of the back are common. They do not require radiological evaluation if the clinical findings do not indicate other causes. Cold therapy should be used for 48–72 hours and muscle spasm may be controlled by anti-spasmodics. Rehabilitation is important and aims to restore normal muscle strength and firing patterns. Tight muscles, typically hamstrings, may need to be stretched to prevent recurrence.

Disc disease

Disc disease is a continuum from degeneration to herniation. There is a loss of water content with age and this permits more stress to be transferred to the annulus fibrosis, which may develop radial tears. These tears may give local pain, but have the potential for herniation and consequent nerve root pain. Disc herniation is most common in the 5th decade of life, although up to 2% occur in those under 18 years.

Investigations

Pain from a degenerate disc often precedes activity, but may be aggravated by it. Plain radiographs may show loss of disc height if advanced and there may be associated facet joint arthrosis. MRI reveals loss of disc water content.

Treatment

Treatment involves adequate analgesia and anti-spasmodics if needed and then rehabilitation to improve muscle strength and firing to decrease the load on the disc. If tears are apparent in the disc, thermal coagulation has been achieved by a probe inserted into the disc. The benefits of this treatment are not yet proven.

Disc herniation

In disc herniation, the nucleus pulposis extrudes through the tear in the annulus fibrosis. Such herniation may press on the nerve root causing leg pain, numbness, and weakness. The history may suggest symptoms of disc degeneration before a 'pop' in the back with more acute intense back pain. Over the next 48 hours buttock and leg pain develops. If bilateral leg numbness or weakness is present, we should consider the possibility of 'cauda equina syndrome' and ask about *loss of visceral function* (e.g. *bladder and bowel,* faecal or urinary incontinence or retention) *and saddle anaesthesia.* Appropriate treatment of cauda equina is urgent. Patients with disc herniation are usually most comfortable lying down.

Examination

Examination reveals they may stand with a list away from the side of the leg pain and flex asymmetrically away from that side too. Muscle weakness, sensory loss and reflex changes in the lower limbs may give an indication of the level of the herniation. Sciatic or femoral nerve tension signs should be positive. In cauda equina syndrome, perianal and scrotal sensation may be lost and sphincter tone may be lost. MRI is the investigation of choice, though CT and CT myelography have previously been useful.

Treatment

Treatment of disc herniation involves analgesia and anti-spasmodics and often bed rest if severe pain on movement. However, activity should be encouraged as soon as the patient can cope with it. Back extension exercises may be useful. An epidural injection may be effective in reducing pain, but does not improve neurological deficit. In persistent cases (e.g. 6 weeks with no response) microdiscectomy may be performed, although studies suggest the long term results are no better than with continued conservative management. Rehabilitation of flexibility and strength must be complete before return to sport. Cauda equina syndrome requires early surgical decompression.

Pars interarticularis and spondylolysis

Definition

Pars interarticularis—bridge of bone between inferior and superior articular process of vertebra (also called 'isthmus').

Spondylolysis—separation in the pars interarticularis of the posterior elements of the spine.

The pars interarticularis is vulnerable to stress fracture in those engaging in repeated hyperextension, rotation, and side flexion of the spine. This occurs in many sports but, because of the nature of the sport, occurs particularly in fast bowlers in cricket and in gymnasts. Imaging with bone scan and CT reveals a continuum of mild stress reaction to complete fracture with potential for non-union. The lower 3 lumbar vertebra are most at risk. The term spondylolysis covers separations in the pars interarticularis, but separations have also been described in the pedicle and other posterior elements of the spine.

Posterior element pain is characterized by pain on extension and particularly a positive one legged hyperextension test (stork test). Pain is usual when the foot of the ipsilateral side to the pars lesion is on the ground. Adding rotation towards the affected side is more sensitive of a stress lesion (Fitch test).

Investigations

Plain radiography, even the oblique view which may show a 'collar' on the Scottie dog, lacks sensitivity and triple phase bone scan with SPECT is the optimal first line investigation. The location of 'hot spots' in the posterior elements indicate possible sites of spondylolysis, which can then be identified on reverse gantry CT. Increasingly MRI is used, as this does not pose radiation risks to the patient and shows bone stress as oedema and spondylolysis as cortical separation.

Increased uptake on bone scan or SPECT indicates bone stress and treatment should include rest from pain-provoking activities, which usually is sport. A thoracolumbar corset may be used to prevent hyperextension. Six weeks' rest may be sufficient for those with early bone stress reaction, but 12 months may be required to allow healing of established stress fractures. After the period of rest, a thorough rehabilitation of the spinal and abdominal musculature is necessary. Imaging is not useful in predicting time to return to sport. It is wise to wait until the athlete is pain free before attempting this. Surgical stabilization of spondylolisthesis by Buck fusion (pedicle screws and bone graft) may be considered for those with persistent pain despite adequate conservative treatment.

Established spondylolysis with wide sclerotic bone margins and negative bone scan are unlikely to heal, even with rest. Thus management is designed to allow pain to settle and then rehabilitation to provide dynamic stability though exercises and an earlier (less cautious) attempt to return to sport. Pain preventing successful return to sport could be treated by surgical stabilization. A local anaesthetic 'lysis' block may give useful information regarding the potential benefit of treating the lysis surgically, though patients must be counselled that outcomes are not always favorable.

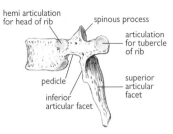

hemi articulation
for head of rib

spinous process

articulation
for tubercle
of rib

pedicle

superior
articular
facet

inferior
articular facet

Fig. 13.3 Superficial muscles of the shoulder girdle and back. Reproduced with permission from MacKinnon P and Morris J (2005). *Oxford Textbook of Functional Anatomy Vol 1*. Oxford University Press, Oxford. ©2005.

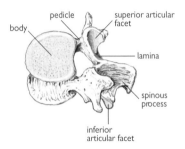

pedicle

superior articular
facet

body

lamina

spinous
process

inferior
articular facet

Fig. 13.4 Vertebal column: (a) lateral view; (b) posterior view. Reproduced with permission from MacKinnon P and Morris J (2005). *Oxford Textbook of Functional Anatomy Vol 1*. Oxford University Press, Oxford. ©2005.

Pars interarticularis and spondylolisthesis

Definition
Spondylolisthesis—anterior displacement of one vertebral body on another.

Classification of spondylolisthesis (Wiltse 1976)
- Dysplastic.
- Isthmic (lytic or elongated).
- Degenerative.
- Traumatic (fractures).
- Pathological.

Staging of spondylolisthesis (Meyerding 1932)
By displacement of vertebral body and relative to the body anteroposterior diameter.
- Stage 1 < 25%.
- Stage 2 < 50%.
- Stage 3 < 75%.

Asymptomatic spondylolisthesis is present in about 5% of the skeletally mature general population. More than 90% of such lesions are at L5. They are not present in the newborn, but have been seen in 6 year olds.

Examination may reveal the step in the spine and hamstrings are often tight, requiring clinical differentiation from sciatic nerve tension. Lateral plain X-rays will demonstrate nearly all spondylolisthesis, but MRI may be useful to assess nerve root foramina and disc quality, which may be compromised in spondylolisthesis.

Spondylolisthesis may progress in the skeletally immature. However, sporting involvement does not appear to be a risk factor and therefore there is no evidence to bar an athlete from participation. Nevertheless it may be wise to avoid gymnastics and weightlifting if at stage 2 or 3. Surgery may be considered for those at Stage 3 or those with nerve root entrapment.

Spondylolysis and spondylolisthesis in the young athlete
- This stress fracture or defect of the pars interarticularis appears to be caused often by activities that require excessive lumbar extension and rotation, e.g. gymnastics, bowling in cricket, and serving in tennis.
- Some children may also have a genetic weakness in the pars interarticularis that predisposes to this condition.
- Most common at L5 (85–95%) and L4 (5–15%) but occasionally occurs at a higher level.
- Can be unilateral or bilateral.
- If the pars defect is bilateral, slippage can occur. This is referred to as a spondylolisthesis (where a vertebra slips forward on the one below) and is graded according to amount of slippage.
- Progression of spondylolisthesis is uncommon but is most likely to occur during the time of peak height velocity.

History and examination

- May be asymptomatic. Do not assume that back pain is due to a radiologically proven spondylolysis or spondylolisthesis unless the clinical picture is consistent.
- Symptomatic pars stress fractures present with an insidious onset of unilateral or bilateral pain in the lumbar region (most commonly at the level of the belt) which may then radiate to the buttocks and leg.
- Pain is worse with activities requiring lumbar extension.
- Clinical findings: may have increased lumbar lordosis and tenderness around the facet joint region at the affected level.
- Pain reproduced by lumbar extension, which is often worse when standing on the leg of the affected side.
- No neurological signs in the lower limbs.

Investigations

- X-ray including oblique view. This gives the classic 'scottie dog' appearance when a pars defect is present.
- Lateral view is also useful to determine whether a spondylolisthesis exists, and its severity.
- Spondylolisthesis is graded 1–4 according to the degree of slip: grade 1: 25%, grade 2: 25–50%, grade 3: 50–75%, grade 4 >75%.
- With recent symptom onset the X-ray is often normal.
- A bone scan including SPECT views is very sensitive for recent stress fractures. A 'hot spot' at the site of the defect suggests that the fracture is recent and active. If no hot spot (i.e. no osteoblastic reaction) is seen, active remodelling is not occurring.
- Bone scan changes often remain positive for many months and are not useful as a means of timing return to sport.
- CT scanning is useful for staging fractures.

Treatment

- Avoid lumbar extension activities.
- Some clinicians recommend the use of a brace to prevent lumbar extension (e.g. modified Boston brace), especially if the child has pain with activities of daily living.
- Use of a brace has not been shown to increase the rate of fracture healing.
- Physiotherapy should include an abdominal strengthening programme and postural retraining to address excessive lumbar lordosis and anterior pelvic tilt.
- A flexibility program to improve hamstring and gluteal flexibility should also be included.
- Return to sport, which usually occurs within 3–6 months, should be based on symptom resolution, absence of clinical signs, and good core trunk strength.

Prognosis

- Fractures treated in the early phase appear to have a good prognosis, especially if they are unilateral.
- Early and progressive stage fractures have a 40–80% chance of fracture healing.

- Terminal stage fractures rarely unite.
- Excellent clinical outcomes can be achieved in the absence of fracture healing.

Management of spondylolisthesis

- Monitor for slip progression during the growing years, as progression may (rarely) require surgical stabilization.
- If persistent pain despite appropriate rehabilitation and in those with a grade 3 or 4 spondylolisthesis (>50% slip), or where the slip is progressing, referral to a specialist is indicated. These children should avoid sports requiring lumbar extension and contact.

Morita T, *et al.* (1995) Lumbar spondylolysis in children and adolescents. *J Bone Joint Surg* (Br) **77B**: 620–625

Scheuermann's disease

Scheuermann's disease is an osteochondrosis affecting the growth plates of the vertebral bodies with Schmorl's nodes, end plate irregularities, and decreased disc water content on MRI, causing vertebral body flattening and wedging. It occurs in the thoracolumbar spine of young adults and sometimes in adolescents and is a cause of kyphosis.

Scheuermann's disease may be a co-incidental radiographic diagnosis, but may be a cause of non-specific low back pain in the adolescent or young adult. Examination findings are usually negative, except the possibility of some axial tenderness and paraspinal muscle spasm. Kyphosis may be noted.

History and examination
- Commonly presents in active adolescent.
- May have mid-thoracic pain with activity.
- May present as a painless thoracic kyphosis in the late teenage years or 20s.
- Tightness of hamstrings and thoraco-lumbar fascia is common.
- Excessive lumbar lordosis often present.

Investigations
- Diagnosis on finding wedging of >5° in three or more consecutive vertebrae on lateral X-ray is diagnostic.
- Schmorl's nodes (irregularities in the cartilage end plate causing irregular ossification) commonly present.

Treatment
Initial treatment should be with analgesia and back flexibility and strengthening exercises. If kyphosis is greater than 50° bracing should be used in addition to exercises. However, if kyphosis is greater than 70° and bracing and exercises have failed, posterior instrumentation and surgical fusion may be warranted. Sport is allowed during conservative management, but contact sports are prohibited after surgery.

- Osteochondrosis affecting growth plates (ring epiphysis) of vertebral bodies.
- Compressive forces cause wedging deformity of the vertebral bodies, resulting in a thoracic kyphosis.
- Affects thoracic spine predominantly but can occur in the lumbar spine or at the thoraco-lumbar junction.
- Aim to resolve pain and stop progression of deformity.
- Avoid activity until symptoms resolve.
- Hamstrings and thoraco-lumbar fascia stretches.
- Abdominal strengthening programme.
- If symptoms severe or kyphosis is progressing, an extension brace (e.g. a Milwaukee brace) may be required.
- Rarely, surgery is required to prevent progression of kyphosis or when pain and deformity is severe.

Prognosis
- Exercises will ↓ symptoms but will not correct existing deformity.
- Use of brace before skeletal maturity may improve kyphosis.
- Pain usually self-limiting and resolves with skeletal maturity unless kyphosis is severe.

Sacro-iliac joint

Movements of the sacroiliac joint are subtle, but during running the ilium rotates posteriorly from foot contact to midstance, when it rotates anteriorly until toe off.

Sacroillitis is a usually manifestation of seronegative arthrititides, such as ankylosing spondylitis or Reiter's syndrome. Pain from the sacroiliac joint may also come from trauma or perhaps overuse type injuries.

Factors which might predispose to overuse type injury of sacro-iliac joint

- Ligamentous laxity due to hormonal changes of pregnancy.
- Excessive side-to-side movement of pelvis in running.
- Forced extension of hip in gymnastics.
- Decreased hip rotation, e.g. due to degenerative joint disease.
- Leg length discrepancy.
- Running on uneven terrain or cambered road.
- Shoes or orthotics.

History and examination

- Pain in low back and or buttock often in relation to activity. May radiate to posterior thigh, but rarely to knee.
- Unilateral low back pain on hopping.
- Aching rest pain, especially after prolonged sitting.

Clinical findings

- Local pain over joint line (posterior inferior iliac spine).
- Pain on compression or distraction of the iliac crests.
- Pain on FABER leverage test (flexion abduction external rotation).

Investigations

- Plain radiographs may show sclerosis, joint narrowing, and osteophytes in chronic cases.
- Bone scan may be hot at sacroiliac joint raising possibility of systemic disorder.
- HLA_{B27} may be positive in those with ankylosing spondylitis.

Treatment

- Address biomechanical factors, such as leg length discrepancy, hip rotation, footwear, training factors.
- Analgesia, consider NSAIDs and ice.
- Second line treatment might include corticosteroid or sclerosant injections.

Cardiorespiratory

Coronary artery disease

- Coronary artery disease remains a major cause of morbidity and mortality in developed countries.
- One million people in the USA sustain myocardial infarction yearly. A major increase in incidence is occurring in developing countries.
- Death rate has declined in developed countries by 30% in last 10 years.
- 50% of deaths with acute myocardial infarction occur within 1 hour attributable to ventricular fibrillation.

Clinical presentation of coronary heart disease

- Stable angina pectoris; predictable onset of anginal symptoms on exercise or stress following imbalance of increased myocardial demand over supply.
- Unstable angina and non ST elevation myocardial infarction. New onset, changing pattern or episodes of angina at rest. May be associated with release of cardiac enzymes (troponin).
- ST elevation myocardial infarction. Presentation with rest pain, typical serial ECG changes and enzyme release. Complicated by arrhythmias, associated with myocardial damage and LV dysfunction or failure.
- Sudden death associated with acute infarction or as an arrhythmic event.
- Cardiac failure secondary to recurrent infarction or ischaemic cardiomyopathy.

Pathophysiology

Development of atheromatous plaques

- Long pre-clinical phase of development with rapid change at time of plaque rupture.
- Affect principally the proximal portions of coronary arteries therefore large muscle beds influenced by stenosis or occlusion.
- Human coronary arteries are end arteries with little collateral development unless stimulated by reversible myocardial ischaemia or previous occlusion and infarction.
- Distribution of arterial narrowings confers prognosis. Increasing mortality through single, double, and triple vessel or left main disease.

Plaque dynamics

- Thrombogenic lipid rich core covered with fibrous cap of smooth muscle and inflammatory cells.
- Inflammation may occur stimulated by oxidized lipid accumulation in the intima. CRP is an inflammatory marker . If elevated confers increased risk of further events.
- Macrophages and T-lymphocytes are present in fatty streaks and mature plaques, cytokines, and growth factors are secreted.
- Adhesion molecules interact with inflammatory cells.
- Plaque rupture leads to platelet deposition and thrombus formation which may precipitate total obstruction and infarction.
- Unstable plaques may be angiographically insignificant but rapidly progress in significance.

- Plaques may stabilize after rupture. Coronary artery disease is episodic in clinical presentation.

Aetiology

Atheroma associated with risk factors; subject to primary and secondary prevention.

Class 1 interventions
- Hypertension.
- Hypercholesterolaemia.
- Cigarette smoking.
- Cardiac protection with aspirin, beta-blockers, and ACE inhibitors.

Class 2 interventions
- Diabetes.
- HDL and triglycerides.
- Physical inactivity.
- Obesity.
- Moderate alcohol consumption.

Class 3 interventions
- Diet.
- Psychosocial factors.

Investigations

History of cardiac pain
- Resting ECG.
- Exercise stress testing for exercise capacity and evidence of myocardial ischaemia (STdepression).
- Radionuclide scanning for distribution of perfusion defects and assessment of LV function.
- Echocardiography for assessment of LV function. Stress echo techniques may be applied.
- Coronary arteriography to determine anatomical distribution of obstructive lesions and for coronary interventions.

Treatment of coronary heart disease

Pharmacological agents

- *Nitrates*—act as venous dilators, reduce preload and systolic wall stress, used sublingually, orally, or by parenteral route in unstable patients. Tolerance may occur.
- *Beta blockers*—act on cardiac beta receptors, reduce heart rate, contractility, systolic wall stress, and blood pressure at rest and on exercise. Used to alter supply-demand ratio in stable angina, and after myocardial infarction for anti-arrhythmic action.
- *Calcium channel blockers*—vasodilating action on coronary and peripheral arteries.
- *Nicorandil*—potassium channel blocker, vasodilating action but no tolerance. Action may be related to preconditioning.
- *Anti-platelet therapies*—given as long term therapy, (aspirin) as adjunct to coronary artery intervention acutely (abciximab) or as continuing treatment (clopidigrel).
- *Thrombolytic therapy*—administered to patients with ST elevation myocardial infarction presenting early.

Interventions

Coronary interventions may be applied to each of the clinical presentations. Choice of intervention is determined by coronary artery anatomy on angiography.

- Coronary artery bypass surgery generally applied to patients with left main or triple vessel involvement.
- Increasing application of percutaneous coronary intervention with balloon angioplasty and stenting in patients with stable angina with severe symptoms, unstable presentations, or in ST elevation myocardial infarction (primary angioplasty).

Exercise and coronary artery disease

Potential benefits of exercise
- Reduced body weight and component of fat.
- Reduced heart rate, systolic blood pressure, lactic acid production, and muscular blood flow at equivalent work rate.
- Increased VO_2 max by 10–15%.
- Increased A-V O_2 difference at maximal exercise.
- Reduced total cholesterol and LDL.
- Reduction in triglycerides.
- HDL and HDL2 increased reduction in fibrinogen and platelet aggregation at rest.

Exercise prescription
- Used as major component of rehabilitation following acute myocardial infarction.
- May be applied to subjects with stable angina.

Potential adverse effects
- Enhanced catecholamine release, increased heart rate contractility, and systolic wall tension; main determinants of myocardial oxygen consumption.
- Potassium release may predispose to arrhythmias.
- Rise in free fatty acids.
- Enhanced platelet activation.
- May induce onset of angina, myocardial infarction, or sudden death.

Physical inactivity, exercise, and CAD

Epidemiological observations
- Occupational physical activity protective. IHD less in bus conductors than drivers, but drivers obese, raised cholesterol and blood pressure.
- Sedentary workers who participate in vigorous exercise have 50% less CHD events than inactive colleagues.
- Indirect relationship of level of exercise and CHD; 3 times mortality in light workers compared to heavy workers.
- Lifelong exercise protective, late exercisers assume low risk.
- Leisure time vigorous exercise protective.
- General increased level of cardiovascular fitness protective against coronary events.

Cardiac rehabilitation

Definition
A long-term process by which patients with cardiac disease are encouraged and supported by multidisciplinary professionals to achieve optimal physical and psychosocial health.

Evidence of benefit
- Individual studies of exercise-based or comprehensive cardiac rehabilitation programmes are equivocal, but meta-analyses confirm 20–25% reduction in mortality and 28% reduction in fatal reinfarction at 2–3 years, in patients with acute myocardial infarction. No effects on non-fatal reinfarction or revascularization.
- 30–50% increase in exercise capacity and peak oxygen uptake of 10–20%. May not be sustained in long term.
- Improved sub-maximal exercise capacity, reduced rate of perceived exertion, and delayed onset of lactate threshold.
- Delayed onset of angina by reduced rate pressure product.
- Improved physical activity but long term effects determined by compliance.
- Improved psychological well-being and quality of life.

Phases of rehabilitation

Phase 1—in-patient

Key elements are evaluation, reassurance, education, risk factor assessment, mobilization, and discharge planning. Applied after myocardial infarction, unstable angina, cardiac surgery or angioplasty, or cardiac failure. To engage the patient and partner and identify particular problems prior to hospital discharge, and tailor the rehabilitation programme according to individual needs. Can be used after a step change in clinical condition. Encourage a positive attitude and introduce educational material.

Exercise prescription

Engage in self-care activities, general range of motion exercise and walk short distances.

Phase 2—early outpatient recovery after discharge

Programme commencing 2–4 weeks after discharge lasting 4–12 weeks. Support from hospital or community-based health professionals through home visits or telephone contact. Education for risk factor modification and behavioural change. Medical evaluation for future management.

Exercise prescription

Undertake daily living activities and gradually increase the duration, frequency, and intensity of walking to increase functional and endurance activity.

Phase 3—intermediate outpatient

Generally comprises an exercise training programme undertaken in hospital gym with self-monitoring. Can be accommodated in community or home-based setting. Generally up to 12 weeks.

Exercise prescription

20–30 minutes of low to moderate intensity aerobic exercise e.g. walking, cycling, circuit training on 3 days a week and moderate intense physical activity e.g. walking, on days when not participating in formal exercise programme.

Phase 4—long-term maintenance

Continued education after exercise period. Long-term rehabilitation may involve self-help groups, exercise leaders, or buddy programme. Community based programme out of the hospital setting with most care delivered in primary care. Patient's clinical status, medication, and risk factor modification undertaken by GP or other health care professional.

Exercise prescription

A minimum of 20 minutes of moderate intensity exercise on 3 days per week, and/or accumulate 30 minutes or more of moderate intensity physical activity on at least 5 days a week. Use of local facilities.

Components at all phases
1 Education.
2 Smoking cessation.
3 Counselling.
4 Exercise training.
5 Psychology.
6 Secondary prevention.

Initially patient group with myocardial infarction, revascularization with CABG, or angioplasty and valvular patients.

Secondary prevention

Rehabilitation now used as vehicle for delivery, and exercise is one component. Encourage life style changes including diet and smoking.
Target risk factors with pharmacological agents to treat:
- Hypercholesterolaemia.
- Hypertension.
- Diabetes.
- Use of anti-platelet compounds, beta-blockers and ACE inhibitors.

The multidisciplinary team includes doctors, nursing staff, physiotherapists, dieticians, and exercise consultants. Coordinate the programme for maximum benefit.

Adherence strategies

High level of dropouts (9–49% from short supervised programmes). Factors include social class, angina, reduced ejection fraction, inactive leisure habits, current smoking, transport problems, medical problems, work or domestic commitments, lack of motivation, inconvenient timing of programmes, anxiety, and depression.

Factors to improve maintenance of exercise

- Membership of cardiac support groups.
- Community programmes.
- Home based programmes using local facilities.

Exercise referral

Exercise referral has now been widened to a larger group of subjects. With recognition that most individuals do not take adequate exercise, exercise prescription is now more widely applied.

Physical activity guidelines—exercise prescription for healthy adults

- 1990 ACSM exercise recommendation to improve and maintain cardio-respiratory fitness a minimum of 3—20 minutes of continuous moderate to vigorous intensity aerobic exercise per week. (60–90% of maximum heart rate or 50–85% of maximum aerobic capacity).
- 1995 ACSM and CDC physical recommendation to promote health and prevent disease. Accumulate at least 30 minutes of moderate intensity physical activity on five or more days per week. This activity would include alterations of daily routine of walking short distances or climbing stairs, and includes activities such as gardening, housework, or washing the car.

Benefits of exercise

Mechanism of increased exercise capacity

Peripheral effects of skeletal muscle and vascular adaptations; increase in arteriovenous oxygen difference, increased extraction, increased blood flow and aerobic metabolism in skeletal muscle, increased fibre area, capillary density and oxidative activity. Cardiac effects increased ejection fraction, cardiac output, stroke volume.

New patient groups

Sedentary low risk groups have risk factors but no clinical symptoms nor overt disease. After screening for symptoms these patients are seen for exercise consultation.

High-risk patient groups have evidence of previous disease with a previous history of angina, myocardial infarction, or revascularization but no ongoing exercise programme. Appropriate programmes of exercise are prescribed after preparticipation health and symptom questionnaires and exercise testing.

Information regarding facilities and sources.

Exercise networks and sites of delivery are collated and advertized in public places, primary care facilities, and websites to provide the widest possible public access.

Exercise and adult congenital heart disease

The live birth incidence of congenital heart disease is 7–8 cases/1000 and 96% survive into adult life. Survival patterns have changed and exercise plays a role in assessment. Common heart defects include atrial septal defect, ventricular septal defect, patent ductus arteriosis, coarctation of the aorta with or without additional disease, valvular aortic stenosis, pulmonary stenosis, Fallot's tetralogy, and transposition of the great arteries. Many have interventions, but some complicated disease states have palliation and supportive therapy, including those with pulmonary hypertension including Eisenmenger circulation.

Areas for advice include employment, insurance, and driving. In particular we are concerned with advice re exercise, activity level, sports participation, and the risk of sudden death.

Patient groups include
- No previous surgery but may need in future e.g. aortic stenosis.
- Previous surgery with possible risk of arrhythmia e.g. Fallot's tetralogy.
- Patients with palliation, further intervention required e.g. Mustard procedure for TGA.
- Inoperable subjects, consideration of heart-or heart lung transplant.

Uses of exercise testing
- To evaluate symptoms and perception of functional capacity and decide if exercise prescription is indicated.
- To identify underlying cardiac lesion severity.
- To assess effectiveness of treatment or interventions.
- To assess functional capacity prior to recreational or athletic activity.

Information available from exercise testing
- Functional capacity including workload, oxygen consumption and anaerobic threshold.
- Heart rhythm including atrial and ventricular arrhythmias induced by exercise or heart block.
- Blood pressure response on exercise. (May induce fall in obstructive lesions or abnormal rise in patients with coarctation, with or without previous intervention.)
- Induction of myocardial ischaemia in patients with valvular disease.

Limitations of exercise capacity
- Limitations of rise in cardiac output; Fontan repair, obstructive lesions of valves or ventricular outflow tract, or regurgitant lesions.
- Associated with chronotropic incompetence, inadequate stroke volume, and ventricular filling.
- Inadequate peripheral compensation and conditioning.
- Associated pulmonary disease.
- Psychological barriers of perceived limitations.

Guidelines for exercise in congenital heart disease

- Advice should be in keeping with the nature of the exercise challenge, including whether the exercise is recreational or competitive, and also including the personality of the participant.
- Factors will include type, intensity, and duration of training and competition related to individual sports.
- Special consideration of the influence of bodily contact in subjects with valve replacements.
- Special limitation in sports if risk of loss of consciousness.
- Classification of sports is required in terms of isotonic and isometric components.

High risk

- Compromised ventricular function.
- Significant cardiomyopathy.
- Critical obstructive lesions.
- Severe regurgitant lesions.
- Severe pulmonary hypertension.
- Exercise induced ventricular arrhythmias.

Light exercise permitted

- Moderate obstructive lesions.
- Moderate regurgitant lesions.
- Moderate pulmonary hypertension.
- Systemic hypertension.
- Uncorrected cyanotic heart disease.

Minimal restriction to exercise

- Mild obstructive lesions.
- Mild regurgitant lesions.
- Shunts in the absence of pulmonary vascular disease.
- Corrected cyanotic patients with minimal anatomical abnormality.

Factors in individual congenital conditions

Coarctation of the aorta

Rigid proximal aorta leads to inappropriate blood pressure response to exercise. Even after repair, 10% of those normotensive at rest have abnormal exercise or 24-hour blood pressure responses. Nature of repair determines the long-term risk of aneurysm development or risk of rupture.

Pulmonary stenosis

Determine if mild, moderate, or severe. If major obstruction, gradient >50mmHg then recommend mild intensity of exercise and short duration. May be unrestricted post operation.

Atrial septal defect

In those without surgery—a small shunt in absence of pulmonary hypertension, no limitation. If pulmonary hypertension, then low intensity. In those following surgery, if pulmonary vascular resistance remains low, then no restriction. If post-operative pulmonary pressure is elevated then restrict. Atrial arrhythmias may occur on exercise.

Ventricular septal defect.

Advice depends on the size of defect and pulmonary vascular resistance. Post-operative advice depends on pulmonary artery pressure, exclusion of ventricular arrhythmias on exercise, and 24-hour monitoring.

Patients with associated pulmonary vascular disease

If severe, low level exercise may lead to marked dyspnoea. Exercise may increase the left to right shunt. Local tissue acidosis occurs. Exercise induced syncope may occur.

Tetralogy of Fallot

If uncorrected, advice depends on exercise capacity associated with the degree of obstruction to the right ventricular outflow tract and increase in right to left shunt. Particular risks may occur with isometric exercise.

After repair, exercise influenced if residual shunt, induced pulmonary regurgitation following outflow tract repair, stenosis of pulmonary artery at site of previous Blalock shunt, or induction of arrhythmias which may occur in any patient with previous ventriculotomy.

Transposition of great arteries. (Mustard repair)

Venous pathway obstruction may reduce exercise capacity. Baffle leaks may induce desaturation on early phase of exercise.

Depression of systemic right ventricle limits increase in cardiac output.

Sinus node dysfunction. Atrial and ventricular tachyarrhthmias or abnormal AV conduction may occur. General guideline of no more than mild to moderate isotonic exercise.

Fontan circulation

Circulation devoid of a functional sub-pulmonary ventricle. Function depends on nature of sub-aortic ventricle, which may be morphological left or right. Exercise performance reduced with lowered aerobic capacity, heart rate reduction, and post-operative hypoxaemia. Exercise capacity may be improved by total caval pulmonary connection.

Marfan syndrome

- Mutations in a single gene affects components of the extracellular matrix, leading to a disorder of the connective tissue.
- Autosomal dominant disease of connective tissue with variable penetrance. Frequency 1 in 20,000; 25% represent new mutations.
- Mutation on chromosome 15 in fibrillin-1 gene (*FBN-1*) affecting the extracellular matrix glycoprotein present in the aorta, suspensory ligament of lens, and connective tissue of tendons and ligaments.
- Molecular analysis of complement deoxynbp nucleic acid and deoxynbo nucleic acid on fibrillin 1 gene from skin fibroblasts culture shows reduced, absent, or structurally abnormal fibrillin.

Challenges

- Diagnosis made on clinical grounds with abnormalities in two systems.
- Genetic counselling, particular problems with pregnancy.
- Life style advice, body habitus may allow sports participation e.g. basketball or volleyball.
- Cardiovascular surveillance aimed predominantly at aortic size and mitral valve.

Diagnosis

Skeletal system

Major criteria:

- Pectus carinatum, pectus excavatum requiring surgery.
- Reduced upper to lower segment ratio or arm span to height ratio >1.05.
- Wrist and thumb signs.
- Scoliosis of >20 degrees or spondylolisthesis.
- Reduced extension at the elbows (<170°).
- Pes planus.
- Protrusion acetabulae (on X-ray).

Minor criteria:

- Pectus excavatum of moderate severity.
- Joint hypermobility.
- High arched palate with crowding of teeth.
- Typical facial appearance.

Ocular system

Major criteria:
Ectopia lentis.

Minor criteria:

- Flat cornea (keratometry).
- Increased axial length of globe (ultrasound).
- Decreased miosis.

Major criteria:

- Dura.
- Lumbosacral dural ectasia by CT or MRI.

Family/genetic history
Major criteria:
- Having a parent, child or sibling who meets the diagnostic criteria independently.
- Known mutation in fibrillin 1 gene.
- Haplotype of *FBN-1* is inherited and known to be associated with unequivocal Marfan syndrome in the family.

Cardiovascular system

Major criteria:
- Dilatation of ascending aorta including sinuses of Valsalva.
- Dissection of ascending aorta.

Minor criteria:
- Mitral valve prolapse.
- Unexplained dilatation of main pulmonary artery <40 years.
- Calcification of mitral valve annulus <40 years.
- Dilatation or dissection of descending thoracic or abdominal aorta <50 years.

Pulmonary system
Minor criteria:
- Spontaneous pneumothorax.
- Apical blebs (chest X-ray).

Skin and integument
Minor criteria:
- Unexplained stretch marks.
- Recurrent or incisional herniae.

Diagnostic criteria for Marfan syndrome

Negative family/genetic history
Major criteria in at least two different organ systems and involvement of a third system, or known genetic mutations plus one major criterion and involvement of a second organ system.

Positive family/genetic history
One major criterion in an organ system and involvement of a second organ system.

Cardiac problems

- Early mortality in 4th and 5th decades.
- Children are more affected by mitral valve disease.
- Aortic problems progressively more likely in adolescents and older.
- Mitral complications more common in females than males.

Higher risk of deterioration (25%) in this group of mitral valve prolapse than in normal population.

Mitral valve disease

Mitral annulus dilatation stretching may occasionally rupture chordae. 10% have associated calcification. Repair of the valve is often successful.

Factors influencing the results of surgery: Valve cusp extremely redundant, marked chordal damage, degree of calcification. There is an increased risk of dehiscence of prosthetic valve if replacement required.

Aortic root involvement

May be dilated at birth, rate of progression variable. Prediction of dissection is difficult. Screening with trans-thoracic echo sufficient if dilation limited to proximal ascending aorta. Usual rate of change slow. If dilatation of descending aorta, trans-oesophageal echo and serial MRI required. Aortic valve regurgitation usually accompanies dilatation of 50mm. Rupture of aorta infrequent if <55mm.

Positive family history may influence the predisposition.

Treatment

Beta-blockers should be introduced as early as possible at the highest tolerated dose.

Valve surgery

Approach to repair dilated aortic root and preserve the aortic valve to avoid risks of endocarditis and anticoagulation.

Aortic root replacement

Elective root repair low operative mortality. Emergency results much poorer. Operate in patients with aortic roots >65mm.

Aortic dissection

Most arise above the coronary ostium (type A Stanford). Some may extend the entire length (type 1 deBakey scheme). 10% distal to left subclavian. (type B or 111) Rarely may be limited to abdominal aorta. Angiography, MRI, TOE. Follow up for progression. Distal branch occlusion, further aortic dilatation.

Pregnancy

- High risk of affected child.
- Dilatation of aortic root with aortic regurgitation and cardiac failure.
- Heightened risk of dissection. In third trimester, at parturition, and first month post-delivery.
- Risk highest if previous dilatation or dissection.
- Risk much less if aorta <40mm.

Preconception counselling

- If dilated or previous dissection consider termination.
- ʾnid physical activity.
- ʾkade.
- ʾctive section.

Indications for monitoring

- Aortic root size must be monitored by echocardiography or MRI if echo window inadequate.
- If aortic root diameter is 5cm then investigations should be undertaken 3-monthly and if diameter is 6cm then prophylactic surgery is recommended.
- If aortic root is normal and no family history of sudden death then dynamic exercise may be undertaken in low and moderate static/low dynamic competitive sports but isometric exercise should be avoided.

Hypertension and exercise

Prevalence

20% of adults over 40 years have a blood pressure >140/90. Prevalence rises with age to >60% over age 60. Risks rise progressively over whole range of blood pressure.

Diagnosis

- To establish level of blood pressure, 3 readings should be taken over 3 months. If borderline recordings are obtained, 24hr ambulatory monitoring can be performed. These values correlate better with target organ damage.
- Transient or persistent increases in blood pressure may occur associated with stress, but have normal values at other times (e.g. white coat hypertension). This may occur in some 20% of subjects and is not related to cardiovascular events.
- There is considerable variability over 24hrs with a normal nocturnal dip. Loss of dip associated with more serious target organ effects.
- Exercise-induced hypertension may occur. Systolic blood pressure rise >60mmHg after 5mins, >70mmHg after 10min or diastolic rise >10 mmHg at any time is associated with the development of hypertension and an increased risk of cardiovascular events.

Aetiology

- Primary, essential, or idiopathic (90–95%).
- Secondary, associated with (a) renal disease (b) endocrine abnormalities, including Cushing's syndrome.
- Coarctation of the aorta.
- Pregnancy.

Natural history of hypertension and prognosis

- Established increase in diastolic blood pressure (5–10mmHg) associated with a 34–56% increase in cerebrovascular accidents and a 21–37% increase in coronary artery disease.
- Absolute risk small 3.5% over 8yrs.
- Cause of death in hypertension; 50% coronary artery disease, 33% CVA, 10–15% chronic renal failure.

Symptoms and signs
- Uncomplicated high blood pressure asymptomatic.
- End organ complications include left ventricular hypertrophy, abnormalities in renal function, hypertensive and athersclotic retinopathy.
- Decision on treatment is based on the overall cardiovascular risk including total cholesterol, low HDL, cigarette smoking, glucose intolerance and left ventricular hypertrophy.
- Left ventricular hypertrophy is a cardiovascular risk factor. LVH independent predictor of cardiovascular death, cardiovascular events, and all cause mortality. Earliest change in LV is diastolic dysfunction. Then asymmetrical septal change, followed by concentric hypertrophy. Regression can occur with therapy.

Exercise and LVH

- Endurance exercise causes eccentric LVH; isometric exercise leads to concentric LVH.
- Posterior left ventricular wall increases with age, left ventricular hypertrophy more prevalent in some ethnic groups. LVH more common in males than females.
- Complications of hypertension.

Vascular accelerated or malignant phase:
- Haemorrhagic stroke.
- Congestive heart failure.
- Nephrosclerosis.
- Aortic dissection.
- May reflect accelerated atherosclerosis; coronary artery disease including sudden death.
- Arrhythmias.
- Thrombotic stroke.
- Peripheral vascular disease.

Exercise capacity and hypertension

- Gradient in exercise capacity; increased from control, to those with no left ventricular hypertrophy, to those with left ventricular hypertrophy.
- Reduced ejection fraction if left ventricular hypertrophy.
- Significant reduction in exercise capacity, even in moderate hypertensives and reduced oxygen consumption.
- Higher levels of systolic blood pressure at each level of exercise.

Exercise haemodynamics, exercise capacity

- Inverse correlation between oxygen consumption, mean arterial pressure, and age.
- Inverse correlation between stroke volume and cardiac output and mean arterial pressure at rest.
- Cardiac output and heart rate inversely correlated with age.
- Left ventricular hypertrophy not associated with maximum oxygen consumption.
- In hypertensives post-exercise blood pressure reduced for up to 12hrs due to enhanced vascular compliance.

Treatment of hypertension

For mild rise in BP, introduce life-style changes.
- Prevention of obesity.
- Moderate reduction in Na intake.
- Higher levels of physical activity.
- Avoid excess alcohol.

Exercise as treatment for hypertension

Effects of exercise for 20–60 mins at 60–80% maximum heart rate, 3 times weekly.
- Reduction in sub maximum heart rate.
- Increase in peak VO_2
- Reduction in maximum blood pressure (systolic and diastolic and sub maximum blood pressure). Associated with reduction in left ventricular mass and left ventricular mass index.
- Meta-analysis of randomized controlled trials. 29 trials including 1533 subjects. Small consistent reduction in blood pressure with aerobic exercise (systolic 4.7, diastolic 3.1).
- Little difference according to intensity of exercise.
- Little effect of number of training sessions.

Drug treatment of hypertension

Agents and specific indications

Diuretics—heart failure, elderly and systolic hypertension.
Beta-blockers—angina, post myocardial infarction, and tachyarrhythmias.
ACE inhibitors—heart failure, left ventricular dysfunction, post-myocardial infarction, and diabetic nephropathy.
Calcium antagonists—angina, elderly patients, and systolic hypertension.
Alpha blockers—prostatic hypertrophy.
Angiotensin 11 antagonists—ACE inhibitor cough.

Exercise and heart failure

Definition
The pathophysiological state in which an abnormality of cardiac function is responsible for failure of the heart to pump blood at a rate sufficient for the requirements of the metabolising tissues.

Epidemiology
- Prevalence in European population 0.4–2%. The prevalence increases with age: 1% at 25–54 yrs, 4–5% at 64–74 yrs, 6.6–7.9% at 89–90 yrs.
- Five-year mortality 50%. 10 million CHF patients in EU countries (ESC Taskforce on Heart Failure 2001). Frequent hospitalization, requirement for help with daily living, but with high economic cost.

Aetiology and clinical presentation
- High output failure secondary to anaemia, pregnancy, thyrotoxicosis, AV fistula, Paget's disease.
- Low output failure—acute or chronic.
- Volume overload—regurgitant valve or high output state.
- Pressure overload—systemic hypertension, outflow obstruction, e.g. aortic stenosis.
- Loss of muscle—acute following myocardial infarction.
- Chronic cardiomyopathy with longstanding ischaemic heart disease.
- Infective—endocarditis, viral myocarditis, infiltrative.
- Metabolic—nutritional.
- Drug induced adriamycin, 5-fluorouracil and daunorubicin.
- Restricted filling—pericardial disease, restrictive cardiomyopathy.

Classified as per New York Heart Association with increased symptoms on exercise.
- Grade 1—no limitation but objective evidence of cardiac dysfunction VO_2 15–20 ml/kg/min.
- Grade 2—limited on moderate physical exertion, e.g. hills and stairs VO_2 10–15 ml/kg/min.
- Grade 3—limited on normal daily activities e.g. bathing, cooking VO_2 5–10 ml/kg/min.
- Grade 4—limited at rest on minimal exertion e.g. rising from chair VO_2<5ml/kg/min.

Left ventricular failure
Dyspnoea may extend to orthopnoea or paroxysmal nocturnal attacks with pulmonary oedema. Increased respiratory rate, tachycardia, S3, and basal crepitations.

Right ventricular failure
Peripheral oedema—site related to posture. Breathlessness, fatigue. Signs of right ventricular hypertrophy, elevated JVP.

Central haemodynamics
- Systolic dysfunction usually associated with left ventricular dilatation.
- Reduced stroke volume and ejection fraction.
- Reduced cardiac output.
- Elevated end diastolic pressures, with increased preload.
- Compensatory neurohormonal activation:
  - Increased sympathetic activity—increases heart rate and contractility but leads to increased arteriolar constriction and afterload and increases oxygen consumption.
  - Increased renin angiotensin aldosterone—leads to salt and water retention with increased venous return, but associated with vasoconstriction and increased afterload.
  - Increased vasopressin—enhances venous return but increases vasoconstriction.
  - Increased endothelin—vasoconstriction but increased afterload.
  - Increased interleukins and TNF $\propto$.

Investigations
- Clinical examination.
- Electrocardiography including exercise testing.
- Echocardiography TTE, or TOE.
- Chest X-ray.
- MRI.
- Invasive investigations including coronary arteriography.

Treatment of cardiac failure

Drug treatment
- Diuretics.
- ACE inhibitor.
- Beta-blocker.
- Spironolactone.
- Angiotensin receptor blocker.
- Digoxin if atrial fibrillation or severe heart failure.
- Consider aspirin and statin.

Devices: CRT, ICD, and LV assist devices.

Lifestyle modification
- Stop smoking.
- Fluid restriction.
- Reduce salt intake.
- Eat more fresh fruit and vegetables.
- Monitor body weight.
- Reduce alcohol intake.
- Lose weight.
- Regular moderate exercise.

Exercise in CHF

LV performance, cardiac output, and myocardial oxygen consumption are determined by: (a) heart rate, (b) preload, (c) contractility, (d) afterload.

- Preload—in a normal heart, ventricular systolic performance is related to the degree of end diastolic fibre stretch or preload. This is influenced by end diastolic pressure and volume. In heart failure, further stretch is associated with decreased function.
- Contractility—force and velocity contraction can be assessed in isovolumic or ejection phases. May be expressed as the ejection fraction.
- Afterload—force resisting myocardial shortening, i.e. resistance—the left ventricle must overcome to eject stroke volume.

Reduction in exercise capacity in CHF

- Cardiac insufficiency, poor left ventricular function and resulting reduced cardiac output, decreased exercise tolerance, and reduced peak VO_2.
- Pulmonary changes with increased respiratory rate, reduced tidal volume, and ventilation perfusion mismatch.
- Skeletal muscle dysfunction secondary to hyperperfusion with reduced oxidative enzymes, and increased glycolytic enzymes. Impaired oxygen utilization during exercise.
- Further changes due to detraining and development of abnormal mitochondria.
- Metabolic receptor activation may lead to increased ventilation and increased sympathetic tone with vagal withdrawal and reduced baroreceptor sensitivity.

Exercise testing

- Exercise time determined using treadmill or bicycle ergometer protocol. Use of ramp protocol most appropriate with workload increasing continuously. Optimum duration 8–12 min. Breath-by-breath analysis shows that Ve/VCO$_2$ peak exercise: rest correlates with exercise time and anaerobic threshold.
- Peak VO$_2$ is the best indicator of prognosis in heart failure, although correlates poorly with haemodynamic measurements at rest, which do not reflect functional reserve.
- Peak VO$_2$ <10mls/kg/min, 77% 1yr mortality. Peak VO$_2$ 10–18 mls/kg/min, 10.1% 1yr mortality.

Six minute walk test

Simple non-invasive test which is a good predictor of morbidity and mortality in patients with mild-to-moderate CHF.

Distance walked in 6 mins is an independent predictor of mortality and hospitalization in advanced heart failure.

Effects of exercise in heart failure

- No significant change in left ventricular ejection fraction.
- Improvement in diastolic function.
- Increased cardiac output at peak exercise with increased peak leg blood flow.
- Reduced chronotropic response to exercise.
- Minute ventilation reduced, slope of minute ventilation to rate of CO$_2$ production reduced.
- Reduction in activity of ergo receptors with reduction in excessive ventilation.
- Reduced sympathetic tone and increased vagal activity.

Altered skeletal muscle function

- Decreased lactate production at sub-maximal exercise.
- Decrease in early acidosis and phosphocreatinine depletion on exercise. Enhanced capacity for oxidative synthesis of adenosine triphosphate.
- Increased volume density of mitochondria.
- Restoration of flow dependent endothelium mediated vasodilatation.

Exercise and treatment of CHF

- *Moderate exercise training*: improved functional capacity, quality of life, and outcome in patients with stable CHF after 2 months   No further improvement after 1yr. Addition of full cardiac rehabilitation with lifestyle education and behavioural modification associated with improved survival for patients with left ventricular dysfunction.
- *Three months of low level exercise training*: increased peak VO_2. Reduced perceived dyspnoea during exercise and improved quality of life score. Improved exercise tolerance of >2 minutes, peak O_2 uptake of 2ml/kg/min.

Beneficial actions are additional to actions of ACEI and beta-blockers.

- *Randomized trials*. Exercise training in heart failure is beneficial in improving functional capacity. Quality of life improves. Reduced need for hospital admission. Mortality reduction.
- *Cost effectiveness*. Exercise prolonged survival when additional 1.82yrs at a relatively low cost per year of life saved.

AHA exercise recommendation in cardiac failure

- Individualized approach.
- Aim 70–80% peak VO_2 for 20–30 mins.
- Severely debilitated—unaccustomed to exercise. Aim 60–65% PVO_2.
- Builds progression into prescription.
- Include adequate warm up of 15 mins.
- 3–5 exercise periods/week.
- Initial session supervized.

Alternative use of low intensity physical training, home exercise programme and localized arm training programmes.

Sudden death

Sudden death in sport is uncommon, but has major media interest. Two cases occur per 100,000 subject years. Five in 100,000 of the sporting population have a predisposing cardiac condition. 10% of those at risk die suddenly. The causes reflect the age of participant, structural abnormalities in the young, coronary artery disease in older groups.

Pre-participation screening

This remains controversial. The main aim is to identify causes of sudden sporting death, with screening applied to the whole participating population. Alternative strategies have been suggested for those with
- A family history of sudden death.
- Premature coronary artery disease.
- Counselling of patients with known abnormalities—education about warning symptoms including syncope, presyncope, palpitation, chest pain, and dyspnoea.

Guidelines may be required for disqualification from competition.

Methods of pre-participation screening
- Use of health questionnaires; includes symptomatic enquiry for warning symptoms and family history. May include aspects of respiratory and orthopaedic health.
- ECGs may be taken as routine.
- Echocardiography and exercise testing may be used in those with suggestive symptoms or with abnormal ECG. May require tests in 10% of population.

Conditions with known cardiovascular risk <35 years
- Hypertrophic cardiomyopathy.
- Idiopathic concentric LV hypertrophy.
- Anomalies of coronary arteries.
- Aortic rupture.
- Right ventricular dysplasia.
- Myocarditis.
- Valvular disease.
- Arrhythmias and conduction defects.

Hypertrophic cardiomyopathy
- Leading cause of sudden unexpected death in young athletes.
- Autosomal dominant with high degree of penetrance.
- Some echocardiocardiographic features present in 1 in 500 of the population.
- Symptoms may include chest pain, palpitation, syncope, and dyspnoea.
- Predisposition to supraventricular and ventricular arrhythmias.
- Clinical signs include a jerky character pulse, double apex beat, and a fourth heart sound often present.
- Ejection systolic murmur at left sternal border.
- Abnormal ECG in 90%.

Echocardiography—hypertrophied non-dilated left ventricle with no predisposing cause for left ventricular hypertrophy. Chamber size reduced. Impaired diastolic filling.

Left ventricular outflow tract obstruction with hypertrophy of sub-aortic septum and systolic anterior motion of the mitral valve.

Adverse prognostic factors include:
- Family history of sudden death.
- Documented ventricular tachycardia.
- Young age of onset of symptoms.

Concentric left ventricular hypertrophy
- Concentric hypertrophy of left ventricle in the absence of hypertension.
- Associated with cardiac death.
- Significant incidence in black athletes which might reflect athletic training.
- If present, expect deconditioning for 6 months, may show regression.

Coronary artery anomalies
- Significant anomaly of left coronary artery arising from the right coronary cusp maintaining an acute angle with the aorta.
- Aortic dilatation on exercise causes obstruction to flow.
- Other anomalies may include the absence or under-development of major coronary branches.
- Symptoms of chest pain, syncope, or sudden death.

Investigations
- Resting ECG.
- Exercise testing or evidence of exercise-induced reversible ischaemia.
- Radionuclide assessment for regional perfusion.
- Coronary arteriography.
- Treatment and transplantation of coronary artery may be undertaken using cuff of peri-coronary artery tissue.

Marfan syndrome
- Connective tissue derangement if fibrillin reduced or defective.
- Autosomal dominant with variable penetrance, 15% sporadic.
- Gene on the long arm of chromosome 15.
Systems involved:
- Musculoskeletal
- Ocular abnormalities
- Cardiovascular system.

Cardiovascular abnormalities
- Mitral valve prolapse.
- May develop significant mitral regurgitation.
- Aortic root dilatation.
- Aortic regurgitation.
- Aortic dissection may occur in ascending, descending, or abdominal aorta.

Investigation
- Echocardiography for aortic valve and ascending aortic root sizing.
- MRI of individual aortic segments.
- Medical therapy—betablockade shows slowing of aortic dilatation.
- Aortic root 5cm. Screening for change on 3-monthly intervals.
- If >6cm screening for prophylactic surgery.

Right ventricular dysplasia
- Right ventricular cardiomyopathy.
- Unusually high incidence in northern regions of Italy.
- Pathological change of fibro-fatty replacement, with irregular muscle disruption.
- Malignant re-entrant ventricular tachyarrhythmias.
- Symptoms—reflecting right ventricular dysfunction, palpitation, and syncope.

Investigation
- Clinical signs of right ventricular dysfunction.
- ECG shows inverted T waves in right ventricular leads.
- Echocardiography shows global right ventricular enlargement with rigid RV wall motion abnormalities.
- Investigations may include right ventricular angiography and endomyocardial biopsy.

Myocarditis
- Variable illness associated with symptoms of viral infection.
- Myocardial lymphocytic infiltration with focal necrosis leading to cardiac dysfunction and conduction system problems.
- Symptoms non-specific, like cold or flu.
- Clinical examination—tachycardia, supraventricular or ventricular extrasystoles., May progress to cardiomegaly and frank signs of cardiac failure.
- Diagnosis: ECG—non-specific changes with ST-T wave changes, arrhythmias, heart block.
- Echocardiography shows signs of chamber dysfunction.
- Management—broad spectrum of severity. If objective signs present return to sport if ECG normal, left ventricular contraction normal, and absence of arrhythmias.

Valvular disease
- The aetiology may be congenital, acquired, or degenerative (atherosclerotic in older age group).
- Type of valve disease identified clinically.
- Severity assessed on clinical examination.
- Electrocardiography for evidence of atrial or ventricular chamber hypertrophy with ST-T wave changes of strain pattern.
- Chest X-ray for identification of chamber enlargement.
- Echocardiography and Doppler assessment for chamber size, assessment of stenosis, and regurgitation of individual valve, calculated gradients, and regurgitant volume.
- MRI shows detailed assessment similar to echocardiography.

Aortic stenosis

- Valve lesion associated with cardiac sudden death in sport.
- Management depends on presence of symptoms of chest pain, syncope, and breathlessness.
- Advice re exercise. If mild, all sports can be undertaken. If moderate, low intensity or moderate static and dynamic exercise.

Mitral valve prolapse

- Variable condition.
- May be a normal variant in 6% of the population.
- Often with non-specific symptoms.
- Clinical examination: may be evidence of click murmur.
- ECG non-specific.
- Echocardiogram—evidence of 'floppy mitral valve leaflets'.
- Complications—TIAs in small proportion.
- Progressive mitral regurgitation.
- Association with supraventricular and ventricular arrhythmias.
- Predisposition to endocarditis.
- Management—pragmatic. If asymptomatic and no family history of cardiac complications, no limitation in activity.

Arrhythmias and heart block

- The mechanism of sudden death is arrhythmic, almost always ventricular fibrillation.
- Predisposing factors of enhanced automaticity, conduction, or repolarization in the electrophysiological tissues of the heart.
- Autonomic changes may occur during exercise, baseline vagal activity leading to bradycardia and heart block.
- Sympathetic activity during exercise—may lead to catecholamine-induced serious arrhythmias.
- Arrhythmias may be associated with structural abnormalities such as hypertrophic cardiomyopathy, or right ventricular dysplasia. Structural abnormalities associated with valvular and other congenital heart disease including those with previous right ventriculotomy.
- Arrhythmic symptoms include palpitation, syncope or presyncope, breathlessness, sudden death.

Investigations:

- ECG for evidence of pre-excitation, prolonged QRS or evidence of myocardial ischaemia or structural abnormality.
- Exercise electrocardiography used to induce symptoms.
- Continuous ECG monitoring (minimum duration 24hrs) period expanded according to symptoms. If rare occurrence but significant symptoms, use of symptom or event triggering monitoring.
- Invasive investigation by programmed electrical stimulation, with intracardiac sensing electrodes.
- Management—anti-arrhythmic therapy, intracardiac ablation techniques for ectopic sites of electrical activity, or pulmonary vein ablation for atrial fibrillation. Device implantation may be required.

Pre-excitation in Wolff–Parkinson–White syndrome
- ECG confirms short PR interval, <0.12 secs.
- Wide QRS complex, initial slurring of the QRS complex (delta wave).
- Commonest tachycardia 150–250 beats per minute.
- Rarely atrial flutter or fibrillation which may conduct through anomalous pathway to predispose to ventricular fibrillation in those with accessory pathways with short refractory periods.
- If symptomatic, assessment of accessory pathway undertaken. In high-intensity sports, elctrophysiological studies should be undertaken, AF induced and shortest RR interval assessed.
- If rapid ventricular rates drug therapy or ablation.

Prolonged QT syndrome
- Repolarization abnormalities and prolonged QT syndrome. Symptoms associated with emotion or physical stress.
- QT prolongation to more than 0.44 seconds corrected for heart rate in absence of other causes of prolongation (drugs and electrolyte abnormalities) leads to ventricular tachycardia, including torsades de pointes.
- Bradyarrhthmias common on ECG monitoring. T wave alternans may be induced by emotion.
- Therapy betablockade, surgical sympathectomy if treatment failure. Occasional pacing therapy.
- Avoidance of competitive athletics and sympathetic stimuli.

Coronary artery disease
- Major cause of death in those >35yrs.
- Most deaths occur in vigorous sports.
- Previous symptoms suggestive of coronary atherosclerosis may be recognized, including anginal symptoms on exertion.
- Established risk factors for coronary artery disease often present, including hypertension and hypercholesterolaemia.
- Victims often perceived as being very fit with type A personality.
- Pathological studies confirm the presence of obstructive coronary artery disease.
- Myocardium may show previous healed infarction.
- Sudden death is not prevented by extreme forms of conditioning.
- Investigations of resting ECG, exercise stress testing, assessment of left ventricular function, and coronary arterigraphy.
- Management by risk factor modification.
- Education concerning warning symptoms of chest pain, palpitation, or syncope.
- In subjects with structural abnormalities including valvular disease or congenital lesions, operated or not, then advice on exercise participation will be directed by the classification of the physical needs of each activity.

Intensity and type of exercise performed

Type A

1. Moderate or high dynamic and static demands

Boxing, cross country skiing, cycling, downhill skiing, fencing, ice hockey, rowing, rugby, running (sprinting), speed skating, US football, water polo, and wrestling.

2. Moderate to high dynamic and low static demands

Badminton, baseball, basketball, field hockey, lacrosse, orienteering, race walking, racket ball, running (distance), soccer, squash, swimming, table tennis, tennis, and volleyball.

3. Moderate to high static and low dynamic demands

Archery, auto racing, diving, equestrian, field events (jumping and throwing), gymnastics, karate or judo, motor cycling, sailing, ski jumping, water skiing, and weghtlifting.

Type B

1. Low intensity (low dynamic and low static demands)

Bowling, cricket, curling, golf, and shooting.

2. Danger of bodily collision

Boxing, ice hockey, karate or judo, lacrosse, rugby, soccer, US football, and wrestling.

Increased risk if syncope occurs

Auto racing, cycling, diving, downhill skiing, equestrian events, gymnastics, motor racing, polo, ski jumping, water polo, water skiing, and weightlifting.

Exercise-induced bronchospasm

Definition

- Exercise-induced bronchospasm (EIB) or exercise-induced asthma (EIA): A transient increase in airway resistance following vigorous exercise.
- Intrinsic asthma (IA) or allergic asthma: Chronic airway restriction assumed to be due to some endogenous cause such as allergies.

Epidemiology

- Exercise-induced bronchospasm occurs in 80–90% of asthmatic persons and 40–50% of those with allergic rhinitis.
- EIB has an incidence of 5–19% in elite athletes.

Aetiology

The exact cause is not well understood and may have multiple aetiologies specific to the individual. It is understood that the airways are much more sensitive in EIB than normal individuals, though normal people can have an exercise-induced bronchospasm under the right conditions (i.e. respiratory infections, cold air).

- Hyperventilation as a cause of airway drying:
  - EIB is worsened in some when exercising in cold dry air.
  - The increased osmolarity of the mucous somehow causes a release of bronchoconstrictors.
  - Hyperventilation alone can cause bronchospasm.
  - Hyperventilation with moist warm air inhibits the bronchoconstriction (explains why indoor swimming is relatively nonasthmagenic).
- The osmolarity of airways does not recover immediately after exercise:
  - Prostaglandin E2 may be protective.
  - Leukotriene B4 is increased following exercise.
  - Leukotriene inhibitors have been shown to decrease bronchoconstriction during exercise.
- Post-exercise rewarming as a source of bronchoconstriction:
  - Rapid rewarming may cause reactive hyperemia and edema in airway mucosa and submucosa.
  - This may result in luminal narrowing and reactive asthma.
- Air pollution:
  - Primary pollutants and secondary pollutants have been identified (see Table 14.1).
  - Hyperventilation also increases the amount of allergens and pollutants that may reach the pulmonary tree.
- Exercise-induced mediator release from mast cells and basophils.
- Parasympathetic mediation through vagus nerve innervation.

Clinical presentation

- In normal people and those with EIB with no baseline pulmonary function test changes, exercise increases pulmonary functions (PEFR and FEV1) by less than 5%. In those with baseline obstruction it may increase by more than 25%.

Table 14.1 Treatment algorithm for exercise-induced bronchospasm

Non-pharmacologic corrections (see text)

EIA continues

⇩

Beta2 agonist

EIA continues

⇩

Add cromolyn or nedocromil if paediatric, a late responder, or Hx of response to cromolyn (may double B2A and cromolyn if needed)

EIA continues

⇩

Add long-acting beta2 agonist

EIA continues

⇩

Add leukotriene inhibitor

EIA continues

⇩

Add inhaled glucocorticoid

EIA continues

⇩

Add theophylline to attain serum level of 10–20mg/L

EIA continues

⇩

Add ipratropium bromide.
By now most asthmatics should be controlled. If not, consider oral steroid burst, alternative cause, or referral

⇩

Effective control of EIA
(check inhaler technique and lung function regularly)

- 28–52% of those with EIB experience a decline in PFTs by the end of exercise.
  - This may intensify over the next 3–20 minutes and may last 20–30 minutes.
- After exercise there may be a decrease in pulmonary function by up to 10% in normal subjects (this decrease is higher in EIB).

Refractory period
- After exercise, approximately 50% of EIB are resistant to further bronchospasm.
- This usually lasts less than 3 hours.
- Mechanism is not readily understood.

Late phase reaction
- A second increase in airway reactivity may be seen in up to 50% of children 4–12 hours after the acute episode.
- The release of inflammatory mediators by bronchial smooth muscle such as eosinophilic chemotactic factor of anaphylaxis, platelet activating factor, and some leukotrienes have been theorized as a cause.

Diagnosis
History
- The athlete may be unaware of any bronchospasm (see Table xxx)
  - More significant symptoms include shortness of breath, cough, lack of endurance, or wheeze, during or immediately following sustained exercise.
  - They may feel vague chest tightness or feel 'out of shape' with exercise.
  - Children may simply avoid strenuous play, have chest pain, or experience abdominal pain.
- Multiple stimulants have been identified (see Table xxx).

Pulmonary function tests (PFT)
- Medications are withheld for 8–24 hours before testing.
- Baseline PFTs are done first and should be within 80% of predicted values (or intrinsic asthma may be present).
- Use bicycle or ergometer for exercise stress (or whatever activity is most asthmagenic).
- Athlete exercises until 80–90% of maximum heart rate is achieved.
- Heart rate is maintained for 6–8 minutes.
- PFTs are measured immediately after exercise and then every 5 minutes for 20–30 minutes.
- EIB is present if there is a 15% or more decrease in peak expiratory flow rate (PEFR) or forced expiratory volume after one second (FEV1).
  - 15–20% decrease is mild EIB.
  - 20–40% decrease is moderate EIB.
  - >40% decrease is severe EIB.

Methacholine challenge test
- If the suspicion is high for EIB and exercise testing is negative, a methacholine challenge test may be performed.
- More sensitive test, but less specific.
- Must have intubation equipment available.

Table 14.2 Clinical clues to exercise-induced bronchospasm (may be present during or after exercise)

Obvious clinical clues	Subtle clinical clues
• Wheezing	• Abdominal pain
• Cough	• Athlete feels 'out of shape'
• Dyspnoea on exertion	• Cannot run 5 minutes without stopping
• Chest tightness	• Chest congestion
	• Chest discomfort or pain
	• Increased difficulty in cold air
	• Problems with running but not swimming
	• Lack of energy
	• Frequent 'colds'

Table 14.3 Stimulants that can contribute to exercise-induced bronchospasm

• Exercise	• Primary pollutants
• Cold air	• Secondary pollutants
• Low humidity	• Other pollutants
• Respiratory infections	• Strong odors and other airborne irritants
• Fatigue	• Allergens
• Emotional stress	
• Athletic overtraining	

Treatment

Nonpharmacologic

- Regular exercise programmes
  - Regular exercise programmes produce a significant reduction in bronchoconstrictions.
  - Increases tolerance and threshold levels for exercise.
  - Decreased medication needs.
  - Decreased absenteeism.
  - Improvement in aerobic capacity.
  - Enhancement of self-image.
  - Greater recognition and acceptance by peers (removes cripple image).
- Considerations
  - Wearing a facemask for outdoor exercise may increase temperature and humidity of air and filter out allergens and pollutants.
  - A warm shower immediately after exercise may reduce the bronchospasm.
  - Don't exercise in early morning or late evening if conditions are cold.
  - Encourage indoor sport in winter.
  - Avoid areas where pollutants and allergens are high.
  - Encourage water sports or sports that allow intermittent rest periods (most team sports, tennis, weightlifting, racquetball, etc).
  - Short bursts of activity can produce refractory periods that last up to 3 hours.
  - Warm up before any exercise for 10–15 minutes and cool down for 8–10 minutes.
  - Nose breathing may increase temperature and humidity of inspired air.
  - Encourage the athlete to try to 'run through' their asthma to take advantage of the refractory period.

Pharmacologic (consult up-to-date doping guidelines)

- Short acting beta2 agonist, meter dosed inhaler (albuterol, terbutaline, metaproterenol, bitolterol, etc).
  - Drug of choice for prophylactic and acute treatment.
  - Initial treatment is with a beta2 agonist metered dose inhaler (MDI) 15–60 minutes before exercise.
  - Effective in about 95% of patients.
  - May provide protection for 3–6 hours.
  - May cause tachycardia or slight tremor.
- Mast cell stabilizers, meter dosed inhaler (cromolyn sodium and nedocromyl sodium).
  - If paediatric, a late responder, or has responded to cromolyn in the past, add cromolyn 15–30 minutes before exercise.
  - 70–80% are protected.
  - May prevent late phase reaction and therefore may be more effective in children.
  - Decreased duration compared to beta2 agonist.

- Not effective for acute attacks.
- May be most effective in combination with beta2 agonists.
- Long acting beta2 agonists, MDI (salmeterol).
  - Taken 45–60 minutes before exercise.
  - May give protection for up to 6 hours.
  - Cannot be used for acute episodes.
  - Expensive.
- Leukotriene inhibitors, oral (montelukast, zafirlukast, zileuton).
  - Leukotriene receptor antagonists.
  - Shown to improve airway edema, smooth muscle constriction and reduce inflammation
  - Blocks leukotrienes D4 and E4 as well as slow reacting substance of anaphylaxis
  - Recently advocated as treatment for EIB
  - May have some drug interactions and liver toxicity
- Glucocorticoids, oral and inhaled (beclomethasone, flunisolide, fluticasone, triamcinolone)
  - Those athletes with a baseline obstruction on PFT (and maybe late phase reactors) should be on an inhaled bronchodilator and an inhaled glucocorticoid
  - Oral glucocorticoids are used acutely for gaining control in inflammatory asthma
  - Inhaled glucocorticoids are used for maintenance of control
  - Both will decrease the reactivity of the airways
- Theophylline, oral
  - May be of some benefit in some patients
  - Serum levels must be monitored
  - Toxic in high doses
  - Not presently used often for EIB
- Anticholinergic agents, MDI (ipratropium bromide)
  - Add ipratropium bromide 1–2 hours before exercise
  - Not effective in all patients
  - Especially effective for COPD, bronchitis, and emphysema
  - May be used for acute attacks
- Antihistamines
  - No significant role in EIB
- New agents under study
  - Alpha 1 agonists
  - Inhaled calcium channel blockers
  - Inhaled heparin
  - Inhaled diuretics
  - Gene therapy

Abdomen

Abdominal injury

Abdominal viscera are vulnerable in contact sport and although the ribs and pelvis provide some protection, the main protection is by the abdominal musculature. In addition to the abdominal viscera, superficial structures such as skin, subcutaneous tissues, and muscle may be injured. Diagnosis is usually obvious and management as for skin and subcutaneous wounds elsewhere in the body. Nevertheless, rectus abdominus muscle rupture with damage of epigastric artery may produce a large haematoma. The swelling may first be thought of as arising from an abdominal organ, but the later bluish discoloration gives a clue that it does not. The swelling will not cross the midline or extend beyond the lateral border of the muscle. It is relatively immovable due to the rectus sheath. Ultrasound or MRI will confirm if required.

The winded athlete

A blow to the solar plexus, with abdominal muscles relaxed, leaves the athlete temporarily unable to breathe. This is frightening for the athlete and the pitchside doctor should provide confident reassurance, ensure the airway is open and clear, loosen any restrictive clothing or equipment and encourage a slight flexion of the trunk. After the episode has passed, the doctor should consider visceral and rib injury.

History

Location of pathology may be obscure as pain can be referred:
- To shoulder from diaphragm (liver).
- To shoulder blade from gall bladder.
- To left chest from spleen.
- To umbilicus from appendix or pancreas.
- To testis from ureter and groin.

Examination

Signs of serious intra-abdominal injury:
- Absence of normal respiratory movements of abdomen.
- Guarding.
- Rebound pain.
- Absence of normal bowel sounds.
- Referred pain to shoulder or back.
- Falling blood pressure, increased pulse rate.

Delayed or slow haemorrhage from abdominal trauma is possible and so reassessment over several days is warranted.

Immediate management of any abdominal trauma will be assessment and appropriate treatment of haemodynamic shock.

Splenic bleeding

The spleen lies on the 9th to 11th ribs on the posterior wall of the abdomen and thus is unusually injured in sport unless enlarged. The most common cause of splenomegaly in athletes is glandular fever (infectious mononucleosis), and this causes the spleen to be vulnerable in blows to the left upper quadrant. Consequently, athletes should be advised against contact sport whilst the spleen is enlarged. The exact time period following the onset of glandular fever is controversial, although 5 weeks is the minimum. Full blood count, liver enzymes, and abdominal examination should have normalized. Some practitioners recommend 6 months off contact sport and even then athletes should be warned to report any abdominal discomfort for thorough assessment.

The spleen may also be ruptured by a fractured rib. The athlete will have persistent aching in the left flank following the initial acute pain. Sometimes there is an intervening period with no pain. Some have referred pain to the shoulder.

Clinicians need a high index of suspicion for splenic bleeds. CT scan can confirm the diagnosis. Though minor splenic injuries can be treated conservatively and with ongoing observation, rapid blood loss demands splenectomy.

Liver damage

Lacerations of the liver are rare in sport, although subcapsular haemorrhage may occur and give rise to right upper quadrant pain and tenderness. Ultrasound or CT scan may confirm the diagnosis.

Pancreatic damage

The pancreas lies deep at the back of the abdomen and is rarely injured in sport. Epigastric pain radiating to the back after severe blunt trauma, with midline tenderness, distension, and loss of bowel sounds due to reflex ileus, should lead the clinician to consider pancreatic damage. Serum amylase will be elevated and CT will confirm the diagnosis.

Bowel rupture

Rarely the bowel may be ruptured in severe blunt trauma in sport. There will be abdominal pain and blood in the peritoneum may irritate the diaphragm giving shoulder pain. Examination reveals tenderness, guarding, even abdominal rigidity and loss of bowel sounds. Shock may be indicated by clammy skin, tachycardia, and falling blood pressure. Peritoneal lavage may detect blood. Free air may be seen under the diaphragm in the upright plain abdominal X-ray. Prompt surgical treatment is required.

Renal trauma

The kidneys have some protection from blunt trauma from the 11th and 12th ribs, Psoas muscle and surrounding fat, however, renal contusions do occur, particularly in the young where the relative size of the kidney is larger. The kidneys are the most commonly injured abdominal organ in sport and result in many hospitalizations. The kidneys are vulnerable when the abdominal muscles are relaxed, and a typical situation might be leaping high and reaching for a ball, whilst taking a blow from another athlete.

The athlete might experience flank pain, though this may refer anteriorly, and might describe haematuria. Nevertheless, the amount of blood in the urine does not correlate to the seriousness of the injury, e.g. frank haematuria may not follow a vascular pedicle injury. Thus after blunt trauma, the wise clinician will investigate microscopic haematuria if blood pressure is dropping (<90mmHg systolic) or if there is any suspicion of palpable mass. Intravenous pyelogram (IVP) and CT scan are indicated, though the CT has the advantage of providing information about other abdominal viscera that might be injured.

Grading of renal injury

- Grade I—cortical lacerations without extravasation.
- Grade II—deep cortical laceration.
- Grade III—calix laceration.
- Grade IV—vascular pedicle rupture.

Management of renal trauma depends on extent of injury. Few (<10%) require surgery though indications are:
- Persistent retroperitoneal bleeding.
- Urinary extravasation.
- Non-viable renal tissue.
- Renal vascular pedicle injury.

Even for grade I injuries, return to strenuous sport should be delayed 4 weeks to reduce the risk of re-bleeding (maximum at 15–21 days). Contact sport should be avoided for at least 6 weeks and follow-up should be for 6 months with repeat blood pressure and urinalysis. Hypertension and hydronephrosis are late complications.

Ureteric avulsion

Rare in sport, though described in motor vehicle and equestrian sports. Gives rise to severe back pain and peritoneal irritation. Confirmed by IVP, requires surgical management.

Bladder rupture

Bladder rupture may occur with severe trauma of abdomen or pelvis. Suprapubic tenderness and haematuria will be present with contusions, but signs of peritonism (abdominal rigidity or rebound tenderness) indicate rupture and leakage of urine. Rupture requires prompt surgical treatment.

Urethral rupture

Urethral rupture is rare in sport and tends to occur with a straddle injury, cycling, gymnastics, or equestrian, or in association with pelvic fractures. It is a more common injury in men than women and it is the bulbous urethra that is more likely to be injured than the penile, which can move more freely. There will be blood at the meatus as well as signs of perineal trauma. Surgical repair and a suprapubic catheter are required.

Injuries of the scrotum and testes

External to the abdomen, the scrotum and contents are vulnerable to injury from blunt trauma. Some athletes wear protective equipment (cricketers and hockey goalkeepers for example).

Scrotal swelling after trauma suggests a ruptured testis or ruptured pampiniform plexus of veins. In the latter situation a varicocele becomes a haematocele. A haematocele does not transluminate well, but if the testicular shadow is visible through the fluid a hydrocele is more likely. Ultrasound examination is effective at diagnosing the ruptured testis, which requires urgent surgery.

If trauma does not result in swelling and scrotal examination is normal, the athlete may be treated by scrotal support, non steroidal anti-inflammatory drugs, and return to activity when pain subsides.

Diarrhoea (runner's trots)

Urgency to defecate, abdominal cramps, and diarrhoea frequently occur in long-distance runners, called 'runner's trots' and can be related to several factors:
• Athletes may have increased catecholamine levels.
• Athletes tend to have high carbohydrate diets, which can increase intestinal transit time.
• Reduced visceral blood flow leading to relative ischaemia of the bowel, particularly as duration of exercise increases.

Renal physiology and exercise

Renal parameters at rest
- Renal blood flow is 20% of CO (1200ml/min).
- Renal plasma flow—700ml/min.
- Glomerular filtration rate (GFR)—15% of plasma flow—105ml/min.
- Smaller proteins than albumin are filtered but then reabsorbed in proximal tubules.

Renal response to exercise
- Renal blood flow decreases.
- GFR is maintained or decreases.
- Increased filtration of macromolecules (albumin) giving rise to a 'glomerular' pattern of protein loss.
- In intense exercise, reabsorption of small proteins (microglobulins) declines giving rise to a tubular pattern of protein loss.

The decrease in renal blood flow is mediated by catecholamines and the sympathetic nervous system and is related to intensity of exercise, such that it may reduce to 25% of resting flow with strenuous activity. Plasma flow may reduce to 200ml/min in such circumstances, yet GFR is often maintained. With dehydration GFR may drop. With intense exercise anti-diuretic hormone (ADH) and aldosterone levels increase to preserve water and sodium. During such activity more red and white blood cells are found in the urine.

Athletic pseudonephritis

Described by Gardner (1956), athletic pseudonephritis is the presence of red and white blood cells, haemoglobin, myoglobin, protein, and casts in the urine after exercise. This is recognized to be a benign situation and has attracted various names depending on the activity with which the findings are associated:
- Stress haematuria.
- Marathoner's haematuria.
- 10,000m haematuria.
- March haemaglobinuria.
- Jogger's nephritis.

Proteinuria

Common in contact and non-contact sports and between 70–100% of runners are reported to have protein in their urine. This relates to intensity and not duration of event and is maximal within 30 minutes of exercise. The pattern is glomerular (macroglobulins) for moderate exercise, but glomerulo-tubular (macro and microglobulins) for intense exercise. This may be due to hypoxic damage to nephrons due to decreased blood flow, or efferent glomerular arteriolar constriction being greater than afferent, and so increasing filtration pressure.

However there are other causes of proteinuria:
- Physiological proteinuria (<100mg/L).
- Orthostatic proteinuria.

1 Gardner KD Jnr (1956). Athletic pseudonephritis; alterations of urine sediment by athletic competition. *J. Am Med. Assoc* **161**(17): 1613–17.

- Glomerulonephritis (>0.2g/d).
- Nephrotic syndrome (>0.05g/kg body wt/day).
- Cystitis/pyelonephritis.
- Hypertension.
- Diabetes mellitus.

Physiological proteinuria is common in adolescents (60%) and recurs in up to 30%. It is benign.

Orthostatic proteinuria clears with recumbency and so an early morning urine might be negative. Prognosis is good if normotensive and protein loss 750mg/day.

Typically, proteinuria records ++ or +++ on urinalysis corresponding to up to 300mg/L, post-exercise. It is wise not to test an athlete's urine shortly after exercise. If one is faced with a positive urinalysis for protein following exercise and no other symptoms to indicate another cause, repeat the urinalysis after 48 hours of rest. The urine should be negative to protein.

Haematuria

Haematuria may be macroscopic and dramatic after exercise, even with clots being passed. However, microscopic haematuria is almost universal as detected by dipsticks, which may detect as few as 1 million red cells/L. For abnormality it is better to look for 100 million red cells/L. As well as being too sensitive, dipsticks look for the haem group and so show up myoglobinuria and haemoglobinuria similarly.

Haematuria has been reported in high numbers of:
- Ice hockey players (100%).
- Swimmers (80%).
- Boxers (73%).
- US footballers (60%).
- Soccer players (50%).
- Runners (10–25%).

Proportions depend on the definitions used in the studies and on the intensity of exercise, though contact also clearly plays a part in some sports.

Early cystoscopy in females showed 'kissing' lesions, localized bladder contusions, urothelial loss, from trigone and interureteric bar (Blacklock 1977) leading to theories of bladder 'slapping' being a cause of haematuria in sports. However, the red cells seen in the urine of marathon runners are often dysmorphic, suggesting damage at the glomerular level. The explanation may be hypoxic damage to the nephron or increased filtration pressure (see Proteinuria).

Other causes of haematuria:
- Acute glomerular nephritis.
- Pyelonephritis.
- Acute tubular necrosis.
- UTI.
- Stones.

- Cancer (esp >40 year old).
- Haemoglobinuria or myoglobinuria.
- Spurious.

History may include trauma, pain, fever, dysuria, weight or appetite loss. Examination findings may include renal tenderness, oedema, raised temperature, raised blood pressure, cachexia. If these are not present and there is a clear relationship to exercise, it would be wise to repeat the urinalysis after 48 hours rest. Further investigation to consider if haematuria persists would be microscopy and culture (MCS) of mid stream sample (MSU), intravenous pyelogram (IVP), ultrasound examination of the renal tract and cystoscopy. Clotting studies may be performed to exclude a bleeding disorder and full blood count (FBC) performed to rule out anaemia.

If 'athletic haematuria' is the final diagnosis, the prognosis is good and there is no need to restrict sporting activity. Adequate hydration before and during exercise may help preserve glomerular filtration and keep the bladder reasonably full to prevent 'slapping'.

Haemoglobinuria

The urine may be positive for blood on urinalysis, but red cells are not seen on microscopy. Haemoglobin from the breakdown of red cells is present in the urine. This was described in relation to long marches in the military and in contact sports such as karate. It is generally a benign condition

Myoglobinuria/exercise induced rhabdomyolysis

The presence of myoglobin in the urine indicates the breakdown of muscle, 'rhabdomyolysis'. It has been recorded in both endurance sports, such as marathon running, and in contact sports, such as American football. The urine appears tea or coca-cola coloured. The urinalysis is again positive for blood, but negative for red cells.

Myoglobin is broken down to haematin. Haematin is nephrotoxic and so there have been concerns that athletes with myogloinuria may go into acute renal failure. However, the risk of acute renal failure in association with sport appears to be small. Sinert proposed a nephrotoxic factor was missing in the rhabdomyolysis of sport, unlike medical causes of rhabdomyolysis. Nevertheless, it is probably best to avoid myoglobinuria if possible by adequate hydration, nutrition, and conditioning.

Acute renal failure in sport

Though rare in sport, acute renal failure is associated with exercise to exhaustion in hot conditions. Those who are less fit and those who become dehydrated or hyperpyrexial are at risk. Attempts to prevent should consider adequate hydration, nutrition, exercising in cooler environment, not exercising to exhaustion.

Spurious causes of red urine

Medication (e.g. rifampicin, nitrofurantoin) and diet (e.g. beetroot) give rise to red urine, but urinalysis will be negative.

1 Sinert R, Kohl L, Rainone T, Scalea T (1994). Exercise-induced rhabdomyolysis *Ann Emerg Med*, **23**(6): 1301–6.

Infectious disease

Effects of exercise on immunity

Benefits

Regular, moderate levels of exercise improve resistance to most infections, particularly those affecting the upper respiratory tract (URTI).

Possibly because of mild elevations in:
- T-cell lymphocytes.
- Interleukins.
- Endorphins.

Adverse effects

There is good evidence that athletes undertaking intensive training (e.g. endurance runners covering >90km/week) are more prone to minor infection, particularly URTI. This is thought to be due to reduction of:
- Salivary IgA, which plays an important role in resistance to some viruses.
- IgM.
- Natural killer cells, which show increased activity during exercise, only to fall in the first few hours of recovery.

Supplementation with carbohydrate, vitamin C, glutamine, and zinc may reduce the immuno-suppressive effect of heavy exercise.

Why are athletes prone to infection?

Stress/overtraining/under recovery

Symptoms may include:
- Poor performance.
- Depressed mood.
- Insomnia.
- Frequent URTIs.
- Cervical lymphadenopathy may be present.
- Lowered testosterone levels are sometimes seen.
- Lack of recovery time in training programmes can lead to lowered IgA levels, reducing resistance to viral infection and lowered T and B lymphocytes (cortisol driven).

High level and endurance athletes are particularly at risk of training excessively, due to their competitive nature.

Treatment includes rest and education about the need for increased training recovery time, optimization of nutrition, psychological monitoring and support, and gradual reintroduction of training.

Close contact with other athletes

On tours and in training/competition camps, the inevitable close contact between athletes, coaches, and support staff can encourage the spread of respiratory and gastrointestinal infections.

Sexual activity

Like the population as a whole, athletes are at risk of sexually transmitted diseases if practicing unsafe sex.

Trauma

Traumatic injury can predispose to infection, especially if wounds are open.

Foreign travel

Hepatitis B is endemic in many third world countries, and travelling athletes should be considered for immunization (particularly in contact sports). Travel also carries risk of tropical diseases, such as malaria and diarrhoea.

Upper respiratory tract infections (URTIs)

Although a small proportion of URTIs will be caused by group A streptococcus, most are caused by a virus such as:
- Echovirus.
- Adenovirus.
- Coxsackie viruses A and B.
- Influenza.

Investigations may include a throat swab and a Monospot or Paul-Bunnell test for infectious mononucleosis (glandular fever).

Treatment of URTIs
Analgesia—paracetamol—effective and safe in correct dosage.
Decongestants—nasal sprays can help. Doctors and sports people need to be aware that some decongestants are still on the WADA banned list and, if in doubt, the drug should be checked using the UK sport drug information database. Menthol or eucalyptus inhalants will relieve most symptoms of congestion and are not banned.

Prevention
Team groups especially are at risk of outbreaks of influenza, and vaccination can be offered every winter to the team members and attached staff.

Dangers of URTIs
Coxsackie virus can cause inflammation of heart muscle (myocarditis) in exercising athletes. If a sports person has a combination of the following symptoms, they should be advised not to train or play:
- Resting tachycardia (>10 beats per minute above normal).
- Myalgia.
- Lethargy.
- Oral temperature >38°C.
- Cervical lymphadenopathy.

The athlete should be advised that a premature return to training/playing will delay recovery and that there is a small risk of myocarditis and cardiac arrhythmias.

'Neck check' guidelines for athletes
- If all of your symptoms are above the neck (stuffy or runny nose, sneezing, watery eyes, and/or scratchy throat), it is okay to start your usual workout at about half speed.
- Do NOT work out if you have a fever or symptoms below the neck (aching muscles, a hacking cough which seems to resound deep within your chest, nausea, vomiting, and/or diarrhoea). Working out under those conditions is risky, and you'll recover much faster from your illness if you rest.[1]

---

1 Eichner, E. R (1995). Contagious infections in competitive sports, *Sports Science Exchange*, **8** (3).

Common viral infections

These can be caused by several viruses, particularly

- Epstein–Barr virus (infectious mononucleosis).
- Toxoplasma.
- Cytomegalovirus (CMV).
- Primary HIV disease.

They commonly occur in younger age groups, and are linked to the development of chronic fatigue syndrome. Splenomegaly occurs and participation in contact sports carries a risk of traumatic splenic rupture.

Infectious mononucleosis (IM)

- Spread by intimate close contact.
- Symptoms of sore throat, cervical lymphadenopathy.
- Fatigue—can last 2–6 weeks acutely.
- Maculopapular rash sometimes seen.
- Splenomegaly may be present (confirmed on ultrasound).
- 5% can have significant complications.
- Up to 40% of traumatic splenic rupture linked to IM.
- Paul-Bunnell blood test positive.
- 15%+ atypical lymphocytes on blood film.
- Epstein-Barr virus IgM positive for approximately 2 months.
- Most can return to sport at 4 weeks.
- Gradual reintroduction of exercise as symptoms settle.
- Chronic fatigue (>3 months) is a complication especially if recovery is rushed.

Toxoplasmosis

- Fever.
- Hepatosplenomegaly.
- Generalized lymphadenopathy.
- Picked up from cats' faeces.
- 60% with positive serology have no history of illness.
- Recent infection diagnosed on IgM serology.
- Self-limiting. Return to sport usually in 6 weeks.

Cytomegalovirus

Similar symptoms to toxoplasmosis, but less common.

Lyme disease

- Tick-borne, spirochaete infection (Borrelia).
- Common in spring and summer especially in USA.
- Rash (red rings), malaise, myalgia, arthralgia, headaches.
- Diagnosed on serology
- Treatment with doxycycline or amoxycillin orally.

Viral hepatitis

Hepatitis A

- Oro-faecal spread.
- Relatively common especially in travellers.
- Can be sub-clinical, often in childhood.
- Fever, nausea, abdominal pains.
- Jaundice after 3–7 days.
- Hepatosplenomegaly and lymphadenopathy may be present.
- Abnormal LFTs and Hep A IgM positive 20+ days after exposure. Hep A IgG positive lifelong.
- Effective vaccination recommended.
- Treated symptomatically and full recovery ensues.
- Self-limiting illness. No chronic liver disease after infection.
- Safe to return to sport when clinically better, although some derangement of LFTs may persist.

Hepatitis B

- Endemic in Africa and parts of Asia.
- Spread by blood or sexual contact, IV drug use.
- Highly infectious. Incubation period 30–180 days.
- Clinical features similar to Hep A, but may have associated arthralgia and urticarial.
- Most cases will recover spontaneously.
- 5–10% of sufferers will become carriers with high risk of transmission especially in contact sports, and if diagnosed are excluded from boxing, wrestling, and rugby.
- Abnormal LFTs and Hep Bs antigen positive 1–6 months post infection. Hep Be antigen positive suggests high infectivity.
- Treated symptomatically and require careful follow-up
- Graded return to exercise only when LFTs are back to normal.
- Complications include chronic active hepatitis, cirrhosis and liver failure, and hepatocellular carcinoma.
- Vaccination available and strongly advised for all participants in contact sports.

Hepatitis C

- Often transmitted in blood transfusions or from IV drug abuse. Less infectious than hepatitis B.
- May be asymptomatic at time of infection.
- 85% develop chronic infection.
- High incidence of cirrhosis and also hepatocellular carcinoma.
- Same symptoms as other forms of viral hepatitis.
- No available vaccine.
- Treated with interferon-α.

HIV

- Spread by blood or sexual contact, IV drug abuse.
- No risk from sweat.
- Present in saliva but no reports of spread by this route.
- 100 times less infectious than hepatitis B.
- Initial symptoms are 'flu-like'.
- May then be asymptomatic for months/years.
- Eventually develops into acquired immunodeficiency syndrome (AIDS).
- HIV antibodies found in blood at approximately 12 weeks after exposure and infection.

Note

Risk of transmission of Hepatitis B, C, or HIV during sport is extremely low. The viruses cannot be transmitted via showers or shared drinks bottles. Vaccination against hepatitis B and the following infection control measures help reduce risks even further:

- Wear protective gloves when giving first aid to a bleeding player.
- Wipe any blood from the face or limbs of players.
- Bloodstained towels should not be reused. Put bloodstained clothing in a plastic bag for disposal or laundering.
- Players should not be allowed to continue in the game until bleeding has stopped, and the wound is cleaned and covered.
- If there is concern about cross infection, contact a doctor straight away.

Otitis externa

- Inflammation ± infection in ear canal.
- Common in swimmers and can be very painful.
- Moistness of ear canal predisposes to the condition.
- Pseudomonas often grown on swab.
- Treated with antibiotic ± corticosteroid eardrops, though can sometimes require aural toilet by suction to remove debris in canal.
- Prevention using 70% alcohol drops before and after swimming is best.

Malaria

- 2000 new cases/annum in UK after foreign travel (7 deaths).
- Most cases have failed to take adequate prophylaxis.
- Natural immunity wanes on leaving endemic area.
- Prevention is better than cure.
- Obtain up-to-date anti-malarial drug advice before departure to a high-risk area.
- All travellers to be supplied with and comply with prophylaxis advice.
- Anti-malarial drugs can have adverse reactions and any doctor travelling with a team to a high-risk area should be aware of these.
- Advise all competitors and staff to wear long sleeves and trousers in the evening and use DEET mosquito repellents.
- Symptoms can present up to 12 months after return from high-risk area, and should always be considered in cases of pyrexia of unknown origin.

Diarrhoea

Diarrhoea of infectious origin is a major cause of morbidity in sports people who travel the world to compete. These athletes are as much at risk of the development of travellers' diarrhoea as the general population.

Symptoms of travellers' diarrhoea:
- Are defined as passing three or more unformed stools over 24 hours, during or shortly after, a period of travel.
- Can be accompanied by fever.
- Can be very disruptive to training and competition, on average lasting 4 days.

High-risk destinations for diarrhoeal illness include most of Asia, Africa and South America.

In most cases, no pathogen is found and possible causes include:
- Change in diet/fluid intake.
- *E. coli* (commonest bacterial pathogen).
- Rotaviruses.
- *Salmonella* and *Campylobacter*.
- *Shigella*.
- *Giardia* and *Entamoeba*.

Advice for sufferers
- Usually no treatment is required.
- Maintain fluid and electrolyte balance with a replacement drink.
- Stick to simple starchy foods.
- Seek medical advice if diarrhoea is bloody, accompanied by fever, or lasts more than 14 days.

Advice to travellers to prevent diarrhoea
- Wash hands after going to toilet/before eating or handling food.
- Drink only sealed bottled water or boil your own.
- Avoid ice in drinks.
- Avoid salads and cold vegetables.
- Peel all fruits if uncooked.
- Avoid shellfish—seawater may be contaminated by sewage.
- Eat only hot, well-cooked food. Avoid any food that has been kept warm or food from street vendors.

Investigation of diarrhoea
Anyone who suffers from chronic diarrhoea will need investigation to rule out other medical causes such as:
- Infection/food poisoning.
- Inflammatory bowel disease.
- Food intolerances (e.g. gluten or lactose).
- Cancer.
- Irritable bowel syndrome.

History and examination are particularly important.

Initial simple investigations will include:
- Stool microscopy and culture (evidence of infection).
- FBC (check for anaemia and abnormal MCV).
- Vitamin B12/folate and ferritin levels to look for evidence of malabsorption.
- U & E (low K^+).
- CRP/ESR (Inflammation/infection/cancer).
- Anti-endomysial antibodies (suggestive of gluten enteropathy).

Pharmacotherapy

- *Loperamide* can reduce stool frequency and ease stomach cramps in cases of diarrhoea.
- *Codeine* is a narcotic analgesic but is no longer on the WADA list of banned substances. It is a very effective analgesic and anti-diarrhoeal agent but may cause drowsiness.
- *Alverine citrate* is a useful additional treatment in the presence of bloating and cramping symptoms.
- The vast majority do not require antibiotic therapy, but *Ciprofloxacin* 500mg as a single dose has been shown to reduce duration of illness (NB this drug has been linked to the tendinopathies and should be used with caution in sports people). *Trimethoprim* is an alternative.
- *Probiotics*, which contain viable microorganisms, are sometimes taken prophylactically and also to treat diarrhoeal illness. Their mechanism of action is unclear, but their use may reduce the length of acute diarrhoea. The widespread use of probiotics is not advocated at present, but travelling sports persons commonly use them, and they appear to have few side effects.

Tip for doctors travelling to high-risk areas

A useful preventative tip:

In many high-risk countries, river water is used on playing fields and after playing/training, players or competitors should be instructed to wash hands thoroughly before eating. Alcohol-based gel is very useful as a readily available hand sterilizer in the absence of clean running water.

Arithritis

Osteoarthritis (OA)

The term osteoarthritis (OA) refers to a heterogenous group of conditions with similar pathological and clinical features. Osteoarthritis is the most common cause of disability amongst adult populations and exists radiographically in more than 80% of those aged over 75. The association between exercise and osteoarthritis starts with the well documented association between osteoarthritis and joint injury and ends with the evidence that patients with osteoarthritis benefit from exercise therapy.

Definition

Historically arthritic disorders were divided into atrophic and hypertrophic disorders. The hypertrophic group are synonymous with what we think of as osteoarthritis, the atrophic disorders referring to inflammatory arthropathies.

The American College of Rheumatology defines OA as a 'heterogenous group of conditions that lead to joint symptoms and signs which are associated with defective integrity of articular cartilage, in addition to related changes in the underlying bone at the joint margins. In simple terms OA can be thought of as representing age-related joint changes that reflect joint insult or injury. In essence the clinical and pathological consequences of OA are caused by attempted (possibly failed) repair following joint failure (injury).

Prevalence

Hand OA occurs most frequently (75% of women aged 60–70 years). Knee OA occurs in 30% of those over 75, and like hand OA is more common in females with female:male ratios between 1.5 and 4. Although not as common as hand OA it is the most significant cause of disability in elderly populations. Hip OA is least common of the 'big three' and probably occurs equally in men and women, although some studies do suggest a male excess.

Pathogenesis

The aetiology of OA remains obscure, however, it is likely that a combination of local and systemic risk factors are responsible for the structural features and that these, certainly as far as symptom reporting is concerned, are variably influenced by central neurological factors. The importance of individual risk factors on the risk of developing OA will vary from individual to individual and from joint to joint and will partly reflect the interaction between risk factors e.g. meniscectomy is a well known local risk factor for knee OA, but is more likely in those with generalized OA.

Local risk factors

The most important individual local risk factor is joint injury, which may occur in a number of ways including:

- Joint fracture.
- Chondral fracture.
- Ligament tear e.g. cruciate.
- Meniscal injury.
- Developmental injury e.g. slipped femoral epiphysis.

The most prevalent example of trauma causing OA is the relationship between knee OA, cruciate ligament rupture, and meniscal tear. The risk increases with advanced age, time since injury, and any background hereditary predisposition.

In global terms however, altered joint biomechanics play an important role and repetitive 'micro-injury' may be a result of a number of factors which may or may not be a consequence of traumatic injury:
- Joint laxity.
- Joint malalignment.
- Muscle weakness.
- Joint shape e.g. dysplastic developmental abnormalities.

Joint shape
The shape of the hip and knee joint predispose to OA. The most obvious example in is someone with developmental abnormalities e.g. Perthes' disease, slipped femoral epiphysis, or joint dysplasia (e.g. acetabular) predisposing to hip OA. It is probable that some normal variants of joint development contribute to the risk of OA. Premature hip OA in runners may be associated with the so called 'bullet' shaped appearance of the femoral head.

Systemic risk factors
A number of constitutional or generalized risk factors may predispose to OA. The most important of these in impact terms is probably heritability, however, in terms of reversibility the lifestyle and environmental factors listed below achieve greater importance.

Heritability
Strong heritability has been demonstrated for OA of the hand, knee, hip, and spine. This susceptibility likely results from multiple unidentified genes, however, individual genetic abnormalities may cause OA—e.g. abnormalities of the Col2A1 gene predispose to premature widespread OA.

Age
Stating the obvious, but age is clearly an important risk factor for OA, the older you are the more likely you are to have osteoarthritis joints.

Obesity
Obesity is associated with knee OA, there is still debate about its association with hip and hand OA. There appears to be a linear relationship between BMI and the risk of knee OA. Further, the prognosis of knee OA, once developed, is worse in patients with a higher BMI.

Gender
OA affecting the hand and knee is more prevalent in females, although the exact explanation for this has yet to be confirmed. It has been suggested that female sex hormones modify chondrocyte function.

Occupation

Repetitive activity in work has been shown to increase the risk of OA. Examples of this are:

- Increased OA in the dominant or non-paretic hand.
- Knee OA in manual workers, especially those whose work requires prolonged kneeling or squatting. Knee OA has been approved for industrial compensation in coal miners.
- Hip OA in agricultural workers, possibly related to heavy lifting and walking on uneven ground. Again industrial compensation has been approved.

Exercise and sport

Joint movement is essential for normal joint health. There is no evidence that exercise is damaging to a healthy joint. However, as previously discussed, significant injury to a joint e.g. meniscal tear, which may have been sustained through exercise, does predispose that joint to premature osteoarthritis. Exercise, and in particular excessive loading of a damaged joint, almost certainly does further increase the risk of osteoarthritis, although what constitutes excessive loading is unknown. Debate also exists as to whether subtle alterations to biomechanics when exposed to excessive loading, as might be seen in endurance runners, predisposes to OA. Even if a certain form of exercise does predispose a susceptible individual to OA, the well documented benefits of exercise would have to be considered against any perceived risk.

Hypermobility

Hypermobility is found in normal healthy populations as well as being a feature of certain inherited conditions e.g. Ehlers-Danlos. It is uncertain to what effect joint mobility has on the risk of OA.

Bone density

High bone density, while helpful in reducing fracture risk, is associated with OA at the hip and knee.

Smoking

Smoking seems to have a protective effect, not that anyone would advocate this as a preventative strategy.

Systemic illness

In addition to the above factors, a number of systemic conditions are associated with OA e.g.:

- Haemochromatosis—iron overload. Worth checking ferritin levels in younger individuals with OA especially if associated with calcium pyrophosphate deposition (chondro-calcinosis).
- Acromegaly.
- Ochronosis.

History

The typical features of any joint pathology; pain, stiffness, swelling, and loss of function, hold true for OA. In addition, patients frequently complain of instability and crepitus.

Pain

Pain is the most important symptom of OA. Typically pain is activity-related but with variations on a weekly if not daily basis. The nature and severity of pain is poorly correlated with radiographic features of OA but is associated with female gender, evidence of psychological distress, and affected joint; patients are most likely to complain of hip pain and least likely to complain of hand pain for any given severity of X-ray change. Rest and night pain is usually indicative of more severe OA.

OA joint pain is multifactorial and may be influenced by the following physical factors in addition to the psychological factors:
- Altered biomechanics due to structural change e.g. osteophytes.
- Bone pain possibly related to raised intraosseous pressure.
- Synovitis; mild synovitis is common. Occasionally patients will present with severe flares of pain related to significant inflammation—sometimes related to the presence of calcium pyrophosphate crystals (pseudogout).
- Secondary pain from other structures e.g. bursitis, tendinopathy.
- Referred muscular pain, usually involving muscles directly responsible for joint movement.

Examination

The osteoarthritic joint will vary in its appearance depending on the severity. You should assess the joint for the following generic signs:
- Functional movement patterns e.g. gait.
- Appearance (standing and at rest):
  - Deformity.
  - Wasting.
  - Swelling (bony and soft tissue/joint effusion).
  - Scars.
- Active and passive ROM:
  - Pain.
  - Tenderness.
  - Crepitus.
- Palpation. Palpation may be least useful, however, it does help identify those patients with generalized tenderness rather than specific joint tenderness. The former usually have a functional element to their symptoms with evidence of psychological distress.
- Related joints. You will have been taught to examine the joints above and below the painful joint because of the tendency for joint pain to refer—e.g. it is not uncommon for hip OA to present with knee pain. Referred pain is not always as simple as joint above and below, and further you should look for evidence of a more generalized arthropathy.
- Assess joint function e.g. gait for lower limb joints, manual function for hand joints.

Hand osteoarthritis

- More common in women.
- Peak incidence in middle age.
- Predominantly affects DIPJ and 1st CMC joint (base of thumb).
- DIP involvement thought to be attributable to stress through these joints. CMC involvement due to ligament (and thereby joint) instability.
- MCP joint involvement unusual. If present consider traumatic cause e.g. previous fracture.
- Involvement of 2nd and 3rd MCPJs (usually symmetrically) a feature of chondrocalcinosis, consider haemachromatosis.

Knee osteoarthritis

Knee OA commonly affects athletes (or ex-athletes) because of its association with joint injury.

- Three major joint compartments, which can alone or in combination, be affected by OA (medial and lateral tibiofemoral and patellofemoral).
- Strongly associated with previous injury to cruciates or menisci.
- Medial compartment takes greatest load during activity. In flexion patellofemoral joint may take over twice the load of tibiofemoral joint. Medial tibial plateau and lateral patella facet therefore most frequently involved.
- Medial OA causes varus (bow) deformity while lateral causes valgus (knock) knee deformity. Deformity increases asymmetrical load thereby accelerating OA process.
- Complex relationship between knee pain and radiological evidence of OA with psychosocial factors playing an important role.
- Acute effusions may develop and are associated with severe pain. Sometimes these acute flares are triggered by chondrocalcinosis.
- When pain increases acutely consider osteonecrosis.

Hip osteoarthritis

A frequent new presentation of osteoarthritis to a sports medicine clinic. In particular, younger patients complaining of groin pain with markedly restricted hip movement whose X-rays have confirmed premature OA.

- Three different patterns described; superior pole (commonest), medial pole, and concentric (affects whole joint uniformly and more frequently associated with generalized OA).
- Not usually associated with OA in other joints.
- Usually presents as groin pain but referral to the thigh and knee not uncommon.
- Usually develops slowly and may even show spontaneous improvement.
- Rapid clinical deterioration either from onset of first symptoms or after years of clinical stability not uncommon.
- May be complicated by osteonecrosis (bone collapse), which presents as sudden deterioration.

Nodal osteoarthritis

- Hereditary variant strongly associated with women.
- Presents in middle age.

- Characterized by extensive involvement of DIPJ and PIPJ with Heberden's (DIP) and Bouchard's (PIP) nodes.
- Associated with knee OA.
- Joint erosions may be seen in affected joints. Bone characteristically shows hypertrophic change on X-ray (osteophytes), which help differentiate from inflammatory arthritis.

Spine

Spinal degenerative change is common on X-ray and usually bears no relationship to patients reporting to back pain. Osteoarthritis affects the spinal apophyseal (facet) joints and is associated with disc degeneration. C5 and L3–5 most frequently affected. In some patients OA changes are sufficient to cause pressure on the spinal cord (spinal stenosis) or exiting nerve roots.

Other joints

It is possible for any joint to be affected by osteoarthritis. Involvement of other joints e.g. shoulder, elbow, temperomandibular joint is usually a reflection of local factors altering biomechanical stress on the index joint e.g. previous joint injury, abnormal development, avascular necrosis.

Non-osteoarthritic joint pain

Not all joint pain is due to 'wear and tear' yet there is an increasing tendency for doctors to apportion this non-diagnosis to musculoskeletal symptoms that elude an immediate diagnosis. A term like undifferentiated joint pain may be more appropriate. Most people accept that the majority of headaches do not have a pathological or diagnostic explanation, so why not joint pain.

- Osteoarthritis does not cause red flag symptoms and, if these develop in a patient with OA, consider an alternative explanation for a patient's symptoms and investigate appropriately.
- It is increasingly common to see patients with generalized non-inflammatory musculoskeletal pain. While OA may be a contributing factor, such symptoms reflect a tendency to chronic pain and psychological distress. Patients should be advised and managed accordingly.

Radiological features

The radiological assessment of OA is usually confined to X-ray examination. Rarely is there a requirement to proceed to ultrasound, MRI, CT, or isotope imaging unless an alternative diagnosis is being considered. Osteoarthritis is characterized by the following features seen on plain X-ray.

- Normal mineralization.
- Non-uniform joint space narrowing.
- Osteophyte formation.
- Subchondral new bone formation (sclerosis).
- Cyst formation.
- Abnormal bone contour.
- Absence of erosions (although OA of the DIPJ and PIPJ can be associated with joint erosion).
- Joint subluxation.

Practical points

- Ask yourself whether an X-ray will alter your management. X-rays expose a patient to a small amount of radiation and are associated with a cost in terms of time (patient and health care professional) and resources.
- It is important to appreciate that a radiology report is only as good as the clinical information provided.
- Always try to review X-rays that you have requested, although I appreciate this is not straightforward for those working outside of a hospital setting.
- Treat your patients and not their X-rays. Severe knee pain, normal knee movement, and a normal X-ray may be a hip problem.
- Request the correct X-ray and consider function.
  - In the patient described above perhaps if the patient had been properly examined an unnecessary knee X-ray would have been avoided, a hip X-ray requested, and the diagnosis confirmed.
  - There is little point in carrying out non-weight bearing knee X-rays in the context of OA. We don't walk lying down, non-weight bearing films give false reassurance of joint space.

OA: management

The standard response to 'how do you manage OA' is painkillers, and if they don't work, refer to an orthopaedic surgeon. Fortunately for the health care professional with the time, and the patient with the motivation there is considerably more that can be advised to assist the OA sufferer.

The management of the individual patient with OA will clearly depend on a number of variables, including joints affected, functional impact of OA, and patient co-morbidity. Generic treatment principles may be tailored to an individual. Treatment strategies are non-pharmacological, local pharmacological, systemic pharmacological, and surgical.

Non-pharmacological

Education

Patient education is essential.
  Confirm diagnosis:
- Emphasize self-management approach.
- Reassure patient that being active is a good thing.
- Reassure patient that pain is not an indicator of doing harm.
- Do not avoid the thorny issue of weight management. It is vital that your patient is fully aware that being overweight will have a negative impact on their OA.
- Discuss breadth of treatment options.

Weight management

Irrespective of how 'badly' you think your patient will respond to a discussion on weight management, you are doing them a disservice by not drawing their attention to the need to loose weight. You must be supportive and empathetic, it is difficult to break out of the overweight, joints hurt, don't exercise, comfort eat, gain weight vicious circle. Exercise physicians have a considerable role to play in advising on the role of exercise to help manage a weight problem, and there is no better place to start than with your overweight OA sufferer.

Joint rehabilitation

The OA joint should be viewed as a dysfunctional unit in which one or more of the components has failed. In simple terms you have a 2 pronged approach, reduce the stress on the joint e.g. weight management, footwear modification, or increase the capacity of the joint to withstand that stress. Joint rehabilitation to try and restore more normal joint function or to ensure that other structures e.g. muscles are more able to compensate for OA changes, is central to OA management. Basic rehabilitation principles should be followed with, if possible, an achievable functional outcome that is patient-centred.

Exercise

You should differentiate between exercise aimed at joint rehabilitation and general aerobic exercise. Aerobic exercise aims to improve overall fitness and may well have a positive affect on self-esteem, psychological wellbeing, and thereby symptoms. In addition, exercise will help with weight management. Exercise prescription for OA follows generic principles, most important of which is that it must be tailored to the individual.

Footwear

The ground reaction forces going through the lower limb during walking are considerable, as much as 4 times body weight on walking alone. Patients should be encouraged to wear shoes with good shock absorbing properties. Ideally shoes should also have a flat sole (particularly for knee and hip OA). You will not win the battle over fashion shoes but most patients accept the logic of 'sensible' shoes for long-term use and fashion footwear for restricted use at appropriate times.

Orthotics

Orthotics may offer a number of benefits for the patient with OA:
- Shock absorbing insoles may be helpful in improving the comfort of shoes without a specialized insole.
- Heel wedges can be useful in counteracting the effects of either a varus or valgus deformity in knee OA.
- Patients with OA have impaired proprioception and feelings of instability, which might be improved by the use of orthotics.

Aids to daily living

A walking aid (usually a more acceptable term to patients than walking stick) will reduce lower limb joint loading, improve balance and stability, and perhaps most importantly restore confidence. For patients with severe OA, a walking aid can enable modest levels of daily living activity, which would otherwise be impossible. For patients with mild OA who wish to remain active then walking poles are a convenient way of increasing walking exercise capacity particularly where slopes are concerned. An essential part of the ramblers kit.

Some patients find knee braces helpful, particularly if stability is a concern.

Diet

Diet is frequently mentioned by patients. A well balanced diet should provide all the essential nutrients and is sufficient to ensure an ideal weight is maintained. Some patients swear by supplements e.g. cod liver oil, or green lip mussel extract, although there is little evidence of effectiveness.

Acupuncture

Acupuncture undoubtedly helps some patients and may be useful if pain control is proving problematic.

Miscellaneous

Standard 'first aid' approaches with a RICES regimen will help in certain situations. Cooling will certainly help an inflamed joint. Heat will help with joint or muscular stiffness e.g. wax treatment, wheat bag (great for troublesome neck pain).

Relaxtion techniques and similar modalities can prove useful for some patients.

Local pharmacological

Topical NSAIDs

Topical NSAIDs are on the whole safe and well tolerated, and do help some patients.

Capsaicin

Capsaicin is the active ingredient in chilli peppers. It is thought to work as a painkiller by depleting substance P. It has been shown to be effective in patients with knee OA. Patients must be advised that it will sting initially but if used regularly this will resolve. It is very irritant to the eye and care must be taken to wash hands thoroughly after application.

Intraarticular steroid

Corticosteroid injections have their place. They appear to work best for:
- The inflamed OA knee where there is a definite effusion (depomedrone 80mg or triamcinolone 40mg). A joint effusion has a significant negative impact on muscle function and aspiration/injection prior to rehabilitation can prove very useful.
- The massive knee effusion; when a combination of joint aspiration and steroid injection can have a dramatic effect.
- The patient with severe OA of the thumb base (1st carpometacarpal joint). Surgery (trapeziectomy) also offers good results and should be considered in patients requiring repeated injections.

Intrarticular hyaluronic acid

Hyaluronate has been shown to improve symptomatic knee OA. Hyaluronate injections are increasingly used for OA in other joints, however, although anecdotal reports seem favorable, there is no published evidence of their use. A number of different hyaluronic acid preparations exist with varying molecular weights and there is debate about the influence of patient selection and preparation. Most treatments require between 3–5 injections on a weekly basis. The current balance of opinion seems to favour high molecular weight preparations in patients with early to moderate knee OA.

Systemic pharmacological

Pain is generally unpleasant and is associated with negative emotions. Occasional pain e.g. a headache, can be perfectly well treated by occasional painkillers. Patients with regular pain, of which OA is a good example, should anticipate their pain rather than playing catch up. Encourage patients to take regular analgesia to control their pain.

Glucosamine

Glucosamine has been shown to provide patients with knee OA some symptomatic benefit, whether it provides a slowing of the disease process is yet to be proven. The 'therapeutic dose' is 1500mg daily, which is usually greater than is available in OTC preparations. Chondroitin sulphate has also been shown to reduce OA pain and is available with glucosamine as a combination preparation.

Paracetamol

An excellent analgesic but underutilized because it is available OTC. Patients with regular OA pain should be encouraged to take paracetamol regularly up to 1g QID daily. If necessary regular paracetamol can be topped up as required by the use of the following.

Compound analgesia

This term encompasses the wide range of drugs which contain varied combinations of weak opiate based drugs e.g. codeine phosphate and paracetamol. These preparations add little in terms of analgesia to paracetamol alone and can be associated with problematic side-effects.

Opiate analgesia

There are a wide range of opiate based analgesics some of which are used in the treatment of OA e.g. the mid range opiates. Opiate patch technology has advanced in recent years on the basis that they offer the analgesic properties of stronger opioids without the side effects. Low dose patches are now available and are being aimed at the OA market. It is too early to advise on their role.

NSAIDs

If alternative analgesics have been tried then NSAIDs offer the next stage in analgesia. The clinician and patient need to weigh up the relative balance between the benefits and side effects of NSAIDs. Use the lowest dose required, ideally supplementing PRN NSAIDs with regular simple oral analgesia to minimize NSAID requirements. Gastroprotection should be considered in at risk patients. The cardiovascular risks need to be balanced against the potential benefits. In patients requiring chronic NSAIDs an annual FBC and U&E is approrpriate.

DMARDs

The role of disease-modifying drugs in the management of inflammatory arthritis is well established. These drugs have been used in managing patients with OA where there appears to be a significant inflammatory component e.g. nodal/erosive OA. Specific disease-modifying osteoarthritis drugs are in development. They aim to inhibit cartilage breakdown. None has been shown to have a clear benefit in human OA.

Surgical

A variety of surgical approaches are utilized in managing the osteoarthritic joint including arthroscopic washout/debridement, soft tissue procedures, arthroplasty, and arthrodesis. While the success of well-established joint replacement operations e.g. knee and hip is not in doubt, recent evidence suggests that arthroscopic washout/debridement of the knee was no more beneficial than sham procedures. The potential for chondrocyte transplantation remains under investigation in specialized centres.

The surgical approach will depend on the joint concerned and a number of patient specific factors.

Inflammatory arthritis

Athletes frequently present with joint pain, usually attributed to musculoskeletal trauma, but joint inflammation should not be discounted, particularly as management will have to be modified accordingly. A careful history and examination will help the sports physician identify those patients who require referral to a rheumatologist for a second opinion.

Arthritis is simply joint inflammation but, to avoid any confusion with osteoarthritis, the term inflammatory arthritis is used. Inflammatory arthritis may present acutely, acute on chronically, or chronically. Joint inflammation is characterized by:

• Pain
• Swelling
• Heat
• Redness/erythema
• Loss of function.

In addition joint inflammation is usually associated with:

• Prolonged early morning stiffness
• Inactivity stiffness.

History

Most clinicians focus on the musculoskeletal features of inflammatory arthritis, but conditions associated with inflammatory arthritis may have systemic features and therefore a full history is necessary. In particular the following will help in establishing your differential diagnosis:

• Pattern of joint involvement.
• Spinal involvement.
• Red flag signs:
  • Constitutional symptoms (fever, weight loss, night sweats).
  • History of malignancy.
  • Neurological symptoms, in particular bladder and bowel dysfunction.
  • Extremes of age (<16, >65).
• Pre-existing connective tissue disease (CTD).
• Evidence of recent infection, in particular streptococcal infection, infectious gastroenteritis, and sexually acquired infection.
• History of established inflammatory bowel disease (IBD) or symptoms suggestive of IBD.
  • Diarrhoea, rectal bleeding, rectal mucus, abdominal pain, weight loss.
• Psoriasis or 1st degree family history of psoriasis.
• Ocular inflammation.
• Family history of inflammatory arthritis or CTD.

Examination

A good history will direct your examination.

• Pain may be referred.
• The importance of the kinetic chain—the presenting symptom may not be the problem.

- Exercising patients frequently justify musculoskeletal symptoms by recounting an injury.
- The inflammation of inflammatory arthritis is not confined to the intra-articular space, all components of the joint including capsule and bone are involved. Inflammation may be present at the enthesis or within the tendon sheath.
- Systemic features may not be appreciated by the patient e.g. a patient may not be aware they have psoriasis or a sexually acquired infection.
- Inflammatory symptoms fluctuate, asking a patient to provide photographic evidence of joint swelling is frequently helpful.
- Pain is not a good indicator of inflammatory symptoms. A number of chronic pain disorders present with joint pain, the key is usually the presence of definite joint swelling or a proven inflammatory response.

As with the history a thorough examination is usually required given the systemic nature of inflammatory arthritis and CTD.

Investigations

Investigations help in establishing the correct diagnosis, although may require specialist interpretation.

Blood tests

FBC

Joint inflammation may produce an anaemia of chronic disease and a thrombocytosis. This gives some measure of chronicity. Several CTDs are associated with leucopenia, neutropenia, lymphopenia, or thrombo-cytopenia.

ESR

The erythrocyte sedimentation rate is useful as a non-specific indicator of inflammation.

CRP

The C-Reactive protein is an acute phase protein produced by the liver and is a non-specific indicator of inflammation. It is very sensitive to change and will reflect improvement or deterioration more responsively then the ESR.

ESR and CRP are particularly useful in patients with few clinical signs, but the following should be considered when interpreting acute phase markers:

- The ESR normally increases with age.
- An elevated ESR may be seen in patients without inflammatory disease.
- Most patients with inflammatory arthritis will have a raised ESR or CRP, although normal results do not exclude inflammation.
- A single inflamed large joint will affect the ESR and CRP to a far greater degree than 10 inflamed small (e.g. metacarpophalangeal, MCP) joints and therefore, the ESR and CRP are not always indicative of severity.
- A raised ESR and normal CRP may be suggestive of a connective tissue disorder e.g. lupus.

Routine biochemistry

Renal, liver, and thyroid function are all worth checking to exclude conditions that may present with musculoskeletal pain, and prior to starting medication that might affect organ function.

Bone biochemistry

Calcium, alkaline phosphatase (usually included with LFTs), and vitamin D levels are useful in more non-specific musculoskeletal pain. Hypovitaminosis D is increasingly being diagnosed in elderly populations.

Blood cultures

If septic arthritis is suspected, blood cultures are mandatory. They may be positive in 30% of cases.

Creatinine phosphokinase (CPK)

A metabolic or inflammatory myopathy may present with symptoms of inflammatory arthritis. A raised CPK is associated with exercise and elevated levels must be considered in the light of a patients exercise history.

Immunoglobulins (urine for Bence–Jones protein)

Multiple myeloma may present with features of inflammatory arthritis. A polyclonal increase in immunoglobulins is invariably seen in inflammatory arthritis.

Bacterial and viral titres

Reactive arthritis is common. If there is a history of infection then objective evidence of recent infection is useful.

Uric acid

Uric acid levels have poor sensitivity and specificity for gout, and therefore neither confirm nor exclude the diagnosis. However, if gout is confirmed on analysis of synovial fluid, serum uric acid level may help with treatment and its monitoring.

Ferritin

Haemochromatosis may present with acute arthritis related to calcium pyrophosphate crystals (pseudogout). Untreated haemochromatosis is associated with systemic complications including diabetes, hepatic, and cardiac dysfunction and has an autosomal recessive inheritance pattern. Detection is therefore important for the patient and their family.

Autoantibody profile

Autoantibodies have poor specificity and/or sensitivity and therefore there are many patients who will have false negative or positive results. The diagnosis of inflammatory arthritis or connective tissue disease is a clinical one. Autoantibodies only become important in a patient with an appropriate history and examination, but a patient with a definite clinical diagnosis may have negative autoantibody tests.

Radiology

Imaging is an important extension to musculoskeletal examination but never replaces careful examination.

Plain X-rays

Plain musculoskeletal X-rays have traditionally been the first line investigation for a patient with suspected inflammatory arthritis although, with alternative imaging techniques, especially ultrasound and MRI, one could reasonably ask if that should still be the case. If access to MRI and ultrasound were responsive and affordable there are relatively few clinical situations when a plain X-ray would be requested.

The decision to image a potentially inflamed joint is made for the following reasons:
- To exclude serious pathology which may mimic inflammatory arthritis e.g. infection, tumour, or fracture.
- To assess the 'health' of the joint in question and the degree of joint inflammation or damage.
- To identify the differing radiological features of inflammatory arthritis which might help with confirming a diagnosis.
- To reassure the patient, or doctor.

MRI and ultrasound will answer most of these questions and will frequently provide far more information than is available on plain X-ray. However, until MRI and ultrasound is widely available, plain X-rays remain the first line investigation.

Ultrasound

Ultrasound is increasingly used to establish a diagnosis, to direct treatment, and to monitor response to treatment. Ultrasound is far more sensitive to articular cartilage and bone damage than X-ray, and will reveal joint erosions before changes are seen on plain films. This is increasingly useful in the assessment and monitoring of drug treatment. Ultrasound is also useful in assessing inflammation in other synovial lined structures e.g. bursae and tendon sheaths.

MRI

MRI is useful to establish the extent of synovitis and involvement of soft tissue structures e.g. tendons, enthesis, bursa, capsule, and muscle. MRI is also very helpful if tumour or infection is considered, and the location of pathology is known. Like ultrasound, MRI is far more sensitive for articular cartilage and bone damage than X-ray.

Isotope bonescan

Bone scintigraphy is useful if you are unsure where a patients pathology (inflammation, tumour, or infection) is located and the potential area concerned is too large to allow straightforward MRI examination e.g. in patients with pelvic pain, or if multifocal inflammation, tumour, or infection is suspected. In either case you may need to proceed to focused investigation with MRI once the site of pathology has been established.

Bone scintigraphy is also helpful if you wish to exclude significant musculoskeletal inflammation in patients without clear symptoms or signs.

CT

Musculoskeletal CTs are rarely helpful in the assessment of patients with inflammatory arthritis.

Dual energy X-ray absorptiometry (DEXA)

Osteoporosis is a complication of arthritis and its treatment, especially systemic steroids. There are several ways in which bone density can be assessed, although the most validated method in terms of establishing fracture risk is DEXA.

Multi-system examination

Inflammatory arthritides and connective tissue diseases are systemic conditions that will therefore require systemic assessment. A number of radiological techniques may assist in this process.

Synovial fluid analysis

Normal synovial fluid has a very pale yellow hue, is transparent, and has a normal viscosity. Progressive levels of inflammation are associated with increasing levels of cellularity with increasing turbidity, (increasingly yellow with loss of clarity) and loss of normal viscosity. Inflammatory arthritis is usually associated with a deeper yellow colour and some clarity, whereas pus, the hallmark of septic arthritis, is thick, a deep mucky yellow with no transparency. Unfortunately the appearances of synovial fluid from non-infectious synovitis, particularly that associated with crystal arthritis, can be identical to septic arthritis and some forms of infectious synovitis (e.g. tuberculous) which are associated with a minimal cellular response.

The presence of blood is usually due to the leaking of erythrocytes as part of the inflammatory response within inflamed synovial fluid, or a traumatic aspiration, rather than reflecting a bleed into a joint (haemarthrosis). A haemarthrosis is usually a sign of trauma, although consider a bleeding diathesis, over-anticoagulation and minor trauma to intensely vascular synovial hypertrophy e.g. pigmented villo-nodular synovitis.

Microbiological analysis is essential if septic arthritis is considered. A septic joint is not always obvious clinically, and given the consequences to the joint (irreversible joint destruction) of failing to make a diagnosis, send synovial fluid for analysis. This should be done prior to giving antibiotics and be followed by intravenous antibiotics (to cover likely pathogens) until culture results are available. Histological analysis of synovial fluid can be extremely helpful in specialist hands.

Monosodium urate and calcium pyrophosphate crystals in synovial fluid is diagnostic for gout and pseudogout respectively. Urate crystals are usually very obvious (rod shaped strongly negatively birefringant), and their absence almost certainly means the diagnosis is not gout. Calcium pyrophosphate crystals are very difficult to see even in experienced hands.

The acute hot joint

An athlete may present with acute joint inflammation to a team or squad physician. The differential diagnosis includes almost every condition capable of causing synovitis, however, there are a number of simple rules, which will help with your immediate management.

Septic arthritis is a diagnosis of exclusion

- Although septic arthritis is unusual in an otherwise healthy young athlete, the consequences of delaying a diagnosis are catastrophic to the joint and therefore the patient.

History

- Symptoms/signs of localized infection e.g. skin injury or excoriating rash, foreign body injury e.g. urchin spines, wood splinters.
- Symptoms/signs of systemic infection that might cause a bacteraemia or reactive arthritis e.g. URTI, chest, urogenital, gastro-intestinal.
- Constitutional symptoms e.g. weight loss, fever, night sweats.
- PMH of arthritis, psoriasis, systemic inflammation e.g. eyes, bowels.
- FH of arthritis, psoriasis.
- A history of trauma is clearly important but beware the patient who tries to justify acute joint pain and swelling with a history of what sounds like minor trauma.

Examination

- Clinical examination of the joint will rarely add useful information over and above confirming that your patient has an inflamed joint. The degree of inflammation is not a good discriminator of infectious and non-infectious causes. In particular it is impossible clinically to differentiate septic arthritis and gout.
- Systemic examination to look for more generalized signs of infection or systemic illness.

Investigations

- Septic arthritis must be excluded and, unless certain on clinical grounds that a patient does not have septic arthritis, the joint must be aspirated, and a synovial fluid sample sent urgently to a microbiology department for microscopy, culture, and sensitivity. Atypical myobacterial infections may present in this way and you should request mycobacterial cultures.
- An FBC, ESR, and CRP are useful, although they will not always discriminate between septic arthritis and inflammatory synovitis.
- Blood cultures will be positive in about 30% of cases of septic arthritis, even when synovial fluid cultures are negative.
- An acutely inflamed joint in a patient without a history of inflammatory arthritis should be X-rayed.

Immediate management

- If septic arthritis is a possibility then, after synovial fluid aspiration, give high dose intravenous antibiotics until culture results are known. In a non-hospitalized patient who is otherwise well *Staphyloccus* and *Streptococcus* are the most likely infecting organisms and your antibiotic regime should reflect this. (Penicillin V with or without flucloxacillin or a 3rd generation cephalosporin. Erythromycin is a reasonable choice for penicillin sensitive patients.)
- Patients with suspected septic arthritis require hospitalization and specialist review.
- If septic arthritis is highly unlikely or has been excluded then aspirate to reduce intra-articular pressure and at the same time inject the joint with steroid (a TUE required).
- NSAIDs are usually helpful.
- Oral steroids maybe helpful where rapid resolution is desirable, however, this decision should only be reached after discussion with a rheumatologist, and will require the completion of a TUE in a competitive athlete.
- Most cases of monoarthritis should be discussed with a rheumatologist, and certainly in someone whose occupation depends on normal joint function a specialist opinion should be sought.
- Most cases of monoarthritis are iatrogenic, and a good proportion (up to 30% of reactive arthritis) become chronic requiring long-term rheumatological care.

Inflammatory arthritis: management

Inflammatory arthritis is a descriptive term rather than a diagnosis, although sometimes the expression undifferentiated inflammatory arthritis will be used in the absence of clear diagnostic criteria. Many diseases may cause or be associated with an inflammatory arthritis.

Inflammatory arthritis—generic principles

The underlying principle of managing synovitis is that joint inflammation causes irreversible joint damage, which causes disability and handicap.

- An athlete's sport must be considered as their occupation. Whatever the occupation/sport, an individual who aspires to high-level performance will become disabled much earlier than an individual whose physical requirements are less demanding. A professional tennis player with knee synovitis is potentially no different to a self-employed builder. On any given day both individuals may be equally affected by their condition.
- The important difference between the tennis player and the builder rests with the relative importance of that days employment.
  - For the tennis player that day maybe the final of a major tournament, whereas for the builder at worst it might mean a 24 hour delay in completing a job.
  - An average professional tennis players career may span 10–14 years with perhaps only a fraction of that time when the player is truly competitive. An average builder might be expected to have a working life of 40–45 years.
  - The tennis player will require 100% confidence in his knee to be competitive whereas the builder, even if required to climb ladders, may be functional with a partial response to treatment.

It is appreciating these subtle differences between a professional athlete and a non-athlete that is central to the successful management of arthritis, and where the sports physician's skills as the athletes advocate will be required.

Controlling synovitis

The control of joint inflammation is imperative to preserve joint function. Drugs that have been shown to control synovitis and prevent or attenuate joint inflamation and subsequent damage fall into 3 categories; disease modifying agents (DMARDs), biological therapies, and steroids.

NSAIDs reduce pain, swelling, and stiffness but do not influence the underlying inflammatory process in terms of reducing joint damage, and should only be used for symptom control.

Table 17.1 Non-infectious inflammatory arthritis

Descriptive term		Associated conditions	Notes
Seropositive arthritis		Rheumatoid arthritis	RA is not always seropositive
Seronegative arthritis	Monoarthritis	Psoriasis	Seronegative arthritides are frequently associated with characteristic extra-articular features e.g. uveitis, genitourinary symptoms, skin rashes.
	Oligoarthritis (less than 4 joints affected)	Inflammatory bowel disease	
		Reactive arthritis	
	Spondyloarthropathy	Ankylosing spondylitis	Inflammatory arthritis involving the sacroiliac joints and spine in addition to peripheral joints. All seronegative arthropathies are associated with HLAB27.
		Psoriasis	
		Inflammatory bowel disease	
		Reactive arthritis	
Crystal arthropathy		Gout	Confirmation of crystals in synovial fluid is the gold standard for diagnosis.
		Pseudogout	
Connective tissue diseases		Systemic lupus scleroderma	Arthritis is only one feature of these multi-system illnesses but this highlights the importance of taking a full history when presented with an acute arthritis.
Systemic vasculitis		Wegener's granulomatosis	
		Polyarteritis nodosa	
Multi-system illness		Sarcoidosis	

DMARDs

A number of DMARDs have been used to treat inflammatory arthritis, however, the most commonly used drugs in current practice are methotrexate, leflunomide and sulphasalazine. They all broadly share the same characteristics:

- They are slow-acting, may take up to 3–6 months to have their full effect.
- They only work in about 70% of patients.
- Their side effect profile requires the regular monitoring of blood tests (FBC, U&E, LFT).
- They maybe used alone or in combination.
- Treatment is escalated in terms of dose and combinations until control of synovitis is achieved.
- Full remission of arthritis is unlikely.

Biological therapies

Biological therapies are designer drugs aimed at blocking particular components of the inflammatory cascade. The only biologics widely used in clinical practice are drugs that reduce or block tumour necrosis factor (TNF) activity. Three drugs are currently available, infliximab, etanercept and adalumimab. They all share the same characteristics:

- All work quickly (within 4 weeks).
- They are all given by injection (infliximab as IVI, etanercept and adalumimab as SC injection).
- Research suggests that they are effective in 70% of patients although clinical observations suggest a more positive response rate.
- They are more effective if co-prescribed with methotrexate.
- They require monitoring with regular blood tests.
- Their main side effect is an increased risk of serious and non-serious infection and in particular TB.
- In the UK they are currently rationed for use when conventional DMARDs have failed because of their cost, although they are more widely available in the USA.
- Current evidence suggests that they should be increasingly considered as first line treatment with methotrexate.
- Complete remission is achievable in some patients.

Steroids

Steroids can be given as injections (intra-articular, intravenous, intra-muscular) or in oral form. Their use will currently require the completion of either an a TUE or a TUE depending on the route of administration.

- Injectable steroids have a rapid onset of action and are widely used, particularly intra-articular steroids. In the context of mono or oligo (<4 joints) arthritis an intra-articular steroid injection can be extremely effective. Some rheumatologists pulse patients with IM or IV steroids at times of a generalized arthritis flare.
- Oral steroids have been used in rheumatological practice for many years. They are very effective at reducing inflammation but unfortunately their long-term use is limited by dose-dependent side effects. Consequently most rheumatologists would not use long-term doses greater than 5–7.5mg daily. With the advent of anti-TNF treatments, the use of long-term oral steroids will probably decrease.

Medical aspects of managing inflammatory arthritis

Specific medical roles include:
- Prevention of disease or treatment-associated side effects e.g. preserving bone health, pro-actively managing cardiovascular risk factors.
- Liason with surgical colleagues to ensure surgical referrals are made expeditiously.
- Specialist medical referral e.g. GU medicine referral if sexually transmitted infection causing reactive arthritis is possible, dermatology referral for problematic psoriasis, gastroenterology referral if occult inflammatory bowel disease causing arthritis is suspected.

Joint rehabilitation

An inflamed joint will undergo the same functional deterioration as an injured joint and therefore rehabilitation is vital to restoring normal joint function. With the exception of an acutely inflamed joint, when pain rather than any evidence that exercise induces damage is the limiting factor, patients with inflammatory arthritis should be encouraged to rehabilitate pro-actively. The greater challenge is often in trying to control the athlete's enthusiasm to prevent overly aggressive rehabilitation.

Multi-disciplinary care

The doctor is only one member of team which includes nurses, physio- and occupational therapists, podiatrists, orthotists, and psychologists.

Monoarthritis

Patients with acute inflammatory monoarthritis may go on to develop a chronic arthropathy. The management of chronic mono-arthritis follows the principles outlined above. There are a number of differences which can be summarised as follows:
- Initial management will utilize joint-specific rather than systemic treatment modalities e.g. intra-articular steroid, medical or surgical synovectomy, along with physiotherapy modalities.
- Patients who fail to respond to targeted treatment will probably have to consider systemic drug treatments. Depending on the joint concerned the impact of monoarthritis on physical function and athletic performance may be no less than that of polyarthritis. DMARDs are uniformly slow acting, which is very frustrating for any patient but particularly an athlete.
- Current rationing guidelines for the NHS prescription of anti-TNF treatment only apply to polyarthritis (specifically rheumatoid arthritis). The use of anti-TNF treatments for monoarthritis would have to be made on the basis of a case of exceptional need or alternatively paid for privately. I believe anti-TNF treatment offers the individual the greatest chance of returning to full competitive sport.
- The importance of rehabilitation can not be overemphasized.

Oligoarthritis

Oligoarthritis is a term used to describe arthritis that affects no more than 4 joints. It is characteristic of the seronegative arthropathies. The management of an oligoarthritis falls somewhere between that of a monoarthritis and a polyarthritis. Intra-articular steroids are widely used but the early introduction of DMARDs would be normal clinical practice.

Spondyloarthropathy

Spondyloarthropathies are inflammatory conditions of the axial skeleton and in particular the sacroiliac joints. Bilateral sacroileitis is therefore a diagnostic feature. The clinical assessment and management of these conditions differ from peripheral arthritis in a number of ways.

- Symptoms usually start as a young adult.
- Strong predilection for male gender.
- Diagnosis is frequently delayed because symptoms are misinterpreted.
- Inflammatory back pain is characterized by early morning stiffness and improvement with activity, contrary to mechanical pain, which is usually eased by rest.
- Bilateral sacroiliac joint involvement is diagnostic. X-rays taken during the early phase of the condition are frequently normal, MRI is the investigation of choice in early disease if radiological diagnostic confirmation is required.
- Unilateral sacroileitis is unusual and infection should be excluded.
- Peripheral joints may be affected but by definition not in isolation.
- Associated with characteristic extra-articular features (Table 17.1).
- NSAIDs help manage symptoms but do not prevent ankylosis (fusion) of the spine.
- Peripheral arthritis may respond to standard DMARDs, axial symptoms do not.
- Anti-TNF medications have been shown to dramatically improve axial symptoms and reduce spinal damage.

Rheumatoid arthritis

Rheumatoid arthritis (RA) is the most common type of inflammatory arthritis, affecting approximately 1% of the UK population. The following points are worth emphasizing:

- The diagnosis should be made on clinical grounds. Investigations should only be seen as providing supported evidence e.g. elevated inflammatory markers, anaemia suggesting chronicity.
- It usually presents as an acute symmetrical inflammatory polyarthritis affecting most of the large and small joints (classically affecting the MCPs and PIPs).
- It can initially present as a mono- or oligoarthritis but will usually evolve into a polyarthritis.
- It is more common in females and classically presents in middle age, although it can present at any age.
- The cause of RA is unknown. Genetic factors only account for 30% of its aetiology. A family history is interesting but neither confirms nor excludes the diagnosis.
- Rheumatoid factor (RF) is unhelpful in proving the diagnosis but is associated with a worse prognosis. Other genetic and serological diagnostic factors are being investigated for their ability to improve the diagnostic utility of RF and as prognostic markers.
- Systemic features e.g. weight loss, fatigue, and even a low grade fever are not uncommon.
- The management of RA is that of an inflammatory polyarthritis.
- Inflammation produces joint damage (which is largely thought to be irreversible) and therefore the emphasis is on early aggressive treatment to switch off joint inflammation as quickly as possible.
- RA is a multisystem disease and is associated with complications that can affect all of the major organs.
- RA is associated with increased mortality. This seems to be largely attributable to increased cardiovascular mortality, hence there is an increasing appreciation of the importance of managing cardiovascular risk factors.
- The use of anti-TNF medication has revolutionized the management of RA. These drugs will likely be used first line in the future to try and induce remission.

Crystal arthropathy

Gout and pseudogout are the most common forms of crystal arthritis. Gout, in particular, is associated with a number of medical conditions for which exercise should be prescribed or recommended. The most important associated feature of pseudogout is osteoarthritis, which is both a consequence of joint injury and another condition for which exercise has an important therapeutic role. The following may help you assess and manage a patient with crystal arthritis.

- Gout is caused by monosodium urate crystals and pseudogout by calcium pyrophosphate.
- Gout is usually a result of the underexcretion of urate.
- Both conditions cause acute and dramatic joint inflammation with severe pain, marked swelling, and erythema. The clinical features are indistinguishable from septic arthritis.
- The classical presentation of gout is podagra, acute inflammation of the first MTP joint. Pseudogout typically presents with knee involvement. Both conditions may present with acute inflammation of any synovial lined structure including tendon sheaths. It is therefore not uncommon for both conditions to be initially diagnosed as cellulitis and treated with antibiotics.
- Although monoarthritis is typical, polyarticular involvement may occur.
- There are no serological diagnostic tests for gout, or pseudogout. A normal uric acid level does not exclude gout, and a raised level is not diagnositic. Synovial fluid analysis is the gold standard for diagnosis.
- An acute attack is best treated with NSAIDs (with appropriate gastro-intestinal protection). For patients who do not respond or can't take NSAIDs then colchicine is a useful alternative.
- Colchicine causes diarrhoea (use a maximum dose of 500mcg bd or tid to control symptoms.)
- Intra-articular steroids can work extremely well, and unlike NSAIDs and colchicine, are not associated with any systemic side effects. At the same time the joint can be drained to provide immediate comfort and synovial fluid sent for examination under a polarising microscope. Septic arthritis must be excluded.
- In resistant or polyarticular disease the use of a 1–2 week course of low dose oral steroids (10mg) can be extremely effective.
- Both conditions maybe triggered by environmental stress e.g. dehydration and joint injury.
- There is no prophylaxis for pseudogout.
- Gout maybe caused by diet (and in particular alcohol) as well as drugs e.g. diuretics. Patients should be encouraged to reduce alcohol consumption, modify their diet (low calorie and carbohydrate restricted), and where possible drug regimes altered.

- The decision when to introduce gout prophylaxis is best left to the patient given the need for daily treatment (assuming there are no features of articular or non-articular damage, uric acid is associated with a nephropathy and raised serum levels may be a cardiovascular risk factor). Drugs either reduce uric acid production (e.g. allopurinol) or increase its renal excretion (uricosuric drugs). Allopurinol is the treatment of choice.
- In otherwise healthy individuals (normal renal function) it is usual to start allopurinol 300mg daily and increase the dose in 100mg increments every 2–3 months until symptomatic control is achieved. Allopurinol may cause hypersensitivity skin reactions and affect renal function. Patients return for a U&E 1 month after starting or changing dose.
- Paradoxically, allopurinol may cause an attack of gout. This must be explained to the patient and, unless contra-indicated, co-prescribe a NSAID or colchicine for the first month after changing dose.
- Losartan (ACE II inhibitor) and fenofibrate have been found to have uricosuric properties. Gout is associated with diabetes, hyperlipidaemia and hypertension and both drugs may be helpful in patients with dual pathology.

Seronegative arthritides

The sports physician is most likely to encounter athletes with a sero-negative arthritis. Dactylitis, the uniform sausage like swelling of a digit, is diagnostic of seronegative arthritides. Enthesitis is another typical feature and may be overlooked as a mechanical tendinopthy unless an inflammatory cause is considered.

Psoriatic arthritis

- Psoriatic arthritis can present as a monoarthritis, oligoarthritis, spondyloarthropathy, arthritis confined to the DIP joints, and a severely destructive polyarthritis.
- 10% of patients with psoriasis may develop an arthritis.
- There is no association between the severity or location of psoriasis and the nature or pattern of the arthritis. Psoriatic plaques may be well hidden on the scalp or around the umbilicus or confined to nail dystrophy, such that the patient may not even appreciate they have psoriasis.
- To complicate matters further, psoriatic arthritis may precede the development of the rash or only be present in a first degree relative.
- A number of drugs used to treat arthritis are also extremely effective for psoriasis e.g. methotrexate, leflunomide and anti-TNF preparations.

Enteric arthritis

- Arthritis associated with inflammatory bowel disease (IBD) is more common than widely appreciated. It mainly presents as a monoarthritis, oligoarthritis, or spondyloarthropathy.
- Uncontrolled arthritis is frequently an indication of active bowel inflammation, which may not be clinically apparent. (Crohns disease in particular).
- Steroids are frequently used to treat IBD and the arthritic symptoms may only reveal themselves upon steroid reduction.
- NSAIDs may exacerbate IBD so should be used cautiously.
- A number of drugs are effective in the treatment of arthritis and IBD e.g. azathioprine, anti-TNF preparations (Crohn's).

Reactive arthritis

- With an acute arthritis consider an infectious cause.
- Streptococcal infections and those causing infectious gastroenteritis and genitourinary infection are most common, although the viral URTI is probably most often to blame but is usually self-limiting, although potentially devastating to the competing athlete.
- Monoarthritis is the most common presentation.
- Chlamydia infection is often asymptomatic and a careful and sensitive history is essential. Referral to a genitourinary medicine department should be considered in all patients, a history of monogamy does not exclude polygamy in the partner!

- Treatment of the infectious cause does not enhance resolution of the arthritis or improve long-term prognosis of the arthritis, with the possible exception of Lyme disease. In some series up to 30% of patients developing reactive arthritis may develop chronic synovitis.

Miscellaneous inflammatory arthritis

The aetiology of inflammatory arthritis is too diverse to discuss fully in this context, however, there are a number of other potential causes that deserve mention.

- Red flag conditions—the importance of local sepsis (e.g. osteomyelitis) or tumour (primary, secondary, and haematological) presenting as an arthritis is worthy of emphasis.
- Erythema nodosum—usually associated with troublesome lower and sometimes upper limb distal arthritis.
- Pigmented villonodular synovitis—usually presents with a blood stained effusion, MRI is diagnostic.
- Osteoid osteoma—still overlooked in patients with chronic joint/bone pain. Triple phase bone scan, CT, and MRI all have diagnostic utility.

Dermatology

Problems caused by friction

Blisters

Description
- Fluid filled bullae that form at the site of friction.
- Usually caused by a change in training pattern, or ill-fitting equipment.
- Location and history are main clues to the diagnosis.

Risk factors
- Early in the workout season.
- Hard playing surfaces.
- Repetitive activities.

Treatment
- Treat 'hot spots' with ice and protection.
- May use protective socks, petroleum jelly, or mole skin for treatment and prevention.
- Superglue may be painted on hot spots for protection from irritation, but may increase traction on the site.
- Drain in a sterile manner only if tense.
- Antibiotic ointment or hydrocolloid if open.

Differential diagnosis
- Pemphigus.
- Pemphigoid.

Calluses

Description
- Thickening of the outer layer of skin (hyperkeratosis) with no central core as seen in verruca vulgaris.
- Skin lines are maintained.
- Caused by repetitive friction.
- Possibly ill-fitting equipment.
- May be painful and lead to blisters or subdermal hematomas.

Risk factors
- Hard playing surfaces.
- Repetitive activities.

Treatment
- Properly fitting shoes and equipment.
- Pumice stone.
- Paring.
- Salicylic acid preparation.
- Use gloves or equipment to protect skin.
- May use protective socks, petroleum jelly, or mole skin.

Differential diagnosis
- Warts.
- Bunion.

Subungual haematoma (black toe, runners toe, tennis toe)

Description
- Splinter haemorrhage of the nail bed usually involving the first or second toe.
- Develop acutely after pressure from tight shoes or from sudden deceleration.

Risk factors
- Most often seen in racquet sports, football, and distance runners.
- Downhill running.
- Long or malformed toenails.
- Tight shoes, especially the toe box.

Treatment
- Close trimming of toenail proximal to the distal aspect of the toe.
- Properly fitting shoes with adequate room in the toe box.
- Change of running style/route.

Differential diagnosis
- Subungual melanoma.

Plantar petechiae (black heel, black dot syndrome, talon noir)

Description
- Intra-epidermal bleeding and petechiae of the heel.
- Occurs on the heel at the edge of the foot pad.
- Caused by sheering forces and sudden stops.
- With paring, skin lines are maintained and no additional bleeding is seen.

Risk factors
- Seen in volleyball, racquet sports, running, lacrosse, and basketball.
- Poor fitting shoes.
- Repetitive trauma (cutting or stops).

Treatment
- Properly fitted shoes.
- Use of a 'soft' shoe.
- Thick socks.
- Heel pads.

Differential diagnosis
- Melanoma.

Sun and heat-related problems

Sunburn

Description
- Excessive exposure to UV light.
- May cause up to second degree burns.
- Increases risk of skin cancers.

Risk factors
- Water sports, outdoor sports.
- Early during the warm season.
- Medications (tetracycline, sulfa, phenothiazines.)
- Fair complexion, blue eyes.

Treatment
- Cool compresses.
- Aloe vera lotions.
- Topical anaesthetics and/or antihistamines.
- Antibiotic ointments if second degree burns.
- Oral fluids.
- Maintain the integrity of the overlying skin.
- Oral and topical steroids may be required for moderate to severe burns, to control inflammation and discomfort.

Prevention
- Sun screen/sun block (sweatproof/waterproof).
- Protective clothing and hats.
- Avoid midday sun.
- Gradual exposure to develop protective tan (tanning booths may be a more controlled environment).
- Provide shade near workout area.

Differential diagnosis
- Sun sensitizing medication.
- Flushing.

Photodermatitis
Ranges from nodular (sun poisoning) to solar purpura, to solar urticaria.

Description
- Immune reaction directed against the skin caused by sun exposure.
- Often requires a co-factor to trigger the reaction (medications, etc).
- May present as hive-like lesions, nodules, purpura, to generalized oedema.

Risk factors
- Outdoor sports.
- Medication use.

Treatment
- Difficult to treat.
- Avoidance of sun exposure is best.
- Psoralen with UVA (PUVA).

- Antihistamines.
- Severe cases may require IV steroids.

Differential diagnosis
- Sun sensitizing medication such as tetracycline, sulfonamides, griseofulvin, diuretics, phenothiazides, first generation sulfonylurea agents, diphenhydraminel, and some cosmetics.

Atopic dermatitis
Description
- Eczematous eruption that is itchy, recurrent, flexural, and symmetric.
- It generally begins early in life, follows periods of remission and exacerbation, and usually resolves by the age of 30.
- Infants have facial and patchy or generalized body eczema.
- Adolescents and adults have eczema in flexural areas and on the hands.
- Polygenic inheritance.
- May be aggravated by heat, sweat, or exertion.

Risk factors
- Exposure to heat, sweat, allergens, and exertion.

Treatment
- May be improved by sun exposure.
- Emollients.
- Avoidance of radical temperature changes.

Differential diagnosis
- Seborrheic dermatitis, psoriasis, contact dermatitis, tinea corporis.

Hyperhidrosis
Description
- Excessive perspiration.
- May be congenital or stress-related.
- May cause problems with grip, vision, self confidence.

Risk factors
- Exposure to heat, physical exertion, and stressful situations.

Treatment
- Aluminum chloride.
- After several weeks, may only need application 1–2 times per week.
- Iontophoresis units.

Differential diagnosis
- Anxiety.
- Excessive heat exposure.
- Hyperthyroidism.

Cold-related injuries

Frostnip

Description
- Involves the superficial layer of skin only (first degree frostbite).
- May appear flushed or have rosy cheeks.
- Affects nose, cheeks, and ears most often.
- Will usually result in flaking of epidermis.

Risk factors
- Outdoor sports.
- Winter sports.

Prevention
- Cover all exposed skin when conditions are poor.
- Petroleum jelly for protection of face and ears.

Treatment
- Treat symptomatically.
- Prevention is the best treatment.

Differential diagnosis
- Viral exanthum.

Frostbite

Description
- Extended exposure to freezing temperatures.
- Results in a freezing injury to the blood vessels, nerves, and soft tissue.
- May cause first, second, or third degree injuries.
- First and second degree injuries most commonly seen in athletes.
- Most often affects the ears and penis.

Prevention
- Recognition and avoidance of unsafe conditions.
- Proper dress.

Treatment
- Rapid rewarming with warm water immersion. Use caution if coexisting hypothermia.
- Treat like burns.

Chilblains

Description
- Chronic exposure of extremities to sub-freezing temperatures.
- Results in breakdown of the dermis with resultant irritation and discomfort.
- Predisposes to future cold intolerance.

Treatment
- Protection from further trauma and cold.
- May require antibiotics.

Prevention
- Recognition and avoidance of unsafe conditions.
- Proper dress and hygiene.

Fungal infections

Tinea pedis (athlete's foot)

Description

- Erythematous, often scaling eruptions on the plantar surface of the foot and between the toes.
- Caused by a variety of dermatophytes and yeasts. Most commonly caused by *Trichophyton rubrum*, *T. mentagraphytes*, and *Epidermophyton floccusum*. Sometimes *Candida*.
- Yeasts do not respond to some over-the-counter preparations.
- Diagnose using skin scrapings, clinical presentation, or fungal cultures.

Risk factors

- Chronically wet feet.
- Locker rooms and public showers.
- Diabetes.
- Immune system failure.

Treatment

- Over-the-counter preparations:
- Prescription antifungal topical preparations: are effective against both fungi, are once daily preparations, and may deliver cure within a week.
- Difficult cases may require oral antifungal agents.

Prevention

- Remove wet socks and use breathable shoes.
- Keep feet clean and dry.
- Drying powders.
- Wash with benzoyl peroxide bar.

Differential diagnosis

Pitted keratolysis, psoriasis.

Tinea cruris (jock itch)

Description

- Begins in the moist, warm crural folds and spreads out to become fan-shaped as it spreads to the thighs.
- Rarely involves the scrotum (see erythrasma).
- Reddened scaly patches with sharp margins.
- May be painful, pruritic, and weeping.
- Similar organisms as tinea pedis. Most commonly caused by *Trichophyton rubrum*, *T. mentagraphytes* and *Epidermophyton floccusum*. Sometimes *Candida*.
- May be spread by contamination from infected feet.

Risk factors

- Shared undergarments.
- Tight fitting synthetic garments.
- Prolonged maceration.

Treatment
- Similar to tinea corporis.
- Topical preparations are effective against fungi.
- Difficult cases may require oral antifungal agents.
- Antihistamine or low potency steroid creams may control itch.

Prevention
- Loose fitting absorbent undergarments.
- Change and shower soon after workout.
- Powders to keep dry. Avoid corn starch due to its conversion to sugars that may act as a growth media.

Differential diagnosis
Intertrigo, psoriasis.

Tinea corporis (ringworm, tinea gladiatorum)
Description
- Presents as an itchy red rash on the trunk, leg, arm, or neck.
- Consists of small red papules, or blisters and scales.
- Caused by the dermatophytes *Microsporum*, *Trichophyton*, and *Epidermophyton*.
- Usually seen on hairless portions of skin.
- Usually more tissue reaction at the advancing borders of infection—accounts for the ring-like appearance.
- May be spread from mats, equipment, and clothing.

Risk factors
- Sweating, heat, and physical exertion contribute to fungal growth.
- Sports with close skin contact or communal mats (i.e. wrestling, martial arts, gymnastics).

Treatment
- Similar to tinea pedis.
- Topical antifungal preparations are effective against both fungi.
- To prevent transmission, cover with occlusive dressing for contact sports.

Prevention
- Proper treatment of mats and equipment with fungicidal cleaners after each practice/meet.
- Enforcement of skin infection rules.
- Prompt treatment and isolation.

Differential diagnosis
Contact dermatitis, atopic dermatitis.

Tinea versicolor (pityriasis versicolor)
Description
- Common fungal infection of the skin.
- Most commonly noted as macular hypopigmented or hyperpigmented lesions on the nape of the neck extending onto the trunk and arms.
- Pathogens include *Pityrosporum orbiculare* and *P. ovale* (both were previously called *Malassezia furfur*).

- Usually painless and does not itch.
- Diagnosis is by scrapings and pathopneumonic spaghetti and meatball appearance.

Risk factor

May affect any athlete.

Treatment

- Treatment consists of topical antifungal or selenium based over–the-counter shampoo on the skin and hair, or topical antifungal medication.
- Oral antifungal agents may be needed in the more difficult cases. Application prior to workouts may increase skin concentrations.
- Hypopigmented regions may take 6–8 weeks to resolve.

Prevention

- Good hygiene with showering immediately after workouts, clean dry undershirts, and use of selenium–based or antifungal shampoo daily

Differential diagnosis

- Vitiligo, guttate psoriasis, nummular eczema.

Onychomycosis (tinea unguium)

Description

- Fungal infection of the nails of the fingers or more commonly the toes.
- Pathogens include many dermatophytes most commonly *Trichophyton rubrum* and *Candida*.
- May cause disfiguring thickening, and discoloration of the nails.
- Predispose to hang nails and secondary bacterial infections.

Risk factors

- Poor circulation.
- Diabetes.
- Poor hygiene.

Treatment

- Very refractory to treatment.
- Oral antifungal agents have been shown to have the best cure rates.
- May require removal of the nail for cure.

Differential diagnosis

- Psoriasis, Reiter's syndrome, nail dystrophy, nail injury.

Intertrigo

Description
- Red, macerated, half-mooned shaped plaques found in the moist body folds.
- Caused by moist irritation allowing mixed infections of dermatophytes, bacteria, and yeast to infect the superficial layer of skin.

Risk factors
Obesity, sweating, poor hygiene.

Treatment
- Similar to tinea cruris.
- Avoid corn starch due to its conversion to sugars that act as a growth media.

Prevention
Weight loss and good hygiene.

Differential diagnosis
Tinea infections.

Bacterial infections

Acne vulgaris

Description
- Typical infections consist of papules, pustules, comedones, nodules, and cysts.
- Located primarily on the face, back, shoulders, and chest.
- Caused by a variety of bacteria.

Risk factors
- 70–80% of adolescents have some degree of acne.
- Worsened by sweat and occlusion from equipment that irritate the skin. Commonly seen under helmets, chin straps, shoulder pads, jock straps, etc.

Treatment
- Topical antibiotics (erythromycin, clindamycin), tretinoin, benzoyl peroxide.
- Oral antibiotics when severe.
- Retinoic acid.

Prevention
- Good hygiene.
- Bathe immediately after workouts.
- Avoid overdrying or scrubbing the skin.
- Protect from equipment.
- Properly fitted equipment.

Differential diagnosis
- Folliculitis, rosacea.

Furuncle (boil, carbuncle, abscess)

Description
- Usually begins as a *Staphylococcus* infection of the hair follicle then invading the surrounding tissues causing a collection of pus.
- Usually located on the upper extremity, buttocks, groin, axilla, neck, waist, or chest.
- Boils on the face are of particular concern because of venous access to the brain.
- Multiple boils is called furunculosis and if they interconnect, a carbuncle,

Treatment
- Boils will usually rupture on their own.
- If persistent, large, painful, or signs of sepsis, they should be lanced and appropriate antibiotics started.

Risk factors
Diabetes mellitus, obesity, poor hygiene

Differential diagnosis
- Epidermoid or pilar cyst, hydradenitis suppurativa.

Folliculitis

Description
- Common infection of the hair follicles often by *Staphylococcus aureus* or other skin bacteria.
- May present as macules, papules, pustules or sometimes crusted lesions at the base of the hair shaft that may produce boils or carbuncles.
- Often seen on the back, thighs, or buttocks.
- May be due to friction from pads or shaving.
- Tend to be worse in the summer and with spandex clothing.
- Hot tub folliculitis caused by a *Pseudomonas aeruginosa* infection from exposure to infected water in hot tub or whirlpool. Generally affect the axillae, breast, and pubic area but occasionally the trunk. Usually resolves on own after 7–10 days.
- Steroid folliculitis is associated with use of anabolic steroids. Usually affects the trunk and occasionally the neck and face. Treatment is with cessation of steroids and treat like folliculitis.

Risk factors
- Sports that require/promote shaving of the body.
- Running sports, wrestling, football, swimming.

Treatment
- Usually resolve on their own once the irritating source is removed.
- Use of antibacterial soaps or topical antibacterial ointment.
- Benzoyl peroxide.
- Refractory cases may need oral antibiotics (tetracycline or erythromycin).

Prevention
- Shower immediately after workouts.
- Keep areas clean and dry.
- Shave in the direction of hair growth.
- Application of alcohol-based aftershave after shaving.

Differential diagnosis
- Acne vulgaris, rosacea, hydradenitis suppurativa.

Impetigo (ecthyma)

Description
- Highly contagious *Streptococcus* or *Staphylococcus* infection of the skin.
- Characterized by small vesicles which form pustules and eventually become honey-colored weeping crustations.
- Transmitted by direct contact of infected skin, towels, or equipment.
- May cause problems with the kidney and doubtfully the heart.
- Should be treated immediately.

Risk factors
Close contact sports such as martial arts, wrestling, rugby, etc.

Treatment
- Topical antibiotics are usually sufficient.

- If in difficult areas to treat topically or if extensive, may treat with oral antibiotics.

Prevention
Same as tinea corpus.

Differential diagnosis
Seborrheic dermatitis, contact dermatitis, herpes simplex, scabies, bullous pemphigoid.

Cellulitis (erysipelas, Ludwig's angina, etc.)
Description
- Infection of the dermis and subcutaneous tissue by group A *Streptococcus* and *Staphylococcus aureus*.
- May be life threatening if it involves the face, airway, or leads to sepsis.

Risk factors
Any skin condition that may allow a portal of entry for infection.

Treatment
Should be treated immediately with appropriate antibiotics, warm compresses, pain medication, and if extensive, irrigation and drainage.

Differential diagnosis
Deep venous thrombosis, contact dermatitis, gout, peripheral vascular disease, insect bite.

Onychocryptosis (ingrown toenail, felon, paronychia)
Description
- Infection of the subcutaneous tissue beneath the toe nail.
- Usually caused by *Streptococcus* species and *Staphylococcus aureus*.

Risk factors
Improper trimming of the nails.

Treatment
Should be treated immediately with appropriate antibiotics, warm compresses, pain medication, and if extensive or very painful, toenail removal.

Prevention
Proper trimming of nails.

Differential diagnosis
Onychomycosis.

Pitted keratolysis (stinky foot, tennis shoe foot)
Description
- Characterized by many circular or longitudinal, punched-out depressions on the sole of the foot.
- Most cases are asymptomatic, but painful, plaque-like lesions may occur.
- *Dermatophilus congolensis* and *M. sedentarius* produce and excrete exoenzymes (keratinase) that are able to degrade keratin and produce pitting in the stratum corneum.

Risk factors
Hyperhidrosis, moist socks, or immersion of the feet favors its development.

Treatment
- Treatment consists of promoting dryness.
- Socks should be changed frequently.
- Rapid clearing occurs with application of 20% aluminum chloride twice a day.
- Application twice a day of alcohol-based benzoyl peroxide (Panoxyl 5) may also be useful.
- Treatment with topical erythromycin is also curative.

Prevention
Keep feet clean and dry.

Differential diagnosis
Tinea pedis.

Erythrasma
Description
- Bacterial infection (*C. minutissimum*) may be confused with tinea cruris because of the similar, half moon–shaped plaque.
- Non-inflammatory, it is uniformly brown and scaly, it has no advancing border, and it fluoresces coral-red with the Wood's light.

Risk factors
- Occlusive clothing/shoes, obesity, hyperhidrosis.

Treatment
- Responds equally well to erythromycin orally 250mg four times a day for 2 weeks or topically twice a day for 2 weeks.
- The topical erythromycins contain alcohol and may be irritating when applied to the groin.

Differential diagnosis
Dermatophytosis, pitted keratolysis, seborrhea.

Viral infections

Verruca vulgaris (warts)

Description
- Due to a viral infection of the epidermis.
- May occur anywhere on the body.
- Presents as a rough hyperkeratotic area that may become quite large

Diagnosis
- Importantly, they lack normal skin lines and can be differentiated from other lesions by this fact.
- May have black dots in the centre from the ruptured blood vessels present there.

Risk factors
Skin to skin contact, immunocompromise.

Treatment
- Usually will regress spontaneously.
- May treat with cryotherapy, topical abrasives, laser, or immunotherapy.
- Should be covered to reduce the low risk of transmission.

Differential diagnosis
- Molluscum contagiosum, actinic keratosis.

Verruca plantaris (plantar wart)

Description
- Caused by a viral infection of the plantar surface of the foot.
- May be painful and cause gait abnormalities.

Diagnosis
Similar to warts.

Differential diagnosis
Public showers and locker rooms.

Treatment
- Treat early rather than late.
- May use a doughnut-shaped pad during the season and definitively treat at the end of the season.
- Topical over-the-counter preparations may take weeks for cure.
- Can be treated with liquid nitrogen, or 40% salicylic acid.
- Duofilm with 17% salicylic acid nightly can be used during the season.

Differential diagnosis
Corns, calluses.

Condyloma acuminatum (genital warts)

Description
- Caused by human papilloma virus (HPV).
- May cause cervical cancer in females.

Diagnosis
- May go unnoticed in females, and may be diagnosed on cervical smears.
- Diagnosed by appearance and location as well as sexual activity.

Risk factors
Unprotected sex, multiple sexual partners.

Treatment
- Prevented by use of condoms.
- Can be treated with topical salicylic acid, cryotherapy, or laser.
- Treatment is imperative to prevent transmission.

Differential diagnosis
Skin tags, moles, seborrhea, molluscum contagiosum, folliculitis

Molluscum contagiosum (water warts)

Description
- The viral pathogen is much more infectious than normal warts, thus its name.
- Transmission is through close physical contact or autoinoculation.
- Presents as a flesh or yellowish colored papular lesion with a collapsed centre especially on the hands, face, and upper body.
- More prevalent in contact sports such as wrestling, boxing, and rugby.

Diagnosis
- Typical appearance.
- Usually do not give a history of contact with infected person.

Risk factors
Exposure to virus, skin to skin contact.

Treatment
- Usually resolve spontaneously after 6–9 months.
- Cryotherapy, topical salicylic acid, or even excision.

Differential diagnosis
Flat wart, condyloma acuminatum, syringoma.

Varicella (chicken pox)

Description
- Vesicular lesions that begin as papules, evolve to vesicles, and rapidly evolve to pustules and crusts.
- Spread by respiratory secretions and contact with weeping lesions.
- Preventable with new immunization.

Diagnosis
- Made by clinical history and typical lesions that begin on the face and scalp and spread to the trunk and extremities.
- Lack of exposure or immunization.

Risk factors
Lack of immunization or disease history, exposure.

Treatment
Symptomatic treatment with isolation until all lesions are crusted over.

Differential diagnosis
Disseminated HSV, eczema, enterovirus infection.

Herpes zoster (shingles)
Description
- Reinfection by Varicella Zoster virus (VZV).
- Virus lies dormant within the ganglion cells and may be reactivated at any time.
- Unilateral dermatomal development of papules (24 hours), to vesicles. (48 hours), to pustules (96 hours), to crusts (7–10 days).
- New lesions may continue to develop for up to 7 days.
- Prevalent in the elderly.
- May be very painful and appear in any dermatome (most commonly on the thorax).

Risk factors
Previous infection of chicken pox, immunocompromise, age.

Treatment
- Pain management.
- Prevent viral transmission.
- Prevent secondary infections.
- Antiviral treatment (acyclovir, valacyclovir, famcyclovir).

Herpes gladiatorum (traumatic herpes)
Description
- Caused by herpes simplex virus (HSV).
- HSV is directly inoculated onto the skin or may recur in cervical and lumbosacral dermatomes.
- Present as blisters that rupture to form a crusted surface.
- May be preceded by an itching or burning sensation.
- Maximally contagious for 5 days after blisters rupture.
- May last for 1–2 weeks.
- Infectious until lesions are crusted over.
- Seen in close contact sports such as wrestling and rugby.

Diagnosis
- Typical lesion and clinical presentation.
- Tzanck smear, viral culture, antigen detection.

Risk factors
- Exposure to virus.
- Skin to skin contact.
- Rugby, wrestling, football.

Treatment
- Prevention of skin to skin contact to prevent transmission.
- Daily disinfection of mats and shared equipment.
- Oral therapy (acyclovir, valacyclovir, famcyclovir).
- Prophylaxis may prevent recurrence.

Table 18.1 Description of terms in dermatology

Terminology	Description	Example
Macule	A discoloured spot or patch on the skin, neither elevated nor depressed, of various colours, sizes, and shapes.	Vitiligo Café au lait spots Petechiae
Papule	A solid lesion elevated above the plane of the surrounding skin. Often precede vesicles and pustules. Generally considered less than 1cm in diameter.	Measles Acne vulgaris
Ulcer	An open sore or lesion of the skin or mucous membranes where there has been destruction of the overlying epidermis and upper papillary layer of the dermis resulting in the formation of a crater.	Decubitus ulcers Venous stasis ulcers Aphthous ulcers
Nodule	A palpable solid round or ellipsoidal lesion deeper than a papule and present in the dermis, subcutaneous tissue, or epidermis. The depth rather than the diameter differentiate it from a papule.	Bouchard's and Osler's nodes Warts Squamous cell carcinoma Basal cell carcinoma
Wheal	A rounded or flat-topped pale red elevation in the skin that is evanescent, disappearing within hours, and often intensely pruritic. A result of oedema in the upper layer of the dermis.	Urticaria Insect bites
Bulla	A large blister or skin vesicle filled with serum, lymph fluid, blood, or extracellular fluid. They are located within the epidermis, or the epidermal-dermal interface. Usually more than 0.5cm in diameter.	Blisters Pemphigus
Vesicle	A small blister filled with serum, lymph fluid, blood, or extrac lular fluid. They are located within the epidermis, or the epidermal-dermal interface. Usually less than 0.5cm in diameter.	Herpes zoster Herpes simplex Variola Varicella

Table 18.1 (*Contd.*)

Terminology	Description	Example
Pustule	A circumscribed elevation of the skin that contains a purulent exudate that may be white, yellow, or greenish-yellow. May be associated with a hair follicle. Vesicles may become pustules.	Acne vulgaris Impetigo
Plaque	An elevation above the skin surface that occupies a relatively large surface area in comparison with its height above the skin. It may be formed by a confluence of papules.	Psoriasis Mycosis fungoides
Lichenification	Like a plaque, but the elevation above the skin surface is due to proliferation of the keratinocytes and stratum corneum due to continued irritation. The skin appears thickened, and skin lines are accentuated.	Eczematous dermatitis
Scales	Due to an increased rate of proliferation of epidermal cells the stratum corneum is not formed normally, causing the skin to peel in visible sheets or flakes.	Eczema Seborrhea Psoriasis
Crusts	Result when serum, blood, or purulent exudate dries on the skin surface. They may be thin, delicate and friable, or thick and adherent.	Impetigo Ecthyma

Disability

What is a disability?

The Disability Discrimination Act of 1995 defines it as 'physical or mental impairment which has a substantial and long-term adverse effect on his ability to carry out normal day-to-day activities.'

Sport and disability evolution

Sport for people with disabilities evolved rapidly over the last century, from an archery tournament at Stoke Mandeville hospital on the opening day of the Olympic Games in London in 1948, to over 4000 athletes from over 120 countries competing at the Sydney 2000 Paralympic Games in 18 different sports.

Reasons for increased participation

- Increased acceptance of rights of people with disabilities within society e.g. Disability Discrimination Act 1995.
- Increased recognition of sporting capability of people with disabilities:
  - High jump >2 metres by a single leg amputee.
  - Wheelchair marathon time below 1 hour 30 minutes.
- Increasing recognition of importance of physical activity for health for all the population, including those with a disability e.g. reduced health care costs for active paraplegics vs sedentary paraplegics.

Physical activity recommendations

How much activity?

- The accumulation of at least 30 minutes of moderate intensity activity on most days of the week and at least five days of the week is equally applicable to someone with a disability. ('At least five a week—Evidence of the impact of physical activity and its relationship to health—A report from the Chief Medical Officer, 2004.)
- The same principles of training apply, i.e. the graded increase in duration, intensity, and frequency of activity.
- More thought may be required as to. the mode of exercise according to the disability.
- The social and psychological benefits of exercise and sport participation.
- Major improvements in self-esteem and social integration may occur through an active lifestyle.

Advice on choosing a sport/exercise

It is important to try and marry the potential benefits of exercise participation and enjoyment for maximizing long-term increases in physical activity behaviour, with various aspects of the individual's disability.

- Personal preference of the individual—important for adherence
- Characteristics of the sport:
  - Physiological demands e.g. aerobic, anaerobic.
  - Collision potential—increased risk of injury e.g. osteopenic limbs in paraplegia.
  - Team or individual—preference of individual, social interaction.
  - Co-ordination requirements—e.g. tremor or ataxia would limit performance in some sports.
- Potential effects of the medical condition:
  - Beneficial aspects—e.g. CVD risk reduction, improved bone density.
  - Detrimental—e.g. excess cardiac risk in high intensity sport where a cardiac defect is present, fracture risk .
- Conditions associated with the condition e.g. syndromic conditions may have physical limitations to sport participation but may have other associated medical issues that need consideration e.g. Down's Syndrome and cardiac anomalies or atlanto-axial instability.
- Cognitive ability—impaired cognition may limit participation in certain activities or reduce safety.
- Social skills of the person—ability to follow rules and interact with others.
- Availability of facilities in the locality.
- Availability of appropriate coaching and support staff (e.g. lifting and handling).
- Equipment availability and cost.

Barriers to physical activity

- Cultural.
- Medical or parental over-protection.
- Social factors.
- Lack of opportunity during education.
- Facilities.
- Accessibility.

Organization of sport for people with disabilities

Disabilities may be physical, sensory, or intellectual or a combination of each of these. There are consequently a large number of organizations that promote and support sport for people with disabilities.

These organisations may be:
- Local
- Regional
- National
- International
- Disability specific
- Multi-disability
- Encouraging participation
- Elite sport.

The International Paralympic Committee (IPC)

The IPC unites these disability-specific organizations globally with the exception of the hearing impaired. The hearing impaired hold a games termed the 'deaflympics' every four years and this is held in a non-Olympic Games year. The Paralympic Games involves sport at the elite level and is held just after, and in the same city as, the Olympic Games for the following disability groups:
- Spinal cord related disability.
- Amputee.
- Visually impaired (VI).
- Cerebral palsy (CP).
- Les Autres—other physical disabilities not falling into the other categories e.g. muscular dystrophy, multiple sclerosis.
- Intellectual disability (or learning disability).

Sports

People with disabilities can take part in most sports and activities but the number of sports in summer Paralympic Games is limited to the following:
- Archery
- Athletics
- Boccia
- Cycling
- Equestrian
- Football 5-a-side
- Football 7-a-side
- Goalball
- Judo
- Powerlifting
- Sailing
- Shooting
- Swimming
- Table Tennis

- Volleyball (sitting)
- Wheelchair basketball
- Wheelchair fencing
- Wheelchair rugby
- Wheelchair tennis.

There are also Winter Paralympic Games with Alpine and Nordic events as well as wheelchair curling and sledge hockey—a form of ice hockey using a seated sledge.

The Special Olympics is a separate event which involves people with intellectual disability with less emphasis on elite performance and more on participation.

Technology

Wheelchair design

Initially people with disabilities took part in sports or activities using a standard wheelchair, but became increasingly frustrated at the lack of performance capability and needs for the specific sport. As a result sport-specific chairs developed. Racing chairs owe much of their design to cycle technology, and are ergonomically designed and individually customized for the user. Wheelchair tennis and basketball chairs have a much larger wheel camber to facilitate rapid turning, and may have a rear wheel to prevent tipping over. Rugby chairs have fenders and guards for attacking and defensive manoeuvres. New technological developments will occur to meet the needs of wheelchair users over time to enhance performance.

Prostheses

People are unable to run using the traditional single-axis prosthetic foot as they cannot push off from the foot flat position. To improve function and reduce fatigue an energy-storing, spring action prosthetic foot can be used to simulate normal gait. As the athlete lands on the prosthetic limb energy is stored and released back on push-off much in the same way as the normal achilles tendon would. Computer-controlled knees for above knee amputees can produce automatic swing-phase adjustments relevant to their activity level.

Classification

To enable athletes to compete 'on a level playing' field athletes are classified into groups for competition. In some sports this is disability-specific groups e.g. cerebral palsy or spinal injury. In others, such as swimming, a functional classification system is used so swimmers with different disabilities compete against each other based upon physical disability and functional performance of the sport. The process is not always straight-forward and many medical tests are open to subjective interpretation. Classification for intellectual disability has been based upon IQ assessment and has been open to abuse in the past. For example, the Spanish basketball team in the Sydney Paralympic Games were subsequently found to have no disability and their gold medals were later removed. Intellectual disability athletes have been suspended from Paralympic Games until a more rigorous classification system has been introduced. There are 'minimum disability' criteria within a sport for a person to become eligible to participate in competitive sport. There is nothing to stop able-bodied people taking part in recreational activities e.g. basketball.

Disability groups

Spinal cord related disability

This may be congenital e.g. spina bifida, or acquired e.g. trauma or disease. Of the spinally injured 60% are in the 16–30 age group with a male to female ratio of 4:1. The majority of these are from road traffic accidents with about 15% occurring in sport. Common activities include diving, rugby, horse riding, and skiing. The injuries can be divided by the level of neurological loss and whether the lesion is complete or partial (incomplete paralysis).

The spinal injury results in a number of problems:
- Motor loss—loss of muscle function relating to the level of injury.
- Sensory loss—increasing the risk of pressure sore.
- Loss of autonomic control e.g. sweating affecting thermoregulation (see later).
- Effects on cardiac function in exercise—sympathectomized myocardium in higher spinal lesions gives reduced HR max of 110–130 beats/min. There is limited:
  - Cardio-acceleration.
  - Myocardial contractility.
  - Stroke volume.
  - Cardiac output.
- Respiratory function—loss of intercostal muscle function.
- Recurrent urinary tract infection from a neuropathic bladder.

Amputee or limb deficiency

This may be congenital e.g. developmental or acquired. Acquired lesions are usually due to:
- Disease e.g. tumour, vascular disease.
- Trauma—RTA, workplace injury.

An athlete with a limb deficiency may compete:
1. With a prosthesis e.g. running.
2. Without a prosthesis e.g. swimming, high jump.
3. In a wheelchair e.g. tennis, basketball.

The fitting and alignment of the prosthesis is important for both function and reducing the risk of musculoskeletal injury. Impact injury or skin chafing of the residual limb are common problems. The leg length discrepancy necessary to allow the toe of the prosthetic limb to clear the ground on swing through may cause problems further up the kinetic chain producing hip, pelvic, or back pain.

Cerebral palsy

Cerebral palsy is a group of disorders affecting body movement and muscle coordination, and is due to an insult or anomaly of the developing brain. Any damage to the developing brain, whether caused by genetic or developmental disorders, injury, or disease may result in cerebral palsy. Cerebral palsy may be classified according to the number of limbs affected (see Fig. 19.1) and/or by the type of movement disorder.

- Spastic cerebral palsy—is the most common type and is caused by damage to the motor cortex. Spastic muscles are tight and stiff, which limit movement.
- Choreo-athetoid cerebral palsy—results from damage to the basal ganglia or cerebellum and leads to difficulty in controlling and coordinating movement.
- Mixed-type cerebral palsy—when areas of the brain affecting both muscle tone and voluntary movement are affected.

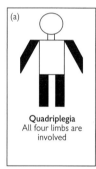

(a)

Quadriplegia
All four limbs are involved

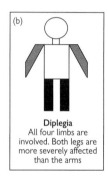

(b)

Diplegia
All four limbs are involved. Both legs are more severely affected than the arms

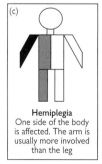

(c)

Hemiplegia
One side of the body is affected. The arm is usually more involved than the leg

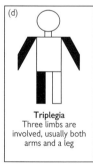

(d)

Triplegia
Three limbs are involved, usually both arms and a leg

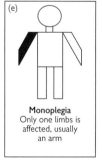

(e)

Monoplegia
Only one limbs is affected, usually an arm

Fig. 19.1 Classification of cerebral palsy.

The classifications of movement disorder and number of limbs involved are usually combined (e.g. spastic diplegia). Athletes with CP may also commonly have associated problems:

- Epilepsy
- Visual defects
- Deafness
- Intellectual impairment.

Approximately half of athletes with CP compete in wheelchairs. The spasticity associated with the condition may be important for function, and without that tone the athlete may not be able to stabilize their trunk. Hence the normal practice of stretching pre-exercise may not be appropriate for all athletes with CP. Maintaining range of movement with flexibility exercises is important, but may have to done away from the competitive environment.

Visually impaired

Visually impaired athletes are classified by ophthalmology examination and the classification reflects both visual acuity and field of vision.

- Class B1—total absence of perception of light in both eyes, or some perception of the light but with inability to recognize the form of a hand at any distance and in any direction.
- Class B2—from the ability to recognize the form of a hand to a visual acuity of 2/60 and/or a visual field of less than 5 degrees.
- Class B3—from a visual acuity of above 2/60 to a visual acuity of 6/60 and/or a visual field or more than 5 degrees and less than 20 degrees.

All classifications must be made by measuring the best eye and to the highest possible correction. This means that all athletes who use contact lenses or correcting glasses normally must wear them during classification, whether or not they intend to use them during competition.

Sports for the visually impaired include athletics, judo, and swimming. In cycling a sighted pilot rider is used on a tandem. Guide runners may be used in athletics where a tie or band is used to link a sighted runner to the athlete. The guide runner cannot run in advance of the athlete and 'pull' them along; doing so brings disqualification for the athlete. In biathlon the skier will follow a guide skier and use a rifle that produces a high tone when aimed at the centre of the target for the shooting component of the event. Injuries in visually impaired athletes often occur following falls, collisions, or misplaced footing.

Les autres

This group encompasses a variety of physical disabilities that does not fit easily within a specific category and encompasses a number of conditions such as:

- Congenital disorders—e.g. spondyloepiphyseal dysplasia, Stickler syndrome.
- Limb deficiencies.
- Muscular dystrophies.
- Multiple sclerosis.
- Arthritis of major joints.

The variety of conditions and in particular the variety of rare syndromes encountered in disability sport makes care of these athletes a challenge for the physician.

Intellectual disability

These athletes are largely able-bodied unless the disability results from e.g. a head injury where there may be physical changes also. As such, they are susceptible to the same sport related injuries as able-bodied athletes. However, the challenge for the treating doctor is in taking the history and then explaining the diagnosis and management of the condition and supervizing the rehabilitation. Training errors are more common and correcting technical problems may be more difficult. Athletes with an intellectual disability may be over keen to please their coach in training and may be susceptible to abusive practices. The duty of care issues are important with these athletes.

Elite sport talent identification and profiling

In able-bodied sport there is a large body of scientific evidence, and profiles of the physical characteristics of the elite athlete help identify the future champions by talent identification. Although elite disability sport is gaining more credibility worldwide, there is still a shortage of research and documentation of these athletes' performance capabilities that makes talent identification and profiling more difficult. This is compounded by:

- Multiple disability groups that may take part within a single sport.
- Wide range of abilities within the same disability e.g. different levels of spinal injury.
- Different physiological responses to exercise e.g. paraplegics vs quadriplegics.
- More research exists for rehabilitation and/or exercise therapy rather than performance-related sport.
- Limited exposure to good quality coaching.

Injury issues

The literature is limited in data on the epidemiology of injuries in disability sport but it is clear there are different aspects:

- Sport-specific injuries similar to able-bodied athletes e.g. shoulder injures in swimmers or throwers.
- Disability sport-related injuries to technical or training factors—wrist injuries from repetitive pushing of the chair e.g. causing nerve compression injuries.
- Disability related injuries—e.g. existing spinal injury aggravated by repetitive strain of training, skin abrasions from rubbing of the chair on skin without pain sensation, osteoporotic fractures from minimal trauma.

Thermoregulation

The spinally-injured athlete has impaired thermoregulation which may impair performance or increase the risk of heat illness. There are several factors contributing to this:

- Loss of peripheral receptor mechanism function.
- Loss of autonomic control on the sweating effector mechanism.
- Loss of control of the ability to appropriately vasoconstrict or vasodilate the peripheral vasculature.

Cold conditions may also adversely affect the spinally-injured athlete—as there is impaired perception of temperature the athlete can become hypothermic without feeling symptoms before an adverse reaction occurs. Precautions regarding wearing appropriate clothing should be taken and a vigilance to consider the possibility of hypothermia developing.

Travel issues

The international nature of disability sport now means that many athletes will face long-haul travel on a regular basis. In addition to the problems of travel fatigue, deep vein thrombosis, and jet lag there can be additional problems that can occur of which the accompanying physician should be aware:

- Skin breakdown of skin pressure areas—prolonged sitting in airline seats.
- Dehydration—increasing the risk of exacerbations of urinary tract infections.
- Dependent oedema—occurs frequently in long haul travel but is worse when there is no active muscle pump.
- DVT—there is no evidence that the incidence of DVT is increased for someone with a disability than an able-bodied person.
- Autonomic dysreflexia—is an exaggerated autonomic response caused by a painful stimulus below the level of the spinal lesion, resulting in high blood pressure that occurs in people with high spinal cord injuries (thoracic level 6 and above). It can cause seizures, cerebral haemorrhage, and death. The stimulus may come from prolonged seating in an uncomfortable position and may occur during travel.
- Medications—the timing of taking medications e.g. anticonvulsants needs to be assessed for athletes crossing multiple time zones.

'Boosting'

Some athletes have intentionally induced the state of autonomic dysreflexia as they found that they had reduced perception of effort during exercise, allowing them to push harder and faster than otherwise. Methods to induce this state may include applying tight straps to the legs or clamping the urinary catheter to distend the bladder. Because of the medical dangers of inducing this response it was originally banned as a 'doping method' by the IPC but is deemed to be a medical safety issue rather than doping. Athletes can have their blood pressure taken during the pre-race period and may be withdrawn from competition if the pressure is above 180mmHg systolic on the grounds of medical safety.

Doping issues

The IPC is a signatory of the world anti-doping code and, as such, the list of substances prohibited by the code are the same as for able-bodied athletes. Athletes with disabilities are more likely to be taking medications for medical conditions as a result of their disability, but the same rules apply for therapeutic use exemption (TUE) where an athlete can apply to take medication on the prohibited list for a specific reason. TUE requires that:

1. The athlete would experience a significant impairment in health if the substance were withdrawn.
2. The substance would produce no additional enhancement of performance.
3. There is no reasonable therapeutic alternative.

Other differences in doping regulations or procedures include:

- Unlike the IOC, the IPC does not require spirometric evidence of asthma for use of beta2 agonists for asthma.
- Sample collection procedures differ where catheter or condom/leg bag urine collection is used.
- Visually impaired and intellectually impaired athletes need to be accompanied by a representative during the procedure.

Useful resources and further reading

International Paralympic Committee—*www.paralympics.org*
CISS—Comité International Sports des Sourds—*www.ciss.org*
CP-ISRA—Cerebral Palsy International Sport and Recreation Association—*www.cpisra.org*
IBSA—International Blind Sport Federation—*www.ibsa.es*
INAS-FID International Sports Federation for Persons with Intellectual Disability—*www.inas-fid.org*
Fallon KE. (1995). The disabled athlete. In *Science and medicine in sport*. Bloomfield J, Fricker PA, and Fitch KD, eds pp.550–551. Blackwell Science, Carlton.
Webborn, ADJ. (2001) Sports in children with physical disabilities/Medical problems of disabled child athletes. In *Sports medicine for specific ages and abilities*. Churchill Livingstone.

Physiology

What happens when we exercise?

The individual response to exercise depends on a number of factors:
- Type of exercise stress encountered.
- Level of training/conditioning/nutritional and hydration status.
- Age/gender/body type/muscle fibre type ratios.
- Genetic factors and environmental conditions.
- Psychological factors.

Physiological responses to exercise stress will vary according to the factors mentioned above. The complex interactions of the body's homeostatic mechanisms and responses can be briefly summarized in a time line:

Short-term—seconds to minutes (stress reaction)

- *Autonomic nervous system response*: sympathetic increase with parasympathetic decrease resulting in the fight or flight response and reduced vegetative functions.
- *Cardiovascular responses*: increased cardiac output to exercising muscles and reduced blood flow to other organ systems. As core temperature increases there is increased blood flow to the skin for thermoregulation.
- *Respiratory responses*: increased rate and depth of respiration to meet demands for gas exchange.
- *Metabolic and respiratory responses*: buffering of lactic acid produced by the active muscles.

Medium-term—minutes to hours (resistance reaction)

- *Hormonal* responses: accentuate and prolong the autonomic neural responses (above); release of catecholamines from the adrenal medulla, ACTH and GH from the pituitary with increased substrate availability for energy metabolism to provide fuel for longer duration exercise. Activation of the renin angiotensin and ADH mechanisms help preserve fluid and electrolyte balance and maintain blood pressure.

Long-term—days to weeks (adaptation)

- Repeated acute bouts of exercise (training) will result in adaptation to the exercise stimulus. Adaptation results from gene activation in various tissues under stress. Cellular structural changes in muscle and other tissues result in strength and endurance changes, changes in neural regulation optimize muscle activation patterns, and renal mechanisms are probably responsible for cardiovascular responses to training through changes in plasma volume and venous return.

Clinical note: overtraining syndrome in athletes is defined by under-performance, and characterized by fatigue, physiological and psychological changes. It has been suggested that this is a maladaptive alternative third stage of adaptation. Long term, such a state may be useful, as a protective physiological mechanism preventing damage from further over-exercise when individual athletes train beyond the limits of physiological compensation.

Components of fitness

Stamina (aerobic conditioning, aerobic power)

All types of exercise require a base level of aerobic conditioning. High levels of aerobic conditioning enable more efficient use of fuel, greater tolerance of environmental extremes, quicker recovery during intermittent exercise and between training sessions, and are essential for long-term cardiovascular health. Important factors are: the hearts ability to pump blood (Q) and muscle extraction and utilization of fuels and oxygen (a-vO$_2$ diff).

Speed and strength (anaerobic power)

Sprint speed, mass of a weight lifted, or the distance of a throw depends on the maximum force that a muscle can exert. Muscle forces depend on body size and type, biomechanics, muscle crossectional area, predominant fibre type, and rate of ATP re-synthesis. Generally the greater the muscle mass the more speed, force, or power that can be generated.

Skill (neuromuscular coordination)

Skills are coordinated neuromuscular patterns of activation, which increase efficiency, speed, and ease of movement. In neurological terms, highly developed skills are implemented subconsciously which involve much quicker neural pathways. Skills can be innate or learned, optimum acquisition is age dependent (9–12yr) with good training practices and high quality coaching.

Suppleness (flexibility)

Flexibility or suppleness is the ability to move a joint through its full range of normal movement. It depends on joint type, joint surface congruity, and tension in capsules, ligaments, and muscles. When a joint is forced outside its normal working range by external forces, greater flexibility may be protective against injury.

Psychology (mental fitness)

When the physiological components of fitness have been optimized, psychological factors become more important. They may be the difference between success and failure at elite level. Mental strength, like skill, may be innate in some individuals, but aspects of psychological preparation can be learned and should be practiced all year round as part of normal training. These include motivation to compete and train, goal setting, mental rehearsal of performance, pre-competition routines to manage anxiety. Coping strategies for success, failure, and injury are all important areas for professional athletes.

Energy for exercise

- Exercise is powered by the high energy phosphate molecule adenosine triphosphate (ATP). Resting cellular energy processes provide a small amount of ATP for normal cellular homeostatic systems. In muscle cells ATP also powers contractile elements, and has to be regenerated rapidly for high-intensity exercise and steadily for long-term exercise. The relative contributions of different energy systems depend on exercise duration, intensity, and individual fitness.

Impulse energy (high energy phosphates/anaerobic)

The small quantity of energy (ATP) present in the cell at rest can provide the initial impetus for a throw, a jump, a punch, a serve in tennis, or the initial reaction off the blocks in a sprint. ATP must be rapidly regenerated if high-intensity exercise is to continue.

Immediate energy (high energy phosphates/anaerobic)

$$CP \rightarrow Creatine + Pi + energy \rightarrow ADP + Pi \rightarrow ATP$$

The phospho-creatine system or ATP-PCR system prevents short-term ATP depletion without the need for oxygen. Phosphate molecules are shuttled from Creatine Phosphate to ADP regenerating ATP rapidly. High energy phosphates can power all out maximum efforts for ~6–7 seconds, after which time high rates of ATP regeneration have to be maintained by metabolism of fuels. Sprint and resistance training, predominance of fast twitch fibres replete with creatine stores (eat more red meat and oily red fish or creatine supplementation) are all factors which optimise function of this system.

Short-term energy (anaerobic glycolysis)

The breakdown of carbohydrate stores or glucose anaerobically yields a small amount of ATP rapidly (substrate phosphorylation).
Glycogen or Glucose $\rightarrow$ Pyruvic Acid $\Leftrightarrow$ Lactic acid $\Leftrightarrow$ Lactate + H+
Its advantage is a high rate of ATP production which can power high-intensity exercise for short periods. Disadvantages are, only small amounts of ATP are generated from fuel stores, it is relatively fast to fatigue, and the end product, pyruvate, is converted to lactic acid. Lactic acid dissociates, the hydrogen ion is buffered and lactate passes out of cell where it is taken up by less active tissues and metabolized aerobically.

In healthy untrained subjects significant blood lactate (BLa) accumulation occurs at ~55% of VO_2 max. In endurance trained athletes significant BLa accumulation does not occur until ~85% of VO_2 max. A shift to anaerobic glycolysis and increased BLa is caused by increased exercise intensity, relative tissue hypoxia, and selection of fast twitch muscle fibres.

ATP-PCR and anaerobic glycolytic systems are the predominant systems for intense exercise lasting from 30–45 seconds to 2 min: e.g. 400m run, 200m swim, or repeated sprints required during field sports. A favourable ratio of fast to slow twitch fibres, correct training methods, and nutritional factors (high creatine level and CHO stores) will optimize function of this energy system.

Long-term energy (oxidative phosphorylation/aerobic)

Prolonged or sustained activity requires metabolism with oxygen and greater energy yield. Breakdown of carbohydrate and free fatty acids (FFA) to produce ATP aerobically also requires the enzymes and cofactors of Krebs cycle, and oxidative phosphorylation present in the mitochondria.

Glucose fully metabolised aerobically yields ~38 moles ATP and glycogen ~39 moles. However, carbohydrate fuel stores are limited and although the rate of energy production is higher than for fat, stores can be exhausted, and must be replenished during endurance activity to avoid depletion or 'hitting the wall'. The energy available from FFA depends on the number of carbon atoms in the chain. E.g. palmitic acid generates 129 moles ATP. There is abundant energy supply and a high yield of ATP, but the disadvantage of fat metabolism is a slower rate of ATP synthesis, and that it requires more O_2 than CHO oxidation. Aerobic metabolism of FFA begins in the Krebs cycle; acetyl co A from glycolysis combines with CH_2 units of FFA. Fat is said to 'burn on a carbohydrate flame'. Aerobic metabolism requires capillaries for delivery of oxygen and fuel, mitochondria, adequate levels of co-factors (NAD/FAD), myoglobin, and glycogen stores to keep Krebs cycle turning.

Factors affecting oxidative capacity

- Environmental effects on PO_2 (altitude or depth).
- Respiratory function (air pollution, bronchoconstriction).
- Oxygen transport (anaemia), delivery (heart disease).
- Extraction of O_2 and fuel (capillary density & myoglobin).
- Predominant muscle fibre types (ST, FOG, FT).
- Speed of utilization of fuel and oxygen (No./size of mitochondria, oxidative enzyme activity, stores/availability of co-factors and fuel).

Muscle function

Muscle function produces force across joints, and this force may provide:
- Primary forces for movement (concentric shortening actions).
- Stabilizing forces (isotonic/isometric static contractions).
- Decelerating movement (eccentric elongating action).
- A combination of all of the above in order to absorb externally applied forces.

The magnitude and direction of the resultant force across a joint depends on the type of contraction, biomechanical effects of joint morphology (articular surfaces), static restraints (ligaments), and dynamic restraints (tendons).

Slow twitch fibres (ST)

Slowly fatiguing aerobic endurance fibres (red), have glycolytic enzyme systems, numerous mitochondria (Krebs cycle and electron transport chain), and small stores of glycogen. They require delivery of FFAs and oxygen (capillarization/myoglobin) for longer term energy production. If provided with constant fuel (FFA or glucose) and oxygen supply, they are slow to fatigue, have low contraction speed, low unit strength, and high number of fibres per motor neuron.

Fast oxidative/glycolytic fibres (FOG/FT_a)

An intermediate fibre type with a mixture of anaerobic and aerobic energy systems. Depending on the training stimulus they may function like ST or anaerobic FT_b fibres.

Fast twitch fibres (FT_b)

Speed and strength fibres (white) with highly developed cytoplasmic anaerobic energy systems: creatine kinase and glycolytic enzymes, stored energy (creatine phosphate), and glycogen fuel stores available for rapid turnover. Oxygen is not required for energy production, and they possess mechanisms to transport and buffer lactic acid, and regenerate creatine phosphate in a small number of mitochondria.

Skeletal muscle actions

- Strength is the force a muscle or group of muscles can generate, and is assessed by a one or three repetition maximum (1 or 3RM). This is the heaviest weight that can be lifted once (1RM) or, in those using resistance training for general conditioning, a three repetition maximum (3RM) is safer.
- Power [(force x distance)/time] is the functional aspect of muscle actions. In most sports it is a combination of strength and speed of movement.
- Muscular endurance is the ability to sustain repeated muscle actions or maintain a single contraction at a given force over a longer duration. It is assessed by counting the number of repetitions possible at any given % of the 1RM or 3RM.

Cardiovascular responses to exercise and training

Structure

- Fluid transport (blood) and central pump (heart).
- Distribution (pulmonary arteries/aorta/arteries/arterioles).
- Exchange (capillaries).
- Collection/return (pulmonary veins/venules/veins).
- Interstitial fluids return system (lymphatics).

Function

- Delivery/removal—*oxygen and nutrients*—*CO_2 and waste products.*
- Transport/immunity—*hormones*—*antibodies and complement.*
- Homeostasis—*temperature, acid/base, fluid/electrolyte balance.*

The system provides constant flow of blood through the exchange vessels (capillaries) to meet tissue demand. At rest ~5% blood volume goes to muscle capillaries rising to ~20–25% blood volume at maximum exercise. Cardiovascular system changes in response to acute bouts of exercise include increased cardiac work, alteration in arteriolar tone, and homeostatic mechanisms which maintain circulating volume and blood pressure. Cardiovascular system changes in part determine the limits of exercise capacity, and adaptation of these responses determine the response to training.

Response to exercise

- Muscle activity creates metabolites, a fall in local tissue PO_2, and a rise in PCO_2. These factors cause capillary beds to open.
- The sympathetic nervous system alters arteriolar tone with a reduction in blood flow to non-essential organs.
- Increased CO and TPR lead to increased blood pressure, which maintains the pressure head driving blood to the active muscles.
- Increased blood flow provides fuel and oxygen, and removes waste products.
- Skin capillaries dilate and the sweat rate increases to dissipate heat.
- Changes in cardiac output and venous tone adjust for sweat losses.
- Fluid and electrolyte homeostatic mechanisms maintain blood volume (ADH) and pressure (renin/angiotensin).

Response to training (at least 3/12 months for significant changes)

- Increase in muscle capillary density leads to increased extraction of O_2 and fuel.
- Increased blood flow to muscle and skin (better arteriolar control).
- Improved heart efficiency (increase in stroke volume and reduced heart rate maintaining the same cardiac output).
- Increased control of skin blood flow with a more efficient thermoregulatory response.
- An increased plasma volume, relative to increased red blood cell production—often leading to pseudo-anaemia.

Respiratory responses to exercise and training

Structure
- Ventilatory mechanism:
  - *Chest wall*: ribs and intercostal muscles.
  - *Pleural cavity*: parietal and visceral layers.
  - *Respiratory muscles*: diaphragm/intercostals.
- Airway: nose/larynx/trachea/bronchi/bronchioles/alveolar ducts.
- Gas exchange: alveoli/pulmonary capillaries.

Function
- Air Movement: pulmonary (V_E) and alveolar (V_A) ventilation.
- Gas exchange: lung ↔ blood ↔ lung.
- Transport of O_2 and CO_2 (CVS).
- Gas exchange: blood ↔ tissues.
- (1 and 2 = external respiration   4 = internal respiration).

Mechanics of ventilation
The lungs lie in the pleural cavity invested in visceral pleura, a small amount of fluid within the pleural space separates the visceral pleura and lung from the parietal layer lining the inner chest wall.

There are two opposing forces acting on the pleural space; (1) elastic recoil of chest wall (ribs and intercostals) acting outwards, and (2) elastic recoil of lung tissue acting inwards. The result is a slight negative intra-pleural pressure which keeps the lung expanded against the inner chest wall. Additional movement of the chest wall therefore, causes small intrapleural and intrapulmonary pressure changes (2–3mmHg), enough to draw air in or expel air from the lungs.

Inspiration is achieved by muscular contraction of the scaleni, external intercostals and diaphragm. Expiration: at rest is a passive action due to elastic recoil of stretched lung tissue, in forced expiration the intercostals and abdominals assist with expulsive effort.

Clinical note: Valsalva manoeuvre; a forced expiration against a closed glottis, increases intrathoracic and intraabdominal pressure, assisting abdominal and back muscles in stabilizing the trunk before heavy lifting. However, during very heavy lifting, increase in intrapulmonary pressure can cause rapid increase in blood pressure, accentuated baroreceptor responses cause a reflex fall in HR, cardiac output is reduced. Clinically this is manifest by dizziness, syncope, and occasional collapse in weightlifters.

Static and dyanamic lung volume measures
The ability to move air in and out of the lungs depends on 2 factors:
- Resistance to airflow in bronchi (proportional to 4th power of radius).
- Resistance of lung tissue to a change in volume (compliance).

Assessments of lung function can measure volume of air, speed of air movement, volume of air moved per unit time, and peak rates of airflow.

Clinical note: objective evidence of a fall in FEV_1 (>10%) is now required for athletes on medications for asthma or EIB. Standard provocation procedures are; exercise of 8–10 minutes duration at 85% of HR max or 6 minutes of eucapnic hyperventilation maintaining V_E at 30 times resting FEV_1. FEV_1 is measured pre, and at 5, 10, 15, and 30 minutes post-exercise or EVH challenge.

Effects of training

There are no differences between the lungs of athletes and the normal population of similar gender, size, and stature. Athletes may wrongly think that static and dynamic lung volumes should be greater than the healthy untrained, and often equate a high FVC value with aerobic endurance capacity. Static lung volumes are genetically determined and in general do not change with training, with the exception of upper body sports like swimming, where muscular development in the chest wall is thought to increase thoracic wall dimensions. However, training does improve ventilatory endurance and endurance trained athletes have a greater ability to sustain ventilation at submaximal workloads, reduced lactate production in respiratory musculature, and report less subjective feelings of breathlessness on exercise. Training makes the work of breathing more efficient.

Pulmonary ventilation (VE) in exercise

Minute ventilation (V_E) is the product of respiratory rate and tidal volume. With a respiratory rate (RR) of 12/min × tidal volume (TV) of 0.5L/breath, the V_E at rest is about 6 litres. With exercise the (RR) increases to 60–70/min and tidal volume can increase to 2.0–3.0L/min, so that at the end of exercise V_E may reach 100L/min in the untrained, 160L/min in the trained, and can exceed 200L/min in highly trained athletes.

Effect of training on ventilation

Training shifts the respiratory responses to exercise by favouring depth of respiration rather than rate, which is much more efficient in energy costs of breathing. Adjustment by alteration of the rate and depth of breathing to meet physiological demands of exercise is exquisitely well controlled. Attempts at readjustment of the rate and depth by entrained breathing are usually futile. At rest and during exercise athletes should be encouraged to breathe naturally.

Gas exchange

Gas exchange is dependent on solubility of gases (CO_2) and their partial pressure gradients. The alveoli provide a large surface area for gas exchange, lungs of mean volume ≈4–6L, contain approximately 300 million thin/elastic walled alveoli, and have a large surface area ≈½ a tennis court!

Approximately 250–300mL of blood is available for gas exchange in the pulmonary capillaries, at rest: 250mL O_2 passes from the alveoli to the capillary and 200mL CO_2 passes from the capillary to the alveoli. On exercise, gas exchange increases 20 fold.

Gas exchange in the lung during exercise

Efficient gas exchange also requires effective matching of blood flow and aeration of the alveoli. In healthy lungs at rest perfusion/aeration mismatch has a negligible effect, and during exercise, opening of upper lobe capillaries and better ventilation of lower lobe alveoli ensure that effects of physiological dead space on gas exchange are minimal or non-existent in most circumstances. The normal lung therefore has more than enough capacity for gas exchange to meet the demands of exercise.

At the alveolar/capillary interface PaO_2 falls little below 100mmHg at maximal exercise and there is little change in $PaCO_2$ (40mmHg). Although at max exercise pulmonary blood flow increases by 50%, opening of many more pulmonary capillaries ensures adequate gas exchange down diffusion gradients. Ventilation is adjusted to maintain alveolar partial pressures of O_2 and CO_2 according to metabolic requirements.

Oxygen transport

Oxygen is predominantly transported bound to the oxygen-carrying pigment haemaglobin, and a small amount is dissolved in plasma. Although O_2 solubility in plasma is very low at 0.3mL O_2 per 100mL plasma, physiologically it is very important as it determines the PO_2 of blood and tissue fluids, in part determines regulation of breathing, and greatly influences O_2 binding to haemaglobin in the lungs and offloading from haemaglobin in the active muscles.

Haemaglobin

Iron-containing pigment inside RBC, increases oxygen-carrying capacity of blood by 60–70 times. Haemaglobin levels; male ~15g/dL, female ~14g/dL. 100mL blood carries 20mL O_2 (19.7mL $O_2 \rightarrow$ Hb + 0.3mL $O_2 \rightarrow$ plasma).

Oxygen binding to Hb is dependent on oxygen dissolved in solution (PO_2).

The PO_2 of alveolar air of 103mmHg fully saturates haemoglobin in blood leaving the lungs. No further change in O_2 saturation of Hb occurs until blood reaches the active tissues where PO_2 falls to <60mmHg and oxygen affinity for Hb drops sharply. PO_2 reduction in active muscle can drop further to 40mmHg as Hb offloads oxygen. Endurance athletes should ensure adequate dietary sources of iron, check iron stores annually (serum ferritin) and should not donate within 6 weeks of important competitions.

Myoglobin

Fe-containing protein found in cardiac and skeletal muscle, facilitates O_2 transfer to mitochondria, especially in early and intense exercise. Myoglobin has a greater affinity for O_2 at lower partial pressures than Hb (myoglobin 95% saturated at PO_2 40mmHg). When tissue PO_2 is less than 5mmHg, myoglobin offloads greatly. Training increases myoglobin levels in slow twitch fibres in $\propto$ to amount of physical activity.

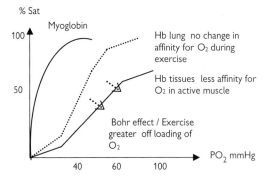

Fig. 20.1

Arterio-venous difference (a-vO$_2$ diff)

At rest~5 mL, i.e. 15mL O$_2$ remains attached to Hb on venous side of capillary, during exercise with ↑metabolic demand for O$_2$ tissue PO$_2$ falls lower, greater offloading of O$_2$ from Hb occurs and greater extraction and utilization by the active muscle is such that (a-vO$_2$) diff → ↑10mL in moderate exercise and → ↑20mL at max. Experimentally after exhaustive exercise, blood taken from the venous side of large muscle groups may contain no oxygen at all.

Oxygen uptake and lactate threshold

Oxygen consumption (VO_2) is the product of cardiac output (Q) and arterio-venous oxygen difference (a-vO_2 diff). VO_2 and associated metabolic variables can now be assessed using on-line cardiopulmonary metabolic carts, with in-built analysers measuring expired gas concentrations on a breath-by-breath basis.

Maximal oxygen uptake (VO_2 max) is a quantitative measure of the ability of lungs to extract O_2 from pulmonary gases, the circulatory system to transport O_2 to the tissues in solution and bound to haemoglobin, and the capacity of exercising tissues to extract and use O_2 in ATP regenerating processes. It is largely a genetic trait. VO_2 max is measured during a graded incremental test to volitional exhaustion, and expressed in $mL.kg^{-1}.min^{-1}$ or alternatively in $L.min^{-1}$ at standard temperature and pressure for a dry gas (STPD). The velocity or load attained by aerobic metabolism is strongly related to an athlete's lactate profile during an incremental exercise test. This lactate profile, together with cardiovascular and metabolic data, is used to design individual training programmes and monitor performance across training cycles.

- Population VO_2 max range from 20–90$mL.kg^{-1}.min^{-1}$, with highest values recorded in endurance trained athletic populations.
- VO_2 max decreases with age and physical inactivity, and is generally higher in males.
- Training can improve VO_2 max by between 5–25%, and the capacity for improvement is dependent on initial fitness level, training frequency, training intensity and duration, and again genetic factors.
- Higher VO_2 max does not necessarily confer competition success. Even among elite athletes with quite similar performance times, VO_2 max can vary significantly.
- Performance differences, despite similar VO_2 max values, are due to better economy of effort. A measure of the efficiency of O_2 utilization and velocity ($mL.kg^{-1}.m^{-1}$) for runners or O_2 utilisation and load ($mL.kg^{-1}.W^{-1}$) for cyclists and rowers, both sub-maximally and at VO_2 max, are important when analysing performance.

Aerobic-anaerobic threshold (TLac)

The aerobic–anaerobic threshold is highly related to performance in endurance events, and is a far better marker of endurance capacity than the traditional 'gold standard' VO_2 max. TLac data provides relevant guidelines for exercise prescription, and with appropriate training the threshold can increase despite little or no change in VO_2 max. Blood lactate accumulation during incremental exercise testing is therefore frequently used to define appropriate training intensities, evaluate the effectiveness of training programmes and predict performance in endurance events by identifying deflection points or transition thresholds on blood lactate versus load/velocity profiles.

Blood lactate concentration (BLa) mirrors muscle lactate and indicates equilibrium between rate of production and utilization. Numerous

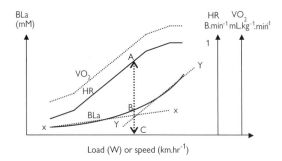

Fig. 20.2 Extrapolation of HR and load or speed at Tlac from an incremental test data plot for an endurance athlete. Intersecting lines XX and YY are drawn through 2 points on the lactate curve below and above lactate threshold respectively. The point of intersection is then used to derive; heart rate at TLac (A), usually 80–90% of HR max; BLa at TLac (B), usually 2–2.5mM; and Load or Speed at TLac (C).

definitions and analytical models are used to assess workload at Tlac, including fixed lactate concentrations (2 and 4mmol.L^{-1}), fixed increases above resting data, maximal lactate steady state models, exponential and logarithmic models, graphical, tangential, and maximum displacement (Dmax) models. Most of these models identify the same transition points: the workload or velocity where there is a sustained increase in BLa- above resting data (generally at BLa > 2mmol.L^{-1}). This part of the BLa response curve to exercise reflects a shift from primarily oxidative to combined oxidative and glycolytic metabolism (BLa 2.5–5.5mmol.L^{-1}).

BLa concentrations are affected by training, recovery, and nutritional status and therefore individualised thresholds are deemed more appropriate. A graphical approach to interpolation of TLac is shown in the schematic figure of endurance performance to a standard laboratory- based incremental test to volitional exhaustion below.

Respiratory-derived anaerobic threshold

Minute ventilation (V_E) increases disproportionately during exercise due to buffering of H+ ions (produced by lactic acid dissociation) by bicarbonate, leading to excess VCO_2. This produces a non-linear increase in V_E relative to VO_2. Ventilatory thresholds are easier to detect using short rapid incremental protocols (40W.min^{-1}), when V_E is plotted as a function of VO_2, the initial non-linear increase (at ~50%VO_2 max) in V_E represents the aerobic threshold, and a second non-linear increase (at ~85% VO_2 max) in V_E represents the anaerobic threshold.

Measuring exercise capacity

Laboratory-based assessment

The purposes of laboratory-based physiological testing include:

- Opportunities for pre-season health check.
- Identification of strengths and weaknesses.
- Design of individualized training programmes.
- Evaluation of effectiveness of the training programme.
- Athlete education (nutrition, hydration, self-monitoring, and assessment).

Sport-specific testing

- The type of ergometer used and variables tested must be relevant to athlete's sport.
- Test protocols used must be highly sport-specific and relevant to the phase of the athlete's season.
- The variables tested must be sufficiently sensitive to infer training-induced adaptations, and data collection methods must be valid, reproducible, and reliable.
- Assessments should be repeated at regular intervals (3–4 months) under identical test conditions, and where possible sub-maximal and maximal field-based self-assessments should be performed at monthly intervals.

Pre-test nutrition, hydration, rest, and exercise performed in previous 24 hours should be strictly controlled and the test administration itself should be carried out by experienced personnel. Test equipment must be regularly calibrated with daily quality control logs maintained to account for equipment variation over time. The athlete's rights should be respected; all test data are treated confidentially, with hard copies and electronic test data storage inline with standard medico-legal recommendations. All test results should be presented and interpreted to the athlete and their coach (if possible) immediately on completion of testing.

Laboratory testing may include the following assessments

- Anthropometric measurement of height, body mass, body composition, % body fat (skinfold thickness technique), and estimation of lean body mass (kg) and body mass index ($kg.m^{-2}$).
- Pulmonary function tests to rule-out pre-exercise respiratory limitation and post-exercise induced broncho-constriction.
- Haematology screen to rule-out sub-clinical infection, anaemia, and dehydration prior to exercise.

Measured variables assessed depend on the athlete's sport and phase of training and competition and may include

- Aerobic assessment to test endurance capacity using either a graded incremental test or a time to exhaustion test at fixed % of VO_2 max or maximum capacity.
- Anaerobic tests of anaerobic power and capacity.

- Strength tests to assess gains induced by resistance training regimens and/or to assess for correction of muscle imbalance.

Anthropometric measurement

Stature

(Height in m) three general techniques: freestanding, stretch (removes the minor effects of daily gravitational compression), and recumbent (used in infants and adults unable to stand). Note: stature in any individual can vary by up to 10mm over the course of the day as fluid is extruded from the intervertebral discs. A wall-mounted stadiometer (measurement range 600–2100mm), can be used for freestanding and stretch methods—the subject stands feet together with heels, buttocks, and upper back touching the scale, head in the Frankfort plane (orbitale in a horizontal plane with the tragion). In the stretch technique the subject inhales maximally while maintaining the head in the Frankfort plane.

Body mass

Measured with a calibrated beam balance (accuracy 0.1kg), assess mass in minimal clothing. Body mass typically exhibits diurnal variation, normally assessed after fasting overnight state and after voiding.

Body mass index

(Units $kg.m^{-2}$), normal range 20–25$kg.m^{-2}$, assessed from height and body mass by formula: BMI ($kg.m^{-2}$) = mass (kg)/height^2 (m^2). Surface area, assessed from height and body mass using a nomogram or by formula: surface area (m^2) = 0.0072 × (mass (kg) × 0.425) × (height (cm) × 0.725). Lean body mass calculated from body mass and estimated fat mass. Lean body mass (kg) = [mass − ((mass × %fat)/100)].

Waist to hip ratio

(Reference data, female 0.7, male 0.8), waist measurement at the level of the umbilicus, hip measurement at the level of the greater trochanter. This ratio is an important predictor of future cardiovascular disease.

Body fat

Skinfold techniques are the most commonly used by most exercise physiologists to estimate % body fat, bioelectrical impedance testing is prone to measurement error, underwater weighing remains the gold standard but may well be superseded by whole body DEXA scanning.

Flexibility

The ability to move a joint through the complete range of motion, maintaining a joint's flexibility facilitates movement. Flexibility assessments routinely undertaken in an exercise laboratory include the active knee extension test at 90° of hip flexion to assess hamstring length and range of active knee extension, and the sit and reach test of low back and hamstring flexibility, a non-specific test of overall flexibility. Active knee extension in the supple athlete should be at least 80° and sit and reach should be beyond the toe line.

Pulmonary function tests

Asthma is one of the commonest medical conditions producing exercise and performance limitation in athletes. Pre- and post-exercise lung function tests should be a routine part of physiological assessment, to detect undiagnosed respiratory limitation prior to exercise testing and/or monitor control in athletes already on inhaler medications for asthma. All subjects with clinical evidence of asthma or exercise-induced bronchoconstriction (EIB), with FEV_1 values of 85–90% of predicted or less pre-exercise, or those who show a 10% fall in FEV_1 from baseline post-exercise, should be further evaluated and assessed.

An exercise challenge of 6–8 minutes running outdoors in early morning cold air at 85% of HR max; or, eucapnic voluntary hyperventilation (EVH), 6 minutes hyperventilation through a mask system of a gas mixture containing 5% CO_2 to prevent hypocapnia, at a minute ventilation (V_E) of 30 times FEV_1, as provocation. Lung function tests are assessed pre-exercise and at 3, 5, 10, 15, and 30 minutes post-exercise. Print outs of data from these tests are now required as objective evidence of EIB supporting applications (a TUE) for permission to use inhaler medications as part of anti-doping regulations.

Routine blood tests

Mild infections, reduced oxygen carrying capacity (↓Hb), and reduced plasma volume due to dehydration will raise resting and sub-maximal HR, and influence exercise test results. Iron deficiency, usually due to vegetarianism and menstrual loss, is fairly common In female endurance athletes. A reduction of as little as 0.5–1.0g in Hb level, even if still within the normal range, can produce significant performance decrements in elite athletes.

Measurement of aerobic capacity

The standard laboratory-based aerobic assessment is a graded incremental test to volitional exhaustion. The following variables are routinely assessed; heart rate, O_2 consumption, CO_2 production, blood lactate concentration, and associated respiratory variables. The normal protocol outline for graded maximal incremental test to volitional exhaustion is as follows:

- All tests preceded by 10 min low intensity warm-up and self-stretching and concluded by 5–10 min low intensity warm-down.
- Following a short period of data recording at rest, the test is started at a low sub-maximal velocity/load.
- Increment duration from 1–3 min, usually 3 min if steady state responses are desired, with average data collected over the final 60–90s of each increment. Fixed increments (W or km.hr^{-1}) for different genders, grades, and sporting disciplines vary accordingly.
- Increased loading or speed (W or km.hr^{-1}) should result in VO_2 increases of ~2–3 MET or ~5–10 mL.kg^{-1}.min^{-1} with each increment.
- Total test time should be between 15–25 min to control for cardiovascular drift, elevation in core temperature, and self-motivation.

Measurement of anaerobic power and capacity

Peak power is the highest power output averaged over short periods of 1 to 3s, whereas anaerobic capacity is defined as the work performed during a short high-intensity sprint test. The main objectives are to accurately measure the rate and quantity of work under circumstances of minimal aerobic contribution.

Vertical jump test
- A measure of 'explosiveness' in physical fitness tests often used as an index of anaerobic capacity.
- Vertical jump height is the difference between standing height and jump height assessed using a vertical jump meter.
- Three jumps are used either from a crouched and held start or with a rapid counter-movement action, from knee angle of ~90° to assess the contribution of the stretch-shortening cycle.
- Power (W) = $21.67 \times$ body mass (kg) $\times v^{0.5}$, where v is jump height (m).
- Following suitable rest periods the test can be repeated with additional loading equivalent to 10, 15, and 20% body mass.

Wingate test
- A supra-maximal 30s cycle ergometer test performed with braking load of 7.5% body mass for females and 8.5% body mass for males.
- Assessment is made of maximum power, mean power, and power decline (fatigue index).
- Mean power data is calculated from pedal cadence and resistance over successive 1s intervals, because of the transient nature of the peak values (longer intervals reduce magnitude of measured data).
- Data for peak and mean power are corrected for body mass ($W.kg^{-1}$) to account for gender, training status, and muscle mass.
- Typical values for peak power range from 9–14 $W.kg^{-1}$.
- Power decline is calculated by expressing the difference between peak and minimum power in reference to peak power, as a percentage.
- Power decline ranges between 35–50%.
- A major limitation is that there is a considerable aerobic contribution (25–30%) to the total work performed.

Margaria stair climbing test
This test purports to assess anaerobic capacity and the protocol involves:
- Sprint up a staircase (~1.8m) as quickly as possible 2 steps at a time.
- Contact mats are fitted at fixed steps on the staircase to measure time.
- Power (W) = [$9.81 \times$ body mass (kg) $\times$ vertical displacement (m)]/ time(s).
- Values for power range from 700W (12 $W.kg^{-1}$) in poorly trained females to >1500W (>18 $W.kg^{-1}$) in male sprint athletes.

Dal Monte sprint test
- This test is designed to assess speed endurance.
- Maximal repeated sprints are performed every 60s over a distance of 50m for male players and 40m for goalkeepers and female players.
- Sprint distance must be completed in <7s.

- Decline in sprint time is computed to assess speed endurance, minimal decline infers excellent speed endurance.

Continuous jump test
- Similar in design to the Wingate test can be used to assess ballistic power and power decline, it involves:
- 10s of maximal counter-movement jumping (knee angle nominally 90°) on a specialized contact jump mat capable of assessing flight times.
- Body mass and flight times are used to compute maximum power and power decline in a similar manner to the Wingate test.

10 by 5m speed/agility test
- A sprinting and turning shuttle test performed at maximum velocity on a slip-proof surface.
- Subject completes 10 shuttles of a 5m distance with both feet crossing end lines at each turn.
- Test is stopped when the subject crosses end line in the final shuttle.
- Performance time is recorded to 0.01s using either a stopwatch or if possible an infra-red beam timing apparatus.

Maximum accumulated oxygen deficit
- An assessment of anaerobic capacity based on extrapolation of the linear relationship between sub-maximal power and O_2 consumption.
- Once sub-maximal relationship has been quantified using loads equivalent to 40–85% VO_2 max, estimated O_2 consumption equivalents at intensities above VO_2 max are calculated.
- Typical values; endurance athletes 2.5–5.0L and sprinters 4.5–7.5L.

Other tests frequently used include sprints through infra-red timing gates over varying distances 10, 30, 50, 100, and 200m, rugby sprint shuttle test, and number of repetitions of exercises such as squat thrusts and push-ups.

Measurement of strength

Strength and power are sport-specific measures. Strength is the maximum force (N) or movement (Nm), whereas power is defined as the rate of work (force by velocity). Strength and power are applied in sport specific movements and postures, and at particular movement velocities.

The following should be considered when assessing strength:
- Reliability of the measurement protocol.
- Degree of correlation between test score and performance indices.
- Sensitivity of the measurement protocol to detect training adaptation.
- Prior effect of acute bouts of exercise.

Strength can be assessed either dynamically (isokinetic or isotonic/isoinertial protocols) or statically (isometric) using open-or closed-chain models; each assessment type has particular advantages and limitations.

Isometric strength measurement
Static assessment of maximum voluntary capacity (MVC) uses strain gauges, load-cells or tensiometers at fixed joint angles. Isometric tests can also be used to assess endurance capacity, the time a fixed % of MVC

can be maintained, and the rate of force development (dF/dT) usually over range of 10–70% of MVC.

Advantages:
- Isometric tests are easily standardized and inexpensive.
- Preferred when joint range of motion is limited by bracing or pathology.

Disadvantage:
- Poor relationship to dynamic performance indices.

Isotonic (isoinertial) strength measurement (gym-based testing)

Isotonic/isoinertial and isokinetic assessment is across the full range of joint motion. Force-generating capacity is measured during both concentric and eccentric actions. Isoinertial assessment reflects effort during a weight lifting task, and implies constant resistance to motion rather than a constant resistance or load throughout the lift. If assessed using free-weights or an elliptical cam loaded variable resistance apparatus, the load applied to a muscle is only maximal at extremes of range, with forces decreasing to 40–50% of maximal capacity in mid range. The maximum eccentric load applied is also limited by maximum concentric load.

Advantages:
- Positive reinforcement from progressive increases in strength.
- Varying exercises can be included to test multiple joints simultaneously.
- Exercises are easily performed in weight bearing closed-kinetic chains.

Disadvantages:
- Unable to quantify movement/torque, work or power.
- Strong muscles may compensate for weak muscle groups during closed-kinetic chain actions.

Isokinetic strength measurement

Using an isokinetic dynamometer, the velocity of joint movement can be controlled by an external motor enabling an accommodating resistance (Newton's 3rd law). This ensures that a maximum force can be applied at all angles both concentrically and eccentrically within the assessed range of movement. Assessment is made of force versus angle profiles at different joint velocities in concentric and eccentric modes, and can also be made of bilateral instability (limb to limb differences) and functional reciprocal muscle group ratios (ratio of concentric agonist to eccentric antagonist).

Advantages:
- Isolation of weak muscle groups.
- Quantification of movement/torque, work and power.
- Accommodating resistance concept in addition to providing maximal resistance also ensures a functionally safe loading mechanism.

Disadvantages:
- Assessment limited to isolated muscle groups acting through cardinal planes in non-weight bearing open-kinetic chains.
- Equipment costs are prohibitive and these assessments are mainly in a hospital-based rehabilitation setting and in academic institutions for research purposes.

- Minor reliability issues associated with subject re-positioning and stabilization in longitudinal rehabilitation and training studies.

Simple field-based tests of exercise capacity

Indirect protocols employing both maximal and sub-maximal effort can be used to predict VO_2 max. These basic predictive tests use steady state heart rate at sub-maximal workloads (exercise HR <85% HRmax) to provide an estimate of VO_2 max using multiple regression equations. HR max may vary depending on body composition and in obese subjects HR max is better predicted by the formula: HRmax= 200 − (0.5 × age).

Indirect sub-maximal tests to estimate aerobic capacity

Single stage walk test

- Walk for 4min at comfortable velocity on a motorized treadmill (nominal velocity 4.8–6.4 km.hr^{-1}).
- Target walking HR of 100–120 beats.min^{-1}.
- Increase treadmill slope to 5% and continue walking for another 4 min but ensure that HR remains below 85% of age predicted HRmax.
- Record steady state HR at 30s intervals in final 2min (steady state HR implies a change of <5 beat.min^{-1}.min^{-1}).
- Use the following multiple regression equation to predict VO_2 max:

$$VO_2max \ (mL.kg^{-1}min^{-1}) = 15.1 + [21.8 \times velocity \ (mph)] - [0.327 \times HR] \\ - [0.263 \times velocity \times age] + [0.00504 \times HR \\ \times age] + [5.98 \times gender] \ (gender \ factor \\ 0=F, 1=M).$$

Single stage jog test

- Walk for 4min at a comfortable velocity on a motorized treadmill (nominally 4.8–6.4 km.hr^{-1}).
- Target walking speed for HR of 100–120 beat.min^{-1}.
- Increase velocity to comfortable jogging speed (range 7–12 km.hr^{-1}) depending on subject's fitness.
- Ensure HR remains below 85% of age predicted HRmax.
- Continue jogging for 4min, record HR at 30s intervals over final 2min while jogging.
- Use the following multiple regression equation to predict VO_2 max:

$$VO_2 \ max \ (mL.kg^{-1}.min^{-1}) = 54.07 - [0.1938 \times mass \ (kg)] + \\ [4.47 \times velocity \ (mph)] - [0.1453 \times HR] + \\ [7.062 \times gender] \ (gender \\ factor \ 0= F, 1= M).$$

Sub-maximal two-stage jog test

This predictive test uses the relationship between sub-maximal VO_2 and HR to predict VO_2 max.

- Subject completes 2 stages each of 3min duration at fixed velocities depending on fitness (8.0, 9.6, 11.2, 12.0, 12.8, 14.4, 16.0 km.hr^{-1}).
- Record HR over final 2min of each stage and convert treadmill velocity to equivalent oxygen cost (see Table 20.1).

Table 20.1 Table for calculation of equivalent O_2 cost of 1st (SM_1) and 2nd (SM_2) stages

Treadmill velocity (km.hr^{-1})	Equivalent O_2 cost (mL.kg^{-1}.min^{-1})
8.0	30.1
9.6	35.7
11.2	40.9
12.0	43.7
12.8	46.5
14.4	51.8
16.0	57.1

Table 20.2 Table of Gender and Fitness Factors for the PWC 170

	Obese/unfit	Normal	Fit
Male <18	0.75	1.00	1.25
Male >18	1.00	1.25	1.50
Female <18	0.50	0.75	1.00
Female >18	0.75	1.00	1.25

- Use equation and age predicted HRmax to predict VO_2 max thus:
  VO_2 max (mL.kg^{-1}.min^{-1}) = SM_2 + [b × (HRmax-HR$_2$)].
  where b= (SM_2 - SM_1) / (HR$_2$ - HR$_1$).
- SM_1 & SM_2 = equivalent O_2 cost of 1st and 2nd stages respectively.
- HRmax= age predicted maxHR, = heart rate during 2nd stage.
- HR$_1$ & HR$_2$ = heart rate during 1st and 2nd stages respectively.
- NB: Test is suitable for semi-sedentary and active populations.

Sub-maximal cycle ergometer test (PWC170)

This predictive test uses the linear increase in HR with load during sub-maximal exercise.
- Exercise load at HR = 170 beats.min^{-1} is the estimated variable [original subject population were age ~20 yr (85% of 220–20=170)].
- Adjust seat height and handlebar position on a stationary cycle ergometer to suit the subject.
- Subject then asked to pedal at a constant cadence (60 rev.min^{-1}) at 3 sub-maximal loads (NB load (W) = cadence × braking mass).
- Steady state HR is measured over last minute of each exercise element.
- Initial load (W.kg^{-1}) is dependent on gender and fitness (see Table 20.2). Multiply body mass by relevant factor according to age and fitness level.
- PWC170 (W.kg^{-1}) = [{((W3–W2) / (HR3–HR2)) × ((170–HR3)} + W3]/BM.
- HR$_2$ & HR$_3$ are the steady state heart rate data at loads 2 and 3.
- W$_2$ & W$_3$ are workloads in Watt at loads 2 and 3 respectively.
- BM is body mass in kg.

- PWC 170 example:
  If HR at load 2 (96W) was 142 beats.min^{-1} and load 3 (136W) was
  163 beats.min^{-1} and BM=65 kg $\Rightarrow$
  PWC170 = [{((136–96)/(163–142)) × (170–163)} + 136]/65=
  2.29 W.kg^{-1}
- NB: Test is suitable for sedentary and semi-sedentary populations.

Indirect maximal tests for estimation of aerobic capacity

The following are all maximal tests for indirect estimation of aerobic
capacity. NB All maximal tests should only be undertaken after medical
clearance.

Maximal cycle ergometer test

This is an incremental cycling test to exhaustion. In non-cyclists, results
for VO$_2$ max on the cycle ergometer are generally lower than for
treadmill tests, due to the involvement of a smaller muscle mass.

- Load (W) = cadence (rev.min^{-1}) x braking mass (kg), e.g. at 60 rev.
  min^{-1} with a frictional braking mass of 2kg the load is 120W.
- Adjust seat height and handlebar position to suit the subject.
- Subject then cycles at pedal cadence at 60 rev.min^{-1} throughout test.
- Subject starts at a low workload 60W for 2min, with load increases of
  30W every 2min until pedal cadence can no longer be maintained or
  volitional exhaustion.
- Load is then reduced to 60–90W for 5–10 min as cool down.
- ACSM cycle ergometer equation is then used to predict VO$_2$ max.
- VO$_2$ max = {12 x load (W) + 3.5 × body mass (kg)}/body mass (kg).
- E.g. If max load achieved was 300W and subject body mass was 80 kg
  $\Rightarrow$: VO$_2$ max = {(300 x 12) + (3.5 x 80)} / 80 = 48.5 mL.kg^{-1}.min^{-1}
- NB: Test only suitable for active subjects who are efficient when
  cycling.

Leger and Lambert 20 metre shuttle test (20 MST)

This is an incremental running test to volitional exhaustion. The test
tends to underestimate VO$_2$ max in individuals inefficient at rapid turning
actions, and is therefore more applicable to games players rather than
distance runners.

- Subjects complete run between 2 lines placed exactly 20m apart in
  time to an audible signal.
- Running velocity is initially slow (8.5km.hr^{-1}) and becomes
  progressively faster by 0.5 km.hr^{-1}.min^{-1}.
- As the velocity increases each minute, the test enters a new level.
- The test stops when the subject can no longer maintain
  synchronization of their turning action at the ends of the runway with
  the audible signal.
- Number of completed levels and shuttles in the final level achieved is
  recorded as the test score.
- Recorded score can be used as a basic measure of fitness or
  alternatively predictive tables can estimate VO$_2$ max in mL.kg^{-1}.min^{-1}.

Cooper 12 minute run test

This is a maximal 12 min running test performed on an all-weather track
with marker cones placed at 10m or 20m intervals.

- Distance completed in km (D) is recorded i.e. number of completed laps plus number of completed 10m or 20m intervals in final lap.
- VO_2 max and velocity at lactate threshold are then estimated from the following equations.
- VO_2max $(mL.kg^{-1}.min^{-1})$ = 22.4 × D − 11.4.
- Velocity @ TLac $(km.hr^{-1})$ = 10.1 − 2.09 × D + 1.03 × D2.

All these predictive tests, both sub-maximal and maximal, for assessing VO_2 max have some degree of predictive error associated with them, usually about ± 5–10%. These predictive errors are due to differences between the population under investigation and the original study population used to derive the empirical formula by simple and multiple correlation analysis.

Basic principles of training

Training is the use of progressive overload to stress the major energy systems used in an activity. Training usually results in adaptation of the energy system and improvement in performance.

Overload

Greater than normal load with appropriate rest leads to adaptation. Exercise intensity should be near maximal and increased as fitness increases.

Progression

Frequency, intensity, time (duration), and type of training are manipulated to create a progression in load. Build up duration or volume of training, and with a basic foundation, reduce volume but increase intensity and speed.

Specificity

The metabolic and neuromuscular demands of exercise are usually specific to the sport or activity, and training must reflect the elements found within the sport, i.e. train rowers in boats not on exercise bikes!

Individuality

Training load should be prescribed according to age, gender, level of skills, experience, and conditioning and then adjusted according to individual response. Elite level training programs should not be imposed on juniors, beginners, or intermediate level athletes.

Rest

Regeneration and adaptation occurs when resting. Rest should be an actively programmed part of training.

Periodization

Plan the season and build the necessary skills, strength, and endurance (distance) or speed systematically in a series of well planned phases.

Table 20.3 Running distance, time and % contributions of energy systems

Event	Time	ATP/CP	Anaerobic	Aerobic
42km	135–180min	–	5	95
10km	28–50min	5	15	80
5km	14–25min	10	20	70
3km	8.5–16min	20	40	40
1.5km	3.6–6min	20	50	30
800m	2–3min	30	55–60	10–15
400m	45–90s	80	15	5
200m	20–35s	>90	<10	–
100m	10–15s	>95	<5	–

Aerobic endurance training

Training aims to maximize base aerobic capacity and develop the ability to maintain high aerobic power outputs without fatigue. Speed or load at threshold and endurance capacity (how long threshold pace can be maintained) can still be improved even after VO_2 max has reached a plateau, and is the most important factor determining success in elite endurance sport.

Build a large aerobic system, by long duration low intensity activity, and then train at an intensity close to, but just below lactate threshold (TLac), for progressively longer and longer periods of time.

Aerobic training intensity, duration and frequency

Training intensity is usually prescribed in 2 or 3 aerobic HR zones, based on the lactate HR data profile from an incremental test (see graph) or empirically at fixed percentages of maximum heart rate or heart rate reserve [Heart Rate Reserve (HRR) = HRmax–HR rest]. In endurance athletes heart rate at TLac ranges from 80–90% of HR max, but prediction of individual zones based on heart rate formulae are prone to error (±10–15 beats.min^{-1}).

TLac for most endurance athletes occurs at BLa of 2–2.5mM, but measuring BLa during training is impractical, and so HR training ranges equivalent to set BLa concentrations are extrapolated from HR Lactate profile recorded in standard incremental tests.

Aerobic base training (A1/A2)

- A1 pace usually HR~120–140 beats.min^{-1} and BLa ≤ 1mM. Train at this intensity for warm up/cool down routines, active recovery and fat burning.
- A2 pace usually HR~145–155, BLa still well below TLac (1–1.5mM) and still predominantly aerobic and fat burning. Training for base aerobic training combines A1/A2 intensities: e.g. 10min warm up A1, 30min steady A2, 10min A1 cool down.

Lactate threshold training (A3)

- A3 pace is set just below TLac; HR ~160–180 beats.min^{-1} and BLa between 2–2.5mM. Training at this pace burns a mixture of fat and carbohydrate fuels, the aerobic system is at its maximum limit.
- A small amount of lactate will accumulate at this pace, and therefore lactate transport mechanisms are also stimulated.

Recommended frequency

- Base aerobic/active recovery (A1/A2) 2–3 sessions per week.
- Aerobic endurance (A3) 2–3 sessions per week on non-successive days.
- Aim for one high quality training session per day, if just starting off; rising to 2 sessions on alternate days for the typical elite athlete.
- NB 2 or 3 sessions per day does not necessarily lead to greater performance gains if of poor quality or if fatigued.

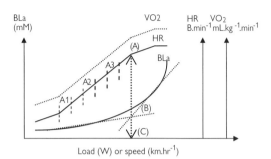

Fig. 20.3 Extrapolation of aerobic training heart rate zones A1 to A3. (A) Heart rate at TLac, (B) BLa at TLac, (C) Load or Speed at TLac. Aerobic training zones A1, A2 and A3

- Incorporate additional early morning easy A1/A2 (45–60min) to increase weekly mileage if needed.

Training duration
- Aerobic base (A1/A2) is built gradually over 3–5 months initially 20–30 minutes per session up to 60–90 minutes for elite endurance athletes.
- Lactate threshold (A3) initially 2 sets of 10min progressing to 2 by 15, 2 by 20, and 3 by 15 etc over 3–5 months.
- Elite endurance athletes would be aiming for 3 by 20 min or 2 by 25 minutes A3 pace by the end of main aerobic winter preparation phase.
- Overall weekly duration for all aerobic training elements should not usually exceed 12–14 hours/week.
- NB excessive endurance training above an optimum 8–12 sessions per week is usually non-productive and will result in overuse injury, athletic staleness, and burnout.

Long-term adaptive responses to aerobic training include;
- Improved O_2 efficiency ($\downarrow O_2$ consumption at fixed velocities/loads).
- Improved HR efficiency ($\downarrow$HR at fixed velocities/loads).
- Increased load/velocity at TLac.
- Decreased BLa data at sub-maximal exercise intensities.
- Increase in maximum load/velocity attained at VO_2 max.

Periodisation for aerobic endurance athletes
Rest phase (normally 3–4 weeks)
Training is generally non-specific to keep generally active and maintain body mass near competition mass. Participation in alternative sporting activities for relaxation.

Preparation phase
Training programme with emphasis on increasing strength and muscular endurance in those muscles most directly involved in sporting activity. Low intensity long distance sessions, two to three times per week will help improve the aerobic base, and shorter sessions should target the lactate threshold—initially 2 per week.

Transition phase (8–12 weeks prior to competition)

A slightly higher intensity program specific to the athlete's sport and predominant energy system. Controlled aerobic (1 to >4hr depending on sport) sessions two to three days per week.

In season training

For the majority of athletes who compete regularly competition itself should maintain the increases in energy systems attained in pre- and off-season, provided they do not over-compete. However, the training programme should contain LSD sessions, 1–2 per week plus sports–specific training sets directed towards upcoming-targeted races.

Resistance training

Resistance training improves athletic performance by increasing muscular strength, power, and speed. Training may induce hypertrophy, increase local muscular endurance, improve motor performance, and also improve balance and coordination.

Resistance training and competition

- *Power lifting*—muscle strength in squat, bench press, and dead lift.
- *Weightlifting*—muscle strength and power in clean and jerk, and snatch type lifts.
- *Bodybuilding*—building optimal muscle hypertrophy for definition and symmetry while reducing % body fat to improve appearance.
- *Strongman*—improve muscle strength, power, and endurance.
- *Athletics*—strength training to improve athletic performance.

Components of a resistance training programme

Programmes usually include dynamic concentric (CON) and eccentric (ECC) actions, isometric actions play a secondary role. Dynamic strength improvements are greatest when ECC actions are included.
When compared to CON actions, ECC actions produce:

- Greater force per unit of muscle size.
- Involve less motor unit activation for a fixed force.
- Require less energy for a fixed force.
- Are critical for optimal hypertrophy.
- Result in greater delayed onset muscle soreness (DOMS).
- Greater potential for injury if done incorrectly.

Types of exercise in resistance training

Free-weights and machine exercises are used in single or multiple joint exercises. Single joint exercises stress one joint or muscle group e.g. leg extension/leg curl and are thought to pose a lower injury risk as less skill is involved. Multiple-joint exercises stress more than one joint and muscle group e.g. bench press, squat, power cleans, they involve complex neural activation and coordination due to the involvement of a larger muscle mass, and are the most effective resistance exercise type for increasing strength and power. Snatch and power clean exercises are the most effective for increasing muscle power because they require fast force production to successfully complete each repetition.

Metabolic and hormonal responses

Exercise stress of multiple large muscle groups will show the greatest acute metabolic responses. Dead lifts, squat jumps and Olympic lifts produce greater testosterone and HGH responses compared with simple bench press and seated shoulder press. Metabolic demand and anabolic hormonal response have direct implications for improvements in local muscle endurance, lean body mass, and reducing % body fat. Sequencing of exercises and number of muscle groups trained effects acute expression of muscle strength.

Basic resistance training workouts

Total body workout (>3 sessions/wk)

- Stress all major muscle groups.
- Normally 1–2 exercises per group.
- Commonly used for general fitness by athletes and Olympic weightlifters.

Upper/lower body routines (2–3 session/wk)

- Exercises are split into upper body during one session, and lower body during the next session.
- Used by athletes for general fitness, in power lifting and body building.
- Large muscle groups before small, multiple joint before single joint, rotate opposing agonist/antagonist exercises.

Muscle group split routines (1–2 session/wk)

- Exercises are targeted at specific muscle groups during the same workout; for example, chest/triceps workout—all exercises for chest performed and subsequently all exercises for triceps are performed.
- Workouts common among body builders or individuals striving to maximise muscle hypertrophy.
- 3–4 exercises performed compared with 1–2 during a total body regimen.
- Multiple joint before single joint, perform higher intensity (higher % of 1RM) before lower intensity exercises.

Exercise sequence

Train large muscle groups before small, multiple joint before single joint, for power training exercise order (most to least complex) before basic exercises such as squat or bench press, rotate upper and lower body exercises or opposing agonist/antagonist exercises.

Loading

Loading describes the amount of weight lifted and is highly dependent on: Exercise order, volume, frequency, muscle action, repetition speed, and rest interval. Optimal strength, hypertrophy, and local muscle endurance training requires the systematic usage of various loading strategies.

Load prescription depends on training status and goals:

- Power training at >85% of 1RM stresses ATP-PC system.
- Hypertrophy training at 70–80% of 1RM stresses ATP-PC and glycolytic systems, with minor contribution from aerobic metabolism.
- Local endurance training <70% of 1RM involves a high aerobic component. Loads <70% of 1RM rarely increase maximal strength, but are effective for increasing local muscle endurance.
- Training continuously at one intensity, high risk of training plateaus or over-training.
- 80% of IRM corresponded to 10RM for bench press, leg extension, and lat pull-down; 6RM for leg curl; 7–8RM for arm curl; and 15RM for leg press.

Rest interval
- Rest interval length is dependent on training intensity, goals, fitness, and targeted energy system utilization.
- The amount of rest between sets significantly affects: metabolic, hormonal, and cardiovascular responses to an acute bout of exercise as well as performance of subsequent sets and training adaptations.
- Rest interval influences relative contribution from the energy systems.
- When training for absolute strength and power rest periods of 3–5min are recommended.
- Rest interval appears to be a potent stimulator for anabolic hormones and local blood flow, and results in significant lactate production.
- Training to increase local muscle endurance requires the athlete to perform high reps, have a long duration workout and minimize recovery between sets. Minimizing recovery between sets is an important stimulus for improving local muscle endurance (increased mitochondrial and capillary number, increased buffer capacity and fibre type transitions).
- Rest intervals vary for each exercise within a training session, consider fatigue associated with previous exercises when performing exercises later in a workout.

Velocity

The velocity that dynamic repetitions are performed at affects responses to resistance training. Moderate velocity training produces the greatest strength increases across all test velocities. Training for local muscle endurance, and in some aspects hypertrophy, may require a spectrum of velocities with various loading strategies.

Frequency/recovery

The number of training sets and number of times certain exercises or muscle groups are trained per week affects subsequent resistance training adaptations. Frequency is dependent on several factors: volume and intensity, exercise selection, level of conditioning/training status, recovery ability, nutritional intake, and training goals.

Heavy ECC training may require 72h recovery, whereas large/moderate loads require less recovery time. Advanced weightlifters and body-builders use high frequency training (4–6 day.wk^{-1}). Double-split routines, 2 sessions per day with emphasis on different muscle groups, are common and this can result in the completion of up to 8–14 sessions.wk^{-1}.

Olympic weightlifters typically do 18 sessions/wk. Short sessions followed by recovery, supplementation, and food intake allows for high intensity training via maximal energy utilization and reduced fatigue during exercise performance.

Anaerobic/sprint training

Anaerobic/sprint training involves a series of repeated bouts of high intensity exercise alternated with periods of relief (rest or low intensity exercise).

Energy system

ATP-PCR supplies more ATP than anaerobic glycolysis, during intermittent short duration efforts when compared to short duration continuous efforts.

Training

- Overload is applied by manipulating intensity, distance, number of repetitions, rest interval between repetitions, activity during rest interval, and training frequency (sets per week).
- Typical anaerobic/sprint training includes:
  - Longer duration intervals at moderate intensity.
  - Medium duration intervals at moderate-high intensity.
  - Very short intervals at close to maximum intensity.
- Longer duration (4–5 min) anaerobic/sprint training sessions are used to induce improved lactate tolerance with HR during exercise > HR at TLac from mid-interval onwards.
- Medium and short (1–2 min) duration intervals; exercise intensity based on recent time-trial (TT) performance time, nominally 92–95% effort during week 1 and 2, and 95–97% effort during week 3, repeat TT at end of recovery week to assess improvement.
- Relief time nominally 1½ times exercise interval, if necessary adjust relief time to ensure that exercise time remains constant across successive repetitions.
- Number of repetitions decreases as exercise duration increases (e.g. 12 by 400m, 6–8 by 800m, 5–6 by 1000m).

Metabolic adaptations

Anaerobic training increases resting levels of anaerobic substrates and key glycolytic enzymes.

- Free creatine ↑32–40%, PCR ↑5–20%, ATP ↑16–18% glycogen ↑30–60%.
- No change or increase in glycolytic enzyme activity (PFK, LDH, HK).
- No change in ATP turnover enzymes (MK, CPK).
- Decrease in mitochondrial volume (density) due to an increase in size of myofibrils and sarcoplasmic volume.
- Selective hypertrophy of FT + FOG and an increase in FT+FOG to ST fibre ratio.
- Increased blood lactate during all-out exercise is probably due to enhanced glycogen storage and increased glycolytic enzymes following anaerobic training, in addition to improved motivation and pain tolerance.
- In addition to the metabolic and biochemical changes noted above, imprecisely identified nervous system changes also occur (better motor unit recruitment patterns and synchronization).

Types of anaerobic training

Strength/Resistance training for speed include short interval sprints, hill training, and weight training: Heavy weights (small number of lifts) or light weights 50–60% 1RM, (large number of lifts with short rests).

- Fartlek—alternating fast and slow running over natural terrain, informal interval training lacking precise control of exercise or relief elements.
- Sprints develop ATP-PCR system, repeat sprints at maximum velocity (duration 5–6s, distance 40–50m to experience running at Vmax), longer relief intervals required to ensure almost complete phosphagen system recovery.
- Interval sprints alternate 50m sprints and 50–70m jog for 3–4 km, because of onset of fatigue after several sprints subsequent sprints are not run at Vmax.
- Acceleration sprints gradual increase in running velocity (from jog-stride-sprint), distance 50–100m followed by 50–100m walk phase, recovery almost complete before successive sprint phase.
- Plyometrics bounding type exercises and drop jumps to improve neuromuscular synchronization and explosiveness.
- Sprint training for games players sprint distance 40–50m, including backward and lateral movement patterns typical of athlete's sport, stop-and-go sprints over 5–10m with sports-specific elements completed during each stop phase.

Short interval sprints (30–50m) facilitate maximum and synchronous recruitment of fibres. Increased recruitment may lead to muscle damage because of force generated, normally prevented via central inhibition initiated by stretch receptors and Golgi tendon bodies. CNS overrides and prevents maximum recruitment, over time sprint training desensitizes central inhibition.

ATP and PCR storage and glycolytic flux increased by inducing biochemical changes in key enzymes in cytosol (phosphorylase, PFK and LDH).

Long interval sprints (100–200m) improved usage of PCR, ↑ATP/PCR and total Cr storage, ↑lactate tolerance and buffering capacity, initial improvements primarily neural—strength gains without muscle hypertrophy.

Gender and performance

Gender issues in sport and exercise embrace genetic, hormonal anatomical, physiological, psychological, and sociological aspects as well as those of sports performance and body image. World record performances in women's sports have been improved rapidly for a variety of reasons, including greater numbers participating and better training practices. Female world record performances are still only 90–95% of that of males, and in all but a minority of sports women will probably never equal or surpass male performance. Anatomical and physiological reasons for this are considered below.

Stature and body mass
- Females are on average of shorter average height—1.6m as opposed to males average height 1.7m.
- Girls are briefly larger and stronger between age 10–12yr, due to earlier growth spurt.

Skeletal differences
- Women have narrower shoulders, shorter arms with a wider carrying angle, broader hips, and shorter legs.
- Shoulder arm difference and smaller muscle mass in women accounts for weaker upper body compared to lower body strength in women than men.
- Broader hips cause greater angle of the femur to the knee (genu valgum), causing many women to throw their heels out when running.

Centre of gravity
- Shorter stature and body shape differences lead to a lower centre of gravity.
- In adults centre of gravity is 55% of standing height in women (S1 level) and 56–57% in men.
- Consequently women have better balance and are better suited to floor exercises and balance beam exercises in gymnastics.

Flexibility
- Women have better flexibility than men.
- Advantageous in gymnastics and dance.
- NB Hypermobility of the joints can bring problems.

Body fat percentage
- Females have higher % body fat (23–28%) than males (12–18%).
- This is advantageous in cold climates, during starvation, and may improve performance in long distance swimming events.
- However greater % body fat is a major disadvantage in weight bearing sports involving running and jumping.

Muscle
- There is little difference in muscle quality between male and females.
- Strength differences in males are due to greater crossectional area, greater overall muscle mass (androgen effects), and longer levers.

- Low grade muscle endurance is better in females e.g. when performing repetitions at 20–30% of 1RM.
- This may benefit women in ultra-distance events, swimming, and cycling.

Cardiovascular system

- Women have proportionately less blood than males ($65mL.kg^{-1}$ vs $75mL.kg^{-1}$) and lower haemoglobin levels (13.9 gdL vs 15.8 gdL).
- Women tend to have smaller hearts, smaller left ventricular mass, and smaller stroke volume.
- Despite female hearts being 8% smaller than males, maximum heart rates are similar.
- At maximum levels of aerobic work women need to pump 7L of blood for every litre of oxygen consumed, whereas men require only 6L.
- This affects maximum oxygen intake, highest recorded values are between 85–$90mL.kg^{-1}.min^{-1}$ for males and 75–$80mL.kg^{-1}.min^{-1}$ for females.

Motor control, vision, and hearing

- Women have better fine manipulative skills but worse visual acuity than men.
- Women have better colour discrimination especially in the blue-grey range, and are able to perceive quieter sounds.

Thermoregulation

Thermoregulation in males and females is slightly different.
- Total body water to body mass ratio is 50–55% in females and 55–60% in males.
- Body temperature is higher in the luteal phase of the menstrual cycle, but this is thought not to have any effect on performance.
- Men sweat more per m^2 of skin (800 $mL.hr^{-1}.m^{-2}$ vs 600 $mL.hr^{-1}.m^{-2}$).
- Women tend to lose more heat through radiation.
- Change in sweat patterns and sweat electrolytes in response to training are similar in both sexes.
- Unfit females lose heat more by radiation and onset of sweating is earlier in trained females.
- Well-trained male and female athletes respond in a similar manner in warm temperatures with low humidity.
- Women therefore are benefited in warm humid conditions and men in warm dry conditions.
- Females may be able to work and survive better in the cold than males because they are better insulated.
- However, surface area to body mass ratio (SA/M) also determines heat loss and women have a larger SA/M ratio than males.
- Women loose heat more rapidly in the cold, especially if immersed in cold water.

Fitness deterioration with ageing

In most humans there is a physiological decline in performance from the mid to late 30s onwards. However, exceptional performance is still possible in later years e.g. men and women over 80 have run marathons in under 5 hours!

Stature
Declines by approximately 1cm per decade after 40yr. This is partly due to degenerative changes in intervertebral discs, and partly loss of vertebral bone height.

Body fat
The body fat % rises steadily to 23–25% in males and 32–40% in females by age 60–70 yr, while lean body mass steadily declines.

Skin
The rete pegs anchoring the epidermis to the dermis become shorter with age, leading to a greater propensity to blister formation and skin tearing. Melanocytes disappear at the rate of 2% per year and the cutaneous inflammatory response diminishes, the elderly are therefore more susceptible to sun burn, and yet show less of the acute effects of sunburn than the young.

Muscle
In comparison with performance matched younger athletes, the muscle of elderly athletes tends towards a predominance of slow twitch type fibres, with greater muscle capillarization. This is thought to be due to re-innervation of muscle by type 1 nerve following type 2 nerve degeneration.

Ageing also causes a decrease in Myosin ATPase levels and size and number of mitochondria. Between the ages of 60–90 yr there is greater loss in muscle power than muscle strength, 3.5% vs 1.8% per year respectively.

In both sexes, decreased strength is not usually apparent until 40yr, with concentric force production lost more rapidly than eccentric. Over 40yr decrement is approximately 25% by age 65, with a further proportionate drop after 65. In women, strength loss is further accentuated by the menopause.

However, these changes are reversible, and an increase in local muscular endurance and doubling of force development with 6–8 weeks of initiation of strength training programmes is well documented in 56–70yr olds. This ability to increase strength with training in the elderly is extremely important for mobility, balance, and independence.

Respiratory
In the lung connective tissue elasticity decreases, alveolar size increases, and the number of pulmonary capillaries decreases, this leads to an increase in the work of ventilation and decreased perfusion quality.

Cardiovascular

Heart rate max declines with age due to decreased sympathetic tone, marked reduction in SA nodal cells, and decreased sarcoplasmic uptake of calcium. Age-related cardiac hypertrophy can paradoxically reduce stroke volume due to decreased chamber size.

Aerobic performance

Oxygen uptake decreases due to the cardio-respiratory factors mentioned previously. From age 20yr the average VO_2 max of ~50mL. $kg^{-1}.min^{-1}$ of an untrained male decreases by approximately 5mL.kg^{-1}. min^{-1} per decade. The same decrements apply to the trained male, but due to higher starting aerobic capacity their VO_2 max values remain consistently higher than the untrained, and are 20mL.$kg^{-1}.min^{-1}$ higher at aged 40yr and 10mL.$kg^{-1}.min^{-1}$ at 70yr.

Response to training

Training effects are still apparent in the elderly and despite the decrements above, the elderly can improve their VO_2 max by 15% and training load by 80% after three months of aerobic training. There are also similar changes seen in lactate threshold and anaerobic performance indices with appropriate training.

Weight training in children

Weight training in children has always been a controversial topic. The detractors say that it is injurious and does not produce strength improvements in the pre-adolescent child, but studies now show that it can produce strength gains even in pre-adolescent children and, when well-supervised, the injury risk is low.

Part of the controversy surrounding weight training in children stems from confusion as to the difference between weight training and weight lifting.

Weight lifting refers to a competitive sport where maximal lifts are performed. Most authorities agree that this sport is unsuitable for children before Tanner stage 5.

Weight training (also called strength training or resistance training) involves repetitive sub-maximal muscle contractions with the aim of improving strength.

Effects

- Weight training has been shown to improve muscle strength in pre-adolescents and adolescents although the mechanism by which it works appears to differ.
- In the pre-adolescent, strength gains are thought to be the result of improved motor co-ordination and neural adaptations which increase motor unit activation and recruitment.
- In the adolescent, muscle hypertrophy is largely responsible for the strength gains which occur.
- There is some evidence that strength training improves aspects of motor performance but no good evidence that it improves overall sports performance or reduces incidence of injuries.

Risks

- When compared with other sports played in the same age group, there is no evidence that a well-supervised strength training program has a greater injury rate than other sports.

Guidelines for weight training in children

- Must be well supervised by an adult familiar with weight training in children.
- Gradual progression of loads.
- Start with low loads and high repetitions (i.e. 2–3 sets of 12–15 repetitions).
- If using weight machines, ensure that the lever length is appropriate for children.
- Train agonist and antagonist muscle groups equally.
- Do not train more than 3 times per week.
- Have 'circuit' set up to encourage cardio-respiratory training at the same time.
- Stress that resistance training should be just one part of overall exercise regimen.
- Avoid lifting maximal loads before Tanner stage 5.

Metabolic

Cellular recovery after exercise

Exercise increases the generation of oxygen free radicals and lipid peroxidation which have harmful cellular effects. The rate of oxygen consumption and the presence of cellular antioxidant systems influence the magnitude of cellular damage occurring as a result of exercise.

Free radicals generated during exercise may arise from three potential sources:
• The mitochondria from which oxygen radicals have escaped.
• The capillary endothelium through hypoxia.
• Inflammatory cells mobilized from tissue damage.

Skeletal muscle has adapted to protect against further cell injury following exercise. Normal cellular adaptation occurs in response to an appropriate stimulus, and ceases once the need for adaptation has ceased. These adaptations include:
• Biochemical changes such as an increase in antioxidant enzymes and production of heat shock proteins.
• Response to increased work demands by changing their size (atrophy or hypertrophy), number (hyperplasia), and form (metaplasia).

Exercise, repair, and recovery

Exercise training reduces the susceptibility of muscles to further damage by:
• Increasing the activity of antioxidant enzymes such as superoxide dismutase, catalase and glutathione peroxidase. The ability of cells to respond to stress by increasing the content of cytoprotective proteins is blunted over time by the ageing process.

Physical damage to muscle cells from repeated muscular contractions (particularly eccentric contractions) is repaired in the following sequence:
• During days 2–4, there is invasion by phagocytic cells and prominent degeneration of cellular structures.
• During days 4–6, regeneration of muscle begins by the activation and migration of satellite cells. These satellite cells migrate into the damaged area, differentiate to form myoblasts, and fuse to form multi-nucleated myotubes which develop into mature skeletal muscle.
• Rapid repair of plasma membrane disruption is essential to cell survival and involves a complex and active cell response that includes membrane fusion and cytoskeletal activation. Tissues, such as cardiac and skeletal muscle, adapt to a disruption injury by hypertrophy. Cells adapt by increasing the efficiency of their rehealing response.

Body weight

Total energy intake must be raised to meet the increased energy expended during training. Maintenance of energy balance can be assessed by monitoring body weight, body composition, and food intake.

Weight gain

For those athletes who wish to gain body weight, caloric intake should exceed energy expenditure. Increased muscle mass, from physical training, can lead to increased body weight even with a reduction in body fat percentage.

Weight loss

For those athletes who wish to lose weight, caloric intake should not exceed energy expenditure. The caloric deficit will dictate the amount of weight that can be lost. To maximize the loss of fat and minimize the loss of lean tissue, weight loss should be limited to 500–1000g per week. This would require an energy restriction of 2–4 MJ per day. Where there is a need to reduce body weight this should be done gradually, and not immediately before competition. The use of diuretics and laxatives should be discouraged.

Fluid status will affect bodyweight. Volume depletion will present as 'weight loss' while hyperhydration can present with body-weight gain. These fluid gains and losses are transient and can be detrimental to health if performed for the wrong reasons (i.e. 'making weight' in sports which require weight classes for competition).

Body mass index (BMI)

BMI is generally used as a descriptive tool for assessing health risks. BMI can be calculated with imperial or metric units.

Weight in pounds / [(height in inches)^2] × 703

or

Weight in kilograms / [(height in metres)^2]

Energy requirements

The main component of daily energy turnover in an average person is the basal metabolic rate (BMR).

Basal metabolic rate (BMR) represents the *minimum* amount of energy expenditure needed for ongoing processes in the body in the resting state, when no food is digested and no energy is needed for temperature regulation. The most variable component of daily energy turnover is the energy expenditure for activity (EEA) which can range between 15–25% of the BMR in moderately active persons.

For sports such as gymnastics, dancing, diving, and running in which a lean physique is desired, athletes will routinely restrict their caloric intake to achieve a leaner body composition. This practice reduces the metabolic rate and may lead to conditions such as menstrual dysfunction (amenorrhea) , iron deficiency (anemia) and a decrease in bone density (osteoporosis/osteopenia).

A chronic negative energy balance will result in a loss of fat free (muscle) mass as well as a loss of body fat. Lethargy from the excessive loss of lean body mass and depletion of glycogen stores generally limits performance and the ability to train properly, making an athlete more susceptible to illness and injury.

An increase in lean body mass will increase energy requirements for basal activities and visa versa. Athletes who sustain hard and vigorous activity for prolonged periods of time must supplement their caloric needs by ingesting more energy to sustain exercise and match energy demands during exercise. While increased energy consumption can be achieved by ingesting primarily more carbohydrate-rich solid food or liquid carbohydrate formulas, increases in fat and protein ingestion are also part of a healthy mixed diet.

The higher the intensity of the exercise and the more muscle groups that are activated, the more the energy requirements of that activity are increased.

Food and exercise

Physically active individuals must meet their energy requirements by ingesting a variety of foodstuffs both before, during, and after exercise.

For most individuals the consumption of a normal mixed diet consisting of 50% carbohydrate and 10–30% fat, with the difference made up with protein, is adequate.

The only reason to consume protein or fat several hours before exercise or exercise performance is to provide satiety, which can influence performance by promoting a sense of well-being. If carbohydrate stores are adequate, the choice of food before exercise should be based on the past experience of the athlete in so much as that the food choice should minimize hunger yet not interfere with the exercise mode and duration.

Habituation to a high-fat diet decreases the amount of muscle glycogen used during exercise by increasing the body's ability to use and mobilize fat. The increased ability to oxidize fat for fuel may enable an athlete to continue exercising for longer periods at intensities of 70% of VO_2 max or less. However, habituation to a high-fat diet is associated with a reduced performance ability during high intensity exercise performance, such as when attempting to elevate power output during hill climbing in endurance cycling or running events.

Carbohydrate needs

The CHO needs of individuals vary depending on their mass and the level of physical activity. Larger and more active individuals will require generally more energy and therefore more CHO. However, in the normal exercising population the CHO needs will be met by consuming a normal mixed diet as described above.

Protein needs

The protein needs of individuals also vary with mass and activity level, but are also generally met when one is consuming a normal mixed diet. Although the RDA for protein is 0.8g per kg of body mass, highly active endurance athletes may require up to 1g per kg of body mass, while those striving to build large amounts of muscle mass may require in excess of 1.5g per kg of body mass. Usually these requirements are adequately covered by the increased energy intake stimulated by physical activity, and it is often unnecessary to increase actively the protein content of the diet by eating selectively protein-rich foodstuffs.

Pre-event diet

Carbohydrate loading has been shown to increase muscle glycogen content before exercise and delay the time at which low muscle glycogen concentrations are reached. The main effect of this practice is to decrease the amount of fat oxidized during exercise. Carbohydrate loading is achieved by eating a high carbohydrate diet (75–90%) for three days prior to the competitive event. To achieve this, athletes should consume approximately 8g CHO or more per kg of body mass.

Pre-event meal

The pre-event diet aims to optimize muscle glycogen and liver glycogen stores which maintain blood glucose levels during exercise. The ingestion of carbohydrate before an event will stimulate carbohydrate oxidation and inhibit fat oxidation. Evidence suggests that performance is improved when 200–300g CHO is consumed 3–4 hours before prolonged exercise, compared to when no food is ingested.

Immediately prior to the event

Foods that are consumed immediately prior to an event should be low in fat, protein, and fibre, and should not cause gastrointestinal distress.

Foods ingested 4–6 hours before an event should be of a low to moderate glycaemic index to minimize the insulin response. If the muscles are not fully stocked with glycogen (because of recent exercise or a low CHO diet), however, then foods with a moderate to high glycaemic index are preferred prior to an athletic event.

Food supplements

Numerous well-controlled studies have concluded that individuals eating a well balanced diet do not need to supplement their diet with vitamins, minerals, or trace elements when undertaking an exercise programme. The ingestion of these supplements on physical performance has not been clearly shown to have benefits.

Vitamins

Vitamins are divided into water- and fat-soluble categories. Water-soluble vitamins such as thiamin, riboflavin, B-6, niacin, pantothenic acid, biotin, and vitamin C are involved in mitochondrial metabolism. Folate and vitamin B-12 are primarily involved in DNA synthesis and red blood cell development. Fat-soluble vitamins include vitamins A, K, E, and D with vitamin E being the most widely studied as an ergogenic aid. Vitamin E has antioxidant properties, as do vitamins C, A, and beta carotene. There is a linear relationship between energy intake and vitamin intake, thus vitamin intake should exceed the recommended daily allowance (RDA) provided that a varied diet is consumed. Mega doses of both fat and water-soluble vitamins have been shown to have toxic effects.

Minerals

Minerals are divided into macrominerals and microminerals (trace minerals). Macrominerals include calcium, magnesium, phosphorous, sulphur, potassium, sodium and chloride with calcium, phosphorus, and calcium each constituting 0.01% of total body weight. Trace minerals include iron, zinc, copper, selenium, chromium, iodine, fluorine, manganese, molybdenum, nickel, silicon, vanadium, arsenic, and cobalt with each constituting less than 0.001% of total body weight. Iron, zinc, copper, selenium, and chromium have been proposed to enhance physical performance and may improve physical performance if an athlete is deficient in that certain mineral, or if an increased level of this mineral would boost the body's natural response to enhance performance.

Amino acids, electrolytes, and herbal supplements have not been shown to improve physical performance in well-controlled scientific studies.

Iron

Iron is a necessary component of haemoglobin and myoglobin and facilitates the transport of oxygen through the bloodstream as well as the transfer of electrons in the electron transport chain system. 60–70% of iron is found in haemoglobin with the remainder found in bone marrow, muscle, liver, and spleen.

Organ meats, black strap molasses, clams, oysters, dried legumes, nuts and seeds, red meats, and dark leafy vegetables are good exogenous sources of iron. Symptoms of an iron deficiency include generalized fatigue and anaemia. Liver damage can occur from iron excess.

Iron deficiency anemia in athletes may result from a poor diet, excess blood loss (through menstruation in females), footstrike haemolysis, and through sweat loss. Although numerous studies have documented that athletes, particularly endurance athletes, are iron depleted, the degree and percentage of iron depletion is similar between athletes and non-athletes.

Pseudoanaemia occurs in athletes secondary to an increase in plasma volume which occurs as an adaptation to training. This increase in plasma volume 'dilutes' an otherwise normal red blood cell count into falsely low levels. Hence, this is an artificial lowering of haemoglobin rather than a true anaemic response which is a common laboratory finding in endurance athletes.

The recommended daily allowance for iron intake for males is 10–12mg/day and 15mg/day for females.

Calcium

Calcium is required for the formation and maintenance of hard bones and for the conduction of nerve impulses. Calcium activates enzymes responsible for the transmission of membrane potentials as well as for muscle contraction. 99% of calcium is found in the skeleton with the remainder found in extracellular fluid, intracellular structures, and cell membranes.

Dairy products, sardines, clams, oysters, turnips, broccoli, and legumes are good exogenous sources of calcium. Osteoporosis and fractures can occur from a deficiency in calcium intake over decades. Constipation, kidney stones, and chelation with antibiotics and other nutrients (such as iron and zinc) can occur with calcium excess.

Weight bearing exercise has been shown to increase bone density, especially when undertaken at critical growth periods (8–14 years of age). Oestrogen has been shown to reduce urinary calcium excretion, increase intestinal absorption of calcium and increase the secretion of calcitonin which reduces bone resorption. Calcium also can be lost through sweat, which may increase an athlete's total daily requirement if exercise is regularly performed in hot and humid environments.

The recommended daily allowance for calcium is 800–1200mg/day for both men and women.

Creatine

Creatine is a naturally occurring compound in the body, specifically in the muscles.

Creatine supplementation is widely practiced by professional and recreational athletes. The benefits and side effects are varied and debatable. Purported benefits include increased mass, improved rate of recovery after exercise, and increased power or speed. Side affects include cramping and water retention.

Although much research has been devoted to creatine and its effects, the real value of creatine supplementation remains uncertain. Untrained persons undertaking a weight training programme for the first time appear to benefit the most. Elite athletes who eat diets with adequate protein intake may benefit less.

Recovery after exercise

Recovery after exercise is most important if another bout of physical activity will shortly follow. Full recovery after exercise is also important in reducing the risk of overtraining, although the training volumes required to produce overtraining are usually achievable only by highly trained individuals.

Recovery is also an important part of adapting to exercise training, because the physical adaptations that are stimulated by exercise training occur during the rest and recovery phase.

Recovery appears to be aided by the ingestion of carbohydrate- and protein-rich foodstuffs within 30–60 minutes after the termination of exercise.

Exercise and the environment

Different environmental conditions will affect exercise tolerance and capacity in different ways. There are three overriding environmental factors to which athletes may be exposed in either training or racing, or both—heat, cold, and reduced oxygen content in the inspired air as occurs at increasing altitude.

In order to survive, humans require to regulate their body temperatures at between 35–41°C and to maintain the partial pressure of oxygen in their blood in excess of about 40mmHg.

Environmental conditions, in particular the environmental temperature, the wind speed, and the water content of the air (humidity) determine the rate at which heat is lost from the body. The normal average human skin temperature is 33°C. At any lower environmental temperature, heat will be lost from the skin to the environment in the process of heat conduction. The rate at which this heat will be lost by conduction from the body will, in turn, be determined by the magnitude of the temperature gradient—the steeper the gradient, the greater the heat loss—and the rapidity with which the cooler air in contact with the skin is replaced by colder air. Continual replacement of warmed air by cooler air causes loss of heat from the body, by means of convection. Convective heat loss rises as an exponential function of the speed at which air courses across the body, in effect the prevailing wind speed. With high humidity, sweat loss by evaporation is reduced.

Body temperature

At rest, humans regulate their body temperatures within a narrow range of between 36.5–37.5°C. During exercise, this safe thermoregulatory range is increased to up to 41.5°C. Heat–acclimatized human athletes have a superior capacity to exercise without apparent distress even up to body temperatures of 41.5°C.

The human body temperature represents a balance between the rate of heat production by, and heat loss from, the body. Hence changes in the rates of either heat production or heat loss, or more commonly both, determine whether an abnormal rise in body temperature (hyperthermia leading to heat stroke) or an excessive fall (hypothermia) is likely to develop and under what conditions. The principal physiological challenge that athletes face during exercise is how to lose the excess body heat produced by muscle contraction.

Hypothermia

When environmental conditions are particularly cold, for example (i) during winter conditions at latitudes above about 50° in either hemisphere, (ii) when cold is associated with windy and especially wet conditions, or (iii) when the athlete exercises in cold water for prolonged periods, the risk arises that the athlete will lose heat faster than he or she can produce it. Under these conditions, the body may be unable to maintain its core body temperature which may fall progressively, leading to hypothermia (core temperature <35°C) and the risk of death from the exposure/exhaustion syndrome.

Low body temperatures of 35°C occur frequently in swimmers exposed to cold water temperatures for many hours, for example, in long distance Channel swims. This occurs because water is an excellent conductor of heat, approximately 30 times more effective than is air. As a result, the naked body exposed to a body of water that is colder than the normal body temperature of 37°C is unable to produce heat as rapidly as it is lost by conduction to the surrounding water. If exposed for sufficiently long, the human body will be cooled to the temperature of the surrounding water which is seldom more than 20°C except at the tropics. Wearing more appropriate clothing, in particular, dry or wet suits that maintain a layer of insulating water or air heated to body temperature, is the only way to prevent the ultimate development of a fatal hypothermia when exposed to cold water for any protracted period (hours).

Prevention of hypothermia

When exercising in cold conditions, hypothermia can be prevented by continued activity, adequate clothing, and the presence of insulating layers. There is a high rate of heat production during exercise. Thus, as a general rule, continuing to move reduces the risk that hypothermia will develop. However, once the subject becomes too exhausted to continue, his or her rate of heat production falls sharply and the risk of hypothermia rises dramatically.

The important practical point is that continuing to exercise will protect against hypothermia if it maintains the rate of heat production that equals or exceeds the heat loss. In contrast, once the hiker, runner, or mountain climber starts to walk or stops walking altogether, the rate of heat production falls dramatically, providing the necessary conditions for hypothermia. The change from running to walking, for example, has a marked effect on the clothing needed to maintain body temperature, even at relatively mild temperatures. Thus, clothing with at least four times as much insulation is required to maintain body temperature at rest at an effective air temperature of 0°C, as when running at 16km per hour. Thus, extra clothing should always be available if there is any possibility that fatigue will develop when exercising in cold conditions.

Whereas air is a poor conductor of heat and hence a good insulator, water is a very poor insulator. Thus, the thin layer of air trapped next to the skin by clothing is rapidly heated to the skin temperature, thereby producing a layer of insulation. But the saturation of clothing with water removes this insulating layer and essentially exposes the skin to whatever the external temperature is. Under these conditions, the exposed human must either find dry, warm clothing and a warm shelter, or he/she will cool to the prevailing environmental temperature. This loss of insulation caused by water explains why saturated, wet clothing experienced by runners, climbers, or hikers in windy, wet conditions or alternatively swimmers in cold water, predisposes to the development of hypothermia.

Experience with the English Channel swimmers has shown that body build, especially the body muscle (but also the body fat) content, is a critical factor determining the rate at which a swimmer will cool down during a long-distance swim in water temperatures below about 24°C. It is probable that the same applies in out-of-water activities; subjects who are more muscular and fatter are likely to cool down more slowly when exposed to very cold conditions.

Thus appropriate fitness, proper clothing including water repellent outer garments, adequate nutrition to prevent premature fatigue, early recognition of danger, and an avoidance of extreme environmental conditions, are crucial to ensure that exercise can be safely undertaken in cold, wet, and windy conditions.

Diagnosis of hypothermia
- Rectal temperature <37°C (usually much lower).
- Exposure to cold conditions for prolonged periods.
- Fatigue.
- Muscle weakness and loss of coordination.
- Desire to stop exercising.
- Disorientation, leading to coma.

Treatment of hypothermia
- Removal from the cold environment, application of dry clothing and/or blankets.
- External heating in the form of hot water bottles, warm water bath, radiant heat, convective heat, or even the body heat of other humans.
- In severe hypothermia, consider using heated intravenous fluids or extra-corporeal blood warming techniques.
- Warming efforts should continue until the body temperature exceeds 35°C since a person with hypothermia is not 'cold and dead' until they are shown to be 'warm and dead'.

Special note
Be aware that ventricular fibrillation is a common complication of treatment for hypothermia, especially during rapid re-warming, and should be treated appropriately.

Hyperthermia

Hyperthermia describes an increase in body temperature above the normal resting upper limit of 37.5°C. Elevated body temperatures of up to 41.5°C are frequently measured in healthy winners of short distance (5–15km) running events contested in hot, humid, windless environmental conditions. Such high body temperatures occur because the rate at which elite athletes produce heat when running at their maximum pace can exceed the capacity of the hot environment to absorb that heat. Fortunately the brain also has protective mechanisms that reduce the allowable rate of energy production (exercise intensity/speed) during exercise in the heat. As a result, incidences of severe heat injury (heatstroke) are remarkably uncommon in sport despite the frequency with which sport is played in severe environmental conditions.

During exercise, the chemical energy stored in the muscles in the form of adenosine triphosphate (ATP), is converted into the mechanical energy of motion. However, this process is inefficient so that only 25% of the chemical energy used by the muscles produces motion; the remaining 75% is released as heat that must be lost from the body if the body temperature is to be safely regulated. Thus, when elite ultra-marathon runners run at an average pace of about 16km per hour during races of 90–100km, they use approximately 56kJ of energy every minute, or about 18,480kJ in the 5.5 hours that they require to complete these races. But, of the total amount of KJ used, only about 4000kJ actually transport them from the start to the finish of their races. The remaining 14,480kJ serve only to overheat the runners' bodies. To prevent their temperatures from rising to over 43°C causing heatstroke, these athletes have to lose more than 90% of the heat they produce.

The humidity of the air determines the extent to which heat can be lost to the environment in the form of sweat, which evaporates from the skin surface and, to a lesser extent, from the respiratory membranes. This process of evaporation is the predominant source of heat loss in exercising humans, especially in the heat since each gram (ml) of water so evaporated removes 1.8kJ from the body. As the humidity of the air rises, the efficiency of heat loss by evaporation falls so that the ease of maintaining heat balance becomes increasingly difficult as the humidity rises above 60–70%.

Sweating is an extremely efficient mechanism for heat loss. Thus, provided the humidity is low, well trained and heat-acclimatized humans can regulate their body temperatures and prevent dangerous hyperthermia even when they exercise at high intensities in hot environmental conditions (up to 34°C).

The brain provides the final mechanism that protects humans from unsafe hyperthermia when exercising in hot, warm, and humid conditions. Feedback from sensors throughout the body to a central regulator in the brain monitor both the extent of the environmental stress to which the body is exposed, as well as the rate at which the body stores heat during exercise in those environmental conditions. Since it is safe to exercise only to a body temperature of less than 42°C, immediately on exposure to the prevailing environmental conditions at the onset of exercise, and on the basis of the rate at which heat will be stored and the expected duration of the exercise, the brain calculates the rate at which work can be safely performed under those specific environmental conditions. This central governor therefore pre-sets the number of motor units in the active muscles that can be recruited in order to ensure that a safe rate of heat production is allowed for the expected duration of the exercise. At the same time, the brain pre-sets the rate at which the perception of effort increases during the exercise bout so that the perceived effort of continuing to exercise becomes intolerable before the body temperature is elevated to dangerous levels.

In this way, the brain ensures that dangerous hyperthermia including heatstroke occurs uncommonly during exercise. When heatstroke does occur during exercise, the presence of pathological precursors must be considered. These include the presence of a pre-existing medical condition including a muscle disorder that predisposes to excessive heat production during exercise (exercise-induced malignant hyperthermia), any condition that elevates the body temperature before the onset of exercise, or the use of drugs, especially amphetamines, that prevent the normal function of the central governor mechanism by reducing the sensations of discomfort during exercise.

Exercise in the heat

Hot (>30°C) and humid (>50% relative humidity) environmental conditions will reduce exercise capacity and performance, although represent no immediate danger to an individual.

Acclimatization and the heat

In addition to the general adaptations that occur with exercise training, individuals can also adapt to exercise in hot and humid environments. This is referred to as heat acclimatization and can be achieved with a specific program of exercise and conditions.

General terminology

Wet bulb

Temperature value derived from specialized thermometer that is used to measure the amount of water vapor pressure in the air. Commonly referred to as the wet bulb (WB) or relative humidity (RH). WB is less than the dry bulb (DB) in proportion to the environmental humidity. When the RH is 100%, the WB and DB are the same.

Dry bulb

Temperature value derived from a normal thermometer, and from which the ambient temperature is obtained. Commonly referred to as the dry bulb (DB).

Black globe

Specialized thermometer to measure the radiant heat load. It consists of a dry bulb thermometer enclosed inside a black, metal sphere. Commonly referred to as the globe temperature (GT).

Wet bulb globe temperature (WBGT)

An index system used to rate the combined environmental variables of temperature, radiation, and humidity, as measured with the above terms. Calculated with the equation

$$WBGT = 0.7 \, WB + 0.2 \, GT + 0.1 \, DB$$

Heat acclimatization

Complete heat acclimatization requires 7–10 consecutive days of low to moderate intensity exercise of 60–120 minutes in ambient temperatures above 30°C and 50% relative humidity. A large proportion of the adaptations occur within the first five days, but 7–10 days are required for full acclimatization. The general adaptations that occur with heat acclimatization include:

Earlier onset of sweating

Sweating begins at an earlier core temperature, representing an increased ability to dissipate heat.

Decreased sweat sodium concentration

- To conserve Na^+, the body produces more dilute sweat. Unacclimatized sweat Na^+ concentration is approximately 75mmol Na^+ per litre. After acclimatization this can decrease to 20–30mmoL Na^+ per litre of sweat.

Cardiovascular adaptations

- After acclimatization, the heart rate and core temperature at the same given exercise intensity will be lower compared to pre-acclimatization levels.

Fluid retention

The amount of fluid in blood (plasma volume) increases.

Heat-related illness in children

Children are disadvantaged compared with adults when exercising in the heat.

The reasons for children's increased susceptibility

- Higher surface area to body mass ratio means that children absorb more heat from the environment in hot conditions.
- Less efficient exercisers i.e. they produce more heat for a given work load.
- Lower cardiac output, therefore less able to divert blood to the skin for cooling.
- Lower sweat rate.
- Higher sweating threshold.
- Slower to acclimatize.

Signs and symptoms of heat-related illness

The signs of heat-related illness represent a continuum from heat exhaustion (at the early stage) to heat stroke (a medical emergency).

Early signs of heat exhaustion include:
- Headache.
- Dizziness.
- Nausea.
- Muscle fatigue.

The signs of heat stroke include:
- Tachycardia.
- May or may not be sweating.
- Altered mental state (confusion → seizures → coma).
- Rectal temp >41°celcius.

Children at particular risk include
- Obese children.
- Children with previous history of heat-related illness.
- Children with diabetes, cystic fibrosis and cardiac conditions.
- Children taking certain medications including antihistamines, phenothiazines, and anticholinergics.

Treatment of heat-related illness in children
- Remove child to shady area and remove unnecessary clothing.
- Measure rectal temperature.
- Give cool fluids if conscious.
- If altered consciousness or rectal temp. >41°C, this is a medical emergency and child should be immediately transferred to hospital facility.
- Cooling and rehydration however should commence immediately.
- Early treatment is important for a favourable outcome.

Prevention of heat-related illness in children
- Avoid scheduling children's events for the heat of the day.
- Ensure adequate hydration by providing cool drinks with flavouring as these appear to be associated with increased consumption.
- Ensure appropriate clothing i.e. light-coloured, permeable materials.
- Early identification of symptoms.

Guidelines for organizers of children's events

Table 21.1 Guidelines for organizers of children's events

Wet bulb globe temperature (WBGT)		Restraint on activities
°C	°F	
<24	<75	All activities allowed, but be alert for prodromes of heat-related illness in prolonged events.
24.0–25.9	75.0–78.6	Longer rest periods in the shade; enforce drinking every 15 minutes.
26–29	79–84	Stop activity of unacclimatized persons and other persons with high risk; limit activities of all others (disallow long-distance races, cut down duration further of other activities).
>29	>85	Cancel all athletic activities.

Committee on Sports Medicine and Fitness, American Academy of Pediatrics: Sports Medicine: *Health Care for Young Athletes*, edn 2. Elk Grove Village, IL: American Academy of Pediatrics; 1991:98.

WGBT is an index of climatic heat stress. It combines air temperature, humidity and radiation and is measured with a special apparatus.

Exercise at altitude

Altitudes exceeding 1500m above sea level will have an effect on exercise tolerance and capacity by reducing the maximal oxygen consumption in a curva-linear fashion. High altitude poses two distinct physiological challenges for the human body:

1. Increasingly lower amount of O_2 in the air as one ascends to higher altitudes

As the altitude above sea level increases, the barometric pressure falls. As a result, the number of oxygen molecules in each litre of air falls. In order partially to compensate for this, humans breathe more often and more deeply at altitude. But as the altitude increases, the partial pressure of oxygen in the blood falls, reaching values that are not compatible with sustained human life at altitudes much above about 7000m. That some humans are able to reach the summit of Mount Everest (8840m) attests to the phenomenal biology of some humans; to the value of oxygen inhalation for others; and the quite remarkable ability of most humans to adapt to the stresses to which they are exposed for weeks to months.

Originally it was argued that exercise performance at altitude was 'limited' by the production of excessive amounts of lactic acid by the oxygen-starved muscles. However, early studies showed that this could not be the case, since blood lactic acid during maximal exercise are as low at the summit of high mountains as they are at rest at sea level. This finding is paradoxical since, according to the traditional understanding, exercise in the increasing levels of hypoxia that occur at altitude should cause an increased skeletal muscle anaerobiosis with an increased production of lactic acid. Elevated lactic acid concentrations would then explain why the capacity to exercise is substantially reduced at increasing altitude. In addition, the maximal cardiac output is also much reduced during exercise at altitude. This too is paradoxical since a higher cardiac output should be advantageous, as it would increase blood and oxygen delivery to the exercising muscles to offset the effects of the progressive reduction in the amount of oxygen stored in each unit of arterial blood.

2. Increasingly harsh ambient conditions due to the cold and wind

Fortunately at the temperatures at high altitude, water exists in the form of ice and snow so that the environment is usually dry. As a result it is easier to keep clothes dry than it is in the cold and wet conditions that predominate at lower altitudes. On the other hand, the presence of high winds at altitude markedly increases the coldness of the environment by increasing the wind chill factor and promoting heat loss by convection to the environment. Many deaths at altitude occur not as a result of fatal falls but are caused by hypothermia.

Studies show that the ability of the brain to recruit the muscles is regulated by a number of variables including, at increasing altitude, the partial pressure of arterial oxygen which is a direct function of the barometric pressure. Thus, as the barometric pressure falls the brain reduces the mass of muscle that it will allow to be activated during exercise. The end result of this control is to reduce the maximal exercise capacity at altitude specifically to prevent a reduction in the arterial oxygen partial pressure to levels that cannot sustain normal brain function.

Hypoxia

As humans ascend to increasing altitude, they are exposed to a progressively lower partial pressure of oxygen in the inspired air. As a result the partial pressure of oxygen in the blood supplying their brains also falls. Whilst there are a number of physiological adaptations that increase this pressure, ultimately each human will reach an altitude at which they are no longer able to survive since their blood oxygen pressure falls below that required for those crucial brain functions necessary for sustaining life. Exercise at altitude is also 'limited' by the brain to ensure that no exercise intensity is undertaken that will produce a blood oxygen partial pressure at which unconsciousness develops.

Altitude acclimatization

Acclimatization to altitude can be achieved with a gradual ascent to higher altitudes over a number of days or weeks. The regulator of exercise at altitude appears to be the partial pressure of oxygen in the arterial blood (PaO_2). When the PaO_2 falls below some critical value (different between individuals, perhaps on the basis of genetic factors or the extent of the adaptation to altitude), the brain prevents the continuing recruitment of motor units in the exercising limbs so that exercise must terminate. Effective adaptations to altitude must increase the PaO_2 at any altitude (barometric pressure), maintain higher PaO_2 during exercise, and adapt the brain so that it is able to maintain the recruitment of an appropriate muscle mass at the same or lower PaO_2, without risking brain damage from hypoxia.

Specific adaptations to altitude:

- Increase ventilation rate.
- Rise in arterial pH as arterial CO_2 is reduced (due to hyperventilation which drives the reaction ($H^+ + HCO_3^- \rightarrow H_2O + CO_2$) to the right).
- Kidney retention of H^+ compensates for this respiratory alkalosis.
- Increased PaO_2 (due to hyperventilation).
- Increase in blood haemoglobin concentration due to an initial fall in blood volume.
- Increased excretion of erythropoietin by the kidneys in response to the reduction in PaO_2.
- Progressive increases in the red cell mass (for up to 3–12 months) with more prolonged exposures above about 3250 m. This is due to increased EPO production at altitude.
- Oxygen dissociation curve of haemoglobin shifts to the left, favouring increased haemoglobin oxygen saturation at any PaO_2.
- No change in pulmonary diffusing capacity at moderate altitude but becomes impaired at very high altitudes.
- Increased pressure in the pulmonary circulation due to pulmonary arteriolar vasoconstriction; develops in proportion to the reduction in PaO_2.
- Potential right ventricular hypertrophy when pulmonary hypertension is sustained.

- Increased cerebral blood flow in response to the reduction in PaO_2. (The extent to which cerebral blood flow increases is limited by the cerebral arteriolar vasoconstriction which occurs in response to the fall in $PaCO_2$ induced by hyperventilation).
- Increased secretion of adrenal cortical hormones and activation of the sympathetic nervous system.
- Increase in the blood concentrations of sodium and water conserving hormones (renin, aldosterone and ADH) especially in response to exercise. These hormones favour increased fluid retention.
- Increased respiratory water losses in response to hyperventilation and the low humidity of the air at altitude.

As a result of these adaptations, exercise performance capacity at altitude improves but is always less at altitude compared to sea-level.

Altitude sickness

Occurs in about 25% of persons unacclimatized to moderate altitude on acute exposure to altitudes in excess of about 2500m. In about 5%, symptoms will be sufficiently severe to require bed rest. The incidence of symptoms, including incapacitation requiring bed rest, increases with increasing altitude and may be 100% in those who ascend rapidly to above 3000m. Although acute altitude sickness is usually no more than an illness of inconvenience, progression to high altitude pulmonary oedema or cerebral oedema can occur. Thus, all persons with the condition must be observed until symptoms disappear.

Symptoms

Symptoms are most intense for the first 48 hours after arrival at altitude, lessening thereafter and disappearing within 5–8 days. Symptoms are worse in the morning, perhaps as a result of increased hypoxaemia during sleep.

- Headache, insomnia, lassitude, anorexia often associated with nausea and vomiting.

Aetiology

- Unknown but may be related to cerebral hypoxia and an increased cerebral blood flow.

Prevention

- Avoid rapid ascension to altitudes above 2000–2500m.
- Ascend slowly with stops at intermediate altitudes.
- Avoid vigorous exercise on the first few days of arrival at altitude. Rather emphasize rest during that period.
- The use of acetazolamide (125–250mg twice daily) beginning 48 hours before ascent to altitude and continued for the first five days after arrival at altitude is the only proven efficacious medication.
- Low flow oxygen at night may be helpful if available.

Treatment

- Treat mild symptoms with appropriate medications.
- If symptoms progress, oxygen at high flow should be administered.
- If available, a hyperbaric bag can be used.
- If symptoms progress further despite these interventions, urgent evacuation to a lower altitude is essential.
- Descent to a sufficiently low altitude cures the symptoms.

Cerebral/pulmonary oedema

A potentially fatal but preventable condition that develops rapidly and with little warning in persons unacclimatized to altitude, but who ascend rapidly to altitudes in excess of about 2500m and who, on arrival at altitude, often partake of vigorous exercise. Easier access to high altitudes for unacclimatized mountain climbers, skiers, and trekkers has increased the incidence of the condition with about 20 deaths per year reported annually around the world.

Aetiology (pulmonary oedema)

Uncertain but probably involves hypoxic pulmonary arteriolar vasoconstriction with thrombotic obstruction of some parts of the pulmonary vascular bed.

- Overperfusion of non-obstructed capillaries increases capillary shear forces.
- Increased shear forces injure capillaries causing leakage of red cells and protein into the alveoli.
- Individual susceptibility (as repeat attacks occur in some individuals).

Aetiology (cerebral oedema)

Increased cerebral blood flow with capillary damage induces leakage of oedema fluid into the brain.

Symptoms (pulmonary oedema)

- Dyspnoea, cough, weakness, chest tightness, and occasionally haemoptysis, usually within the first 3 days of arrival at altitude.
- In more severe cases, alterations in consciousness may occur.

Symptoms (cerebral oedema)

Symptoms of central nervous system dysfunction including ataxia, headache, lethargy, and irrational behaviour indicate the impending development of high altitude cerebral oedema. Coma indicates the presence of advanced cerebral oedema.

Signs (pulmonary and cerebral oedema)

- Cyanosis, tachycardia, tachypnoea, and pulmonary rales.
- Papilloedema.
- Abnormal reflexes.
- Altered level of consciousness.

Treatment

- Oxygen at high flow rates.
- Use of a hyperbaric bag if available.
- Immediate evacuation to lower altitudes.
- Bed rest, oxygen, and nifedipine should be given at lower altitudes if rapid clinical improvement does not occur.
- Descent to lower altitude cures the condition.
- Deaths usually occur only when the initial diagnosis is delayed; the emergency nature of the condition is not appreciated and descent to lower altitude either does not occur, or occurs too late in the course of the illness.

Overtraining syndrome

History and examination

A condition of fatigue and underperformance that occurs following a period of hard training and competition. It affects mainly endurance athletes. The symptoms do not resolve after two weeks adequate rest and may be associated with frequent infections and depression. No causative medical condition can be identified.

Normal training is usually cyclical (periodization) allowing adequate time for recovery, and with progressive overload to improve performance. During these cycles there may be transient symptoms and signs of overtraining known as overreaching.

With overtraining syndrome, there may have been a sudden increase in training, prolonged heavy training, and other physical and psychological stresses. Most athletes recover fully after two weeks of adequate rest but the diagnosis of overtraining syndrome is made when the symptoms and signs persist after two weeks of relative rest. The main complaint is of underperformance but there are other associated features:

- Sleep disturbance is common.
- There may be loss of competitive drive, loss of appetite, and increased emotional lability, anxiety, and irritability.
- Athletes may complain of frequent upper respiratory tract infections or other minor infections, sore throats and lymphadenopathy, myalgia, arthralgia and heavy legs. The athlete may also report a raised resting heart rate.
- There may be symptoms of depression and reduced concentration. There may be loss of libido.

Clinical examination is frequently normal.
- Cervical lymphadenopathy is common but non-specific.
- Increased resting heart rate.
- Increased postural fall in blood pressure and postural rise in heart rate.
- Slow recovery of pulse rate to normal after exercise.
- Reduced sub-maximum oxygen consumption.
- Reduced maximum power output.

Investigations

There is no specific diagnostic test. Clinical investigations exclude other causes of fatigue and reassure the athlete.
- Routine haematological screen. Many athletes have a relatively low haemaglobin and packed cell volume. This athletic anaemia is physiological due to haemodilution and does not affect performance.
- Creatine kinase levels are often high reflecting the intensity, volume, and type of exercise.
- Post-viral illness is confirmed by appropriate viral titres.
- Stress hormones e.g. adrenaline and cortisol are generally higher in overtrained athletes compared to controls. A low testosterone:cortisol ratio has also been noted in underperforming athletes.
- Low levels of glutamine have been found in overtrained athletes compared to controls.

Women

Menstrual cycle

- The normal cycle lasts from 21–36 days. The first day of menstruation is day 1 of the cycle.
- The cycle usually consists of 3–5 days of menstruation. Follicular phase is from last day of menstruation to ovulation which occurs at approximately 14 days, and the luteal phase lasts from ovulation to menstruation which is approximately 15–28 days.
- A cycle lasting fewer than 21 days is polymenorrhea and longer than 36 days is oligomenorrhea. Secondary amenorrhoea is defined as having had no periods for 3–6 months.

Hormonal changes that occur during the menstrual cycle

Gonadotrophin releasing hormone (GnRH) causes the synthesis, storage, and the activation release of follicle stimulating hormone (FSH) and luetinzing hormone (LH).

During the follicular phase, levels of oestrogen increase so that both LH and oestrogen peak just before ovulation. Oestrogen then falls and rises again during the luteal phase. Progesterone is secreted by the corpus luteum during the luteal phase, and both oestrogen and progesterone levels fall if fertilization does not take place. Hormone levels should normally be tested after the 21st day of the cycle, during the luteal phase.

Physical exercise produces marked changes in the post-exercise pulsatile, secretion of LH, FSH, oestrogen and progesterone, and cortisol. The more intense and longer the duration of exercise the greater the effect, resulting in marked changes in the menstrual cycle. Factors associated with changes to the normal menstrual cycle include:

- Psychological stress.
- Physical exercise.
- Seasonal rhythms.
- Circadian rhythms.
- Strenuous exercise causes an increase in dopamine which inhibits GnRH, beta endorphins, catecholamines, oestrogens.
- Beta endorphins stimulate dopamine and combine with noradrenaline receptors in the hypothalamus, which inhibit stimulation of GnRH.

Menarche

The average age for menarche in Europe is 12–13.4 years and in the USA, for Caucasians, it is 12.8 years. Failure to menstruate after 16 years of age is considered to be late menarche and the cause should be investigated. Tall thin girls tend to have a later menarche than small larger girls. In some cases, bone age may be below the chronological age due to illness or inadequate nutrition. To determine this, X-ray the carpal bones of the left hand.

Later menarche tends to occur in gymnasts, ballet dancers, and athletes who start high intensity training early. Girls who have a low caloric intake, low body fat, and high emotional stress are also affected.

Primary amenorrhoea

Any girl, who by the age of 13, has not developed any secondary sexual characteristics, or who has not menstruated by the age of 16 should be evaluated and examined. This should include a detailed medical, family, and nutritional history and, in an athlete, a record of her training and competition. Physical findings will direct the appropriate investigations and may indicate referral to a gynaecologist. The preliminary tests should include hormone levels (FSH, LH, oestrogen, progesterone, testosterone, prolactin, and thyroid function tests), ultrasound of the pelvis, and investigation for chromosomal abnormalities. Treatment for delay of menarche is advised at 18 years because of the risk of osteopenia.

Menstrual irregularities

Menstrual irregularities tend to occur in the athletes with the most intense training schedules or in those who have participated or competed for the longest period of time.

- Vegetarians and people with a low caloric intake have the highest incidence of oligomenorrhea and amenorrhoea.
- Menstrual irregularities are reported in 7% of recreational runners, 12% of swimmers, and 25% of distance runners.
- The incidence depends on how the menstrual irregularities are assessed, and vary in studies by questionnaire or measured hormone levels.

About one third of athletes believe that menstruation affects performance, but medals have been won during all phases of the menstrual cycle. There are no medical contraindications to exercise while menstruating. The effects of menstruation on performance appear to be sports related.

Athletes with menstrual problems often had them prior to training. Many 'normal' cycles show abnormal serum hormone levels after 21st day of cycle. Non-athletes also have problems. A mother's attitude to menstruation is often reflected in the daughter.

Multifactoral causes of all menstrual irregularities include

- Stress, both psychological and physical. Severe emotional stress acts above hypothalamic-pituitary axis.
- Sudden increases in the quantity and intensity of training or increase in the number of competitions.
- Late menarche, irregular cycle prior to sports participation, intense training prior to menarche, and an immature pituitary axis.
- Inadequate nutrition, weight loss. Decreased caloric intake, and a low protein, high fibre diet results in a high serum sex hormone binding globulin and low oestrogen, which predispose to amenorrhoea.

Amenorrhoea

- Higher incidence of musculoskeletal problems and stress fractures in amenorrheic athletes, particularly those with irregular menstrual cycles. Amenorrheic athletes with hyperprolactinaemia have an associated low bone mineral density.
- Cannot assume an amenorrheic athlete is infertile.
- Must rule out pregnancy and other causes of amenorrhoea.

Progression of menstrual changes due to strenuous exercise

- Stage 1. Normal follicular, normal luteal phase.
- Stage 2. Prolonged follicular and a shortened luteal phase results in luteal phase defects which is associated with infertility and premenstrual tension.
- Stage 3. Euoestrogenic anovulatory oligomenorhea, possibility of endometrial hyperplasia adenocarcinoma if this phase persists (Shangold and Mirkin Women and Exercise, 1988).
- Stage 4. Hypo-oestrogenic— amenorrhoea leads to osteoporosis and genital atrophy.

1 Shangold MM and Mirkin G (1988). *Women and Exercise*. FA Davis, Philadelphia, PA.

Dysmenorrhoea

- Dysmenorrhoea is due to the release of prostaglandins and is limited to an ovulatory cycle.
- Exercise has a beneficial effect and dysmenorrhoea is rare in an athlete.
- If dysmenorrhoea is present, look for pathology e.g. fibroid or ovarian cysts, polycystic ovarian syndrome, or endometriosis.

Premenstrual syndrome

- Premenstrual syndrome in athletes may cause problems in sports that require fine judgement; women are more accident prone, and more intolerant to alcohol. It results in irritability, mood swings, and fluid retention.
- Patients with premenstrual tension should not scuba dive. Judgement is poor, more accident prone.
- Diuretics should not be prescribed in athletes. Reduce training.

Treatment

Low dose oral contraceptive pill. It is important not to start the pill just before a major competition but, ideally, several cycles before the competition if possible.

Contraception

Barrier methods include condoms, either on their own, or in conjunction with barrier creams i.e. spermicidal cream or gel. Diaphragm, if correctly fitted, can be worn during exercise with hardly any side effects. Intrauterine devices may cause increased pain and bleeding. Barrier methods are not as reliable as the pill, but have fewer side effects.

It is important to start treatment with the pill, combined or progesterone only, well in advance of any competition due to individual variations in reactions to the pill. Depo-Provera should be used with caution in young athletes, the effect of Depo-Provera on oestrogen levels and bone growth has not been determined. Bone mineral density should be monitored by DEXA to study the effect on bone growth. Particularly in the teens and early twenties.

- The oral contraceptive pill can be prescribed safely from 16 years or three years post menarche.
- Low dose oral contraceptive pill, which consists of a combination of oestrogen and progestogens, can regulate the cycle, control the pain of dysmenorrhoea, and prevent early osteoporosis.
- Progesterone only oral contraceptive pill inhibits ovulation but it is not as effective at reducing pain.

Treatment of menstrual irregularities

The team approach should include the athlete, physician, physiotherapist, nutritionist, physiologist, and psychologist.

- Identify cause.
- Dietary advice, increase caloric intake if necessary.
- Reduce training intensity.
- Monitor hormone levels.
- DEXA scan.
- Low dose pill.
- Monophasic pill or bi- or triphasic. HRT.
- Ultrasound of pelvis.
- Referral to gynaecologist.

Manipulation of menstrual cycle

In an athlete where menstrual problems may affect performance (e.g. premenstrual syndrome, dysmenorrhoea) it may be possible to manipulate the menstrual cycle.

If taking the oral contraceptive pill (OCP) the athlete may stop taking the pill 10 days before sporting event, which will result in a withdrawal bleed. Restart a new packet of OCP at the end of menstruation, or after the sporting event. Barrier methods of contraception will be necessary until two weeks after commencing the pill again. Or, the athlete may continue to take an oral contraceptive pill throughout the period of the sporting event. A monophasic pill is simpler to use if the athlete wishes to manipulate their cycle.

If not taking the oral contraceptive pill, menstruation man be induced 10 days before the event, by giving a progesterone derivative (e.g. progestogen only, norethisterone), for 10 days duration, then stopping the course 10 days before the event when menstruation will occur.

Athletic triad

- Amenorrhoea.
- An eating disorder.
- Osteoporosis or osteopenia (Low bone mineral density).

Each of these conditions can occur on their own or in combination.

Eating disorders or eating distress

Anorexia and bulimia may occur singly or together. There has been a marked increase in the prevalence of eating disorders in the last decade, in both the general public and among athletes. The female athlete is at risk during adolescence and young adulthood. This may be due to psychological, biological, or social pressures at this time. Other factors include poor training programmes, too many competitions and inappropriate goals (a 'win at all costs' approach by athlete, coaches, or parents).

There is an increased incidence in sports with an emphasis on leanness e.g. gymnastics, ballet, long distance running, synchronized swimming, skating, and in weight category sports e.g. judo, light weight rowing, but it can occur in any sport.

It is essential to take an accurate and detailed social, medical, and menstrual history. If there is a history of irregular periods or amenorrhoea, it is essential to do hormone levels and a DEXA scan to out rule osteopenia or osteoporosis. The result of the scan should be explained to the individual and if bone density is low, the patient must be told that it is due to loss of oestrogen because of inadequate calorie intake and that the only way to prevent fractures is for them to take control. Athletes must restore their hormone levels by increasing their body weight and take either hormone replacement (HRT) or the oral contraceptive pill until the bone density has improved.

Osteoporosis

Osteoporosis is characterized by a decrease in bone mass and mineral density and a deterioration in micro-architecture, which results in loss in bone strength and a greater risk of fracture.

Osteoporosis, or in a larger number of cases osteopenia, is associated with low levels of oestrogen, increased bone loss, hypercortisolaemia, low T3 syndrome, and a deficiency in Insulin like growth factor-1 (IGF 1). It is a silent disease which can occur at any age.

Bone is a living tissue which is constantly removed and replaced. The rate of turnover is determined by hormonal and local factors. 60% of bone is laid down during the growth spurt at puberty. Peak bone mass occurs around twenty years. Bone mass plateaus until the age of forty and then declines at menopause. Peak bone mass is affected by genetic factors, environmental factors, mechanical strain, hormones, chronological age, skeletal age, and the stage of sexual maturation.

Weight bearing activity during adolescence and early adulthood is a more important predictor of peak bone mass than calcium intake.

Young women who participate regularly in sports at school demonstrate higher bone mass than those who do not.

Bone requires normal sex hormone levels, adequate nutrition including 1000mg calcium, 800 international units of vitamin D, and regular weight bearing exercise, particularly during the growth spurt. Oestrogen decline affects calcium metabolism and results in increased bone loss—low peak bone mass.

Mechanical stress exerts a positive effect on bone. It increases blood supply and lays down bone. Muscle action is the main stimulus for bone formation. Exercise should be weight bearing, and produce dynamic not static strains. Greater loads with fewer repetitions of a load will result in greater gains in bone mass. Lower loads repeated a greater number of times result in lower gains. The effect of exercise reflects the strains imposed at individual sites. The osteogenic response to mechanical loading is site-specific, so that professional tennis players, for example, have 30% greater bone density in the dominant forearm. Growing bone has a greater capacity to add new bone to the skeleton than mature bone.

Bone mass

Peak height velocity for girls is between 10.5–13 years and the peak height velocity for boys is between 12.5–15 years.

The rate of bone turnover is determined by hormonal and local factors. Osteogenesis is induced by dynamic not static strains. The osteogenic response to mechanical loading is site-specific, so that professional tennis players, for example, have 30% greater bone density in their dominant forearm.

There is a 7–8% gain in bone mass per year during childhood and early adolescence. Daily physical exercise has a positive effect on bone. Weight training should be done for 30 minutes at least three times a week. Weight bearing aerobic exercise should be for 30 minutes daily and this can be divided up into smaller time segments. Weight bearing exercise should be continued throughout the life cycle.

Intensive endurance training and amenorrhoea may be associated with decreased trabecular bone density in young females. Those who have been running for the longest period of time have the highest incidence of oligomenorrhoea and amenorrhoea.

The best predictor of bone mineral density (BMD) of the lumbar spine in women in their thirties and forties (premenopausal) are the years of regular menstruation. The best predictor of BMD of the hip is the number of years of amenorrhoea.

Pregnancy and exercise

Exercise is now an integral part of life and many women wish to continue during pregnancy. Fit women tend to have fewer problems and regain their figure earlier and feel better. They are less likely to be depressed. Exercise helps prevent excessive weight gain, maintains aerobic fitness, and helps sleep.

Musculoskeletal system

The anterior enlarging uterus results in a shift of the centre of gravity posteriorly, resulting in a progressive lordosis and rotation of the pelvis. Increased hormones cause laxity of the ligaments with increased stress on the lumbar spine and ligaments. Back pain occurs in approximately 50% of pregnancies and is more common in the older age group and with increased parity. This may be due to sacroiliac strain or unilateral lumbarization or unilateral sacralization. The increased anterior flexion of the lumbar spine and slumping of the shoulder predisposes to paraesthesia in the distribution of the median or ulnar nerves.

Cardiovascular changes

There is a 30% increase in maternal blood volume during early pregnancy, which peaks at the mid pregnancy, so there is a reduced cardiac reserve during strenuous exercise. There is an increase in cardiac output due to an increase in heart rate and stroke volume. There is a decrease in peripheral resistance due to the vasodilation of vessels in the skin, breast, uterus, GI tract, and kidneys.

Respiratory changes

Pulmonary hyperventilation changes include an increase in vital capacity, increased expansion of the lower ribs, a decrease in residual expiratory reserve, a decrease in arterial pCO_2, and elevation of the diaphragm. There is a reduction in pulmonary reserve in late pregnancy.

Other changes

Additional energy requirements during pregnancy:
- 150 calories a day during the first trimester. 350 calories a day during the second and 300 extra calories needed daily during the third trimester.
- Because of the greater utilization of carbohydrate, there is a greater risk of hypoglycaemia.
- Hyporesponsive to insulin due to somatomammo-trophin.
- Hypoglycaemia occurs if the exercise is prolonged or strenuous.
- Higher risk of dehydration.

Placental hormones

During the first three months of pregnancy the hormones are produced by the corpus luteum, and during the second and third trimester by the placenta. Placental hormones include oestriol, progesterone, chorionic gonadotrophins, and somatomammo-trophin, (which antagonizes insulin).

Exercise increases the catecholamines, prolactin, endorphins, and glucagon. There is a decrease in insulin due to the gonadotrophins.

The placenta metabolizes amines so that only 10–15% of maternal cate-cholamines reach the foetus. Excess catecholamines have an adverse affect on the fetal circulation by reduced fetal breathing and reduced fetal movements.

During exercise there is a major redistribution of blood flow from the uterus to the exercising muscles. There is an increase in fetal heart rate within minutes. But 50% of the uterine blood flow must be diverted before fetal hypoxia occurs. Signs of fetal distress include fetal tachycardia or fetal bradycardia.

Fetal heart rate usually returns to normal 15 minutes after stopping mild or moderate maternal exercise, but it may take 30 minutes after strenuous exercise.

Temperature changes

Maternal body temperature is increased due to fetal and placental metabolism. Under resting conditions, the fetal temperature is 0.5°C above the maternal. Trained athletes have a lower resting core temperature, and a more efficient temperature control. Not all women respond to heat stress in the same way.

During exercise there is an increase in maternal temperature followed by a rise in fetal temperature. Maternal temperature should not exceed 38°C; heart rate should not exceed 140bpm. A core increase of 1–1.5°C in the non-pregnant woman may easily exceed 2–2.5°C, resulting in an increase of 2.5–3°C in the fetus. Heat production and heat loss depends on the intensity, duration, and efficiency of exercise, and environmental factors such as ambient temperature, humidity, and physiological adaptation. In animals a temperature of 39°C has a tetrogenic effect on the neural tube in the fetus during the first trimester. Moderate or strenuous exercise in adverse conditions can increase the maternal temperature above 39°C. The risk of dehydration during exercise is increased in pregnant women.

Type of exercise

The type of exercise depends on their medical and obstetrical history and stage of pregnancy. Recommended exercises include; walking, running, cycling, water aerobics. Swimming can be done throughout the pregnancy. Racquet sports such as tennis, badminton, and squash are suitable provided the patient does not cause too great an increase in body temperature. Sports, to be avoided are water skiing, scuba diving, contact sports, and horse riding. The amount and type of exercise depends on a large number of factors, and recommendations must be individually based.

Contraindications to exercise

- Acute infection.
- Placenta praevia.
- Toxaemia of pregnancy.

- Hydramnios.
- Threatened abortion.
- Premature labour.
- Incompetent cervix.

Warning signs to stop exercise

- Shortness of breath.
- Dizziness.
- Chest pain.
- Headache.
- Muscle pain.
- Decrease in fetal movement.
- Leakage of amniotic fluid.

Maternal exercise

An individualized exercise programme that is closely monitored can improve fitness and help to ensure the safety of the individual.

The intensity and amount depends on the level of fitness of the individual. If they have not exercised for some time, they should start slowly, at a low intensity, always warm up and cool down for at least 5 minutes. Adequate fluid intake to avoid dehydration. Correct equipment and clothing in a well ventilated room. Get up slowly from the floor to prevent postural hypotension.

Regular aerobic exercise lasting 20–40 minutes is preferable to occasional bursts of intense exercise. Exercise should use large muscle groups. Strenuous exercise should not exceed 15 minutes (60–90% of maximum heart rate or 50–85% of VO_2max. Maternal heart rate should not exceed 140bpm Maternal core temperature should not exceed 38°C. No exercise should be performed in supine position after the fourth month. Vigorous exercise should not be performed in hot humid conditions. Ballistic movements should be avoided. Exercises that involve the Valsalva manoeuvre should be avoided.

Adequate caloric intake to meet extra needs of pregnancy and exercise involved.

The first trimester

Exercise is contraindicated in the first trimester in women with a history of spontaneous abortion. This is often associated with a luteal phase defect due to low levels of progesterone. When the placenta takes over the production of hormones, they may be able to exercise, but must be closely monitored.

Fitness can be improved during pregnancy. Pregnant women who do not normally exercise are advised to do so and can start to exercise for the first time. (Walking, cycling, swimming etc). It helps prevent excessive weight gain. Women who normally train may continue and may be monitored using heart rate monitors. The level and intensity must be individually prescribed. A patient with known obstetrical problems should consult a gynaecologist.

The second trimester

Enlarging uterus causes the centre of gravity to be displaced posteriorly. Lumbar lordosis increases, resulting in stress on the sacroiliac joint, lumbar vertebrae, and ligaments. No exercise should be carried out in the supine position after the fourth month, as the uterus may fall back and compresses the aorta and IVC, restricting the arterial blood flow and venous return.

The third trimester

Alterations in neck posture may result in neck pain. Fluid retention may cause carpal tunnel syndrome.

During exercise, the noradrenaline produced increases the frequency and amplitude of uterine contractions. Women with multiple pregnancies should avoid strenuous exercise. Dyspnoea may be due to displacement of the diaphragm causing a reduction in pulmonary reserve which limits exercise. Excessive exercise may cause fetal distress, intrauterine growth retardation, or prematurity.

Pregnant women with a poor obstetrical history should consult a Gynaecologist. Exercise or sport may normally be resumed a few weeks after a normal delivery, depending on the individual, the sport, and type of delivery. They should all do core stability exercises to improve abdominal and gluteal muscles the day after delivery. This may be restricted, if they had a Caesarean section. Walking should start straight away; it takes approximately 6 weeks for the ligaments to recover, so golf that involves rotary movements of the spine should be avoided during this period. Any sport should be started slowly and the amount and intensity should be gradually increased.

Pelvic pain

Pelvis pain is a generic term which covers many causes, some of which may be gynaecological. It may be due to a local cause or referred. It may be acute or chronic. Local causes include the bladder, ureter, uterus, (body or cervix), broad ligament, uterine tube, ovaries, rectum, vagina, or a pelvic appendix.

It is essential to take a detailed history of the pain to include the quality, type, radiation, factors that relieve or aggravate, its relationship to menstrual cycle (to rule out an ectopic pregnancy or pain due to ovulation), associated symptoms, such as nausea, vomiting, and diarrhoea. Infection should be investigated. Routine abdominal and gynaecological examination including a PV/PR combined bimanual. Referral may be appropriate for further investigation including pelvic ultrasound. The pain may be of musculoskeletal origin.

Gender verification

Gender testing is no longer required by the IOC and was not carried out at the last two summer Olympic Games in Sydney (2000) and Athens (2004). Routine sex tests carried out at the previous Olympic Games were not appropriate, and only differentiated between females who had two XX chromosomes and a positive Barr body in the cell from a buccal smear. Individuals with only one X chromosome had no Barr body and were not considered female. The normal male chromosomal count is 46XY, normal female is 46XX.

Gender testing should not be confused with genetic sex as determined by chromosomal tests.

Eight criteria determine a person's sexual status:
- Sex chromosome constitution.
- Sex hormonal pattern.
- Gonadal sex (ovaries or testes).
- Internal sex organs.
- External genitalia.
- Secondary sex characteristics.
- Apparent sex, role in which person was reared.
- Psychological sex or gender identity.

Gender testing for sports only considers the sex chromosome pattern. Chromosomal test discloses the Y fluorescent long arm in males or the second X (Barr body) in a buccal smear in females. If a laboratory test is abnormal, a gynaecological examination is performed.

Disorders of sex chromosomes

Turner's syndrome 45 XO: is a female who has a negative buccal smear. It consists of gonadal dysgensis, primary amenorrhoea, and immature secondary sex characteristics. There may be a mixture or mosaicism, some cells having 46XX.

Disorders of gonadal sex: the chromosomal sex is normal, but the differentiation of the gonads is abnormal.

Pure gonadal dysgenesis: the individual has an immature female phenotype with bilateral streak gonads, with a normal 46XX or 46XY chromosomal complement.

XXX triple X female: has a tendency to secondary amenorrhoea.

Disorders of phenotypic sex

The phenotypic sex is ambiguous or is completely opposite to the chromosomal and gonadal sex.

Female pseudo-hermaphroditism
Congenital adrenal hyperplasia associated with an inherited deficiency of the 21-hydroxylase enzyme, it is the most common cause of virilization in a newborn female.

Male pseudo-hermaphroditism
Defective virilization of the 46XY.

Individuals with deficiency of 5 a-reductase enzyme have a female habitus, plasma testosterone are in normal male range.

Androgen receptor defects, i.e. testicular feminization syndrome is an individual with an XY chromosome and end organ insensitivy to testosterone, who develops as a female; there is no physical advantage in sport, no male muscle development, and a negative buccal smear.

Congenital adrenal hyperplasia (adrenogenital syndrome) The most common cause is 21-hydroxylase, with an incidence of 1:300–1000, there is increased formation of dehydroepiandrosterone. Mild forms of congenital adrenal hyperplasia may only manifest as increased muscular strength in a female, and a positive buccal smear.

Androgen excess in women may be due to drugs e.g. androgens, anabolic steroids, androgenic progestagens. Ovarian causes include polycystic ovarian syndrome, tumours, hyperthecosis.

Adrenal causes: congenital adrenal hyperplasia. Classical or late onset, Cushing's syndrome. Tumours: hyperprolactinaemia.

There have been rare cases of athletes who have competed as one gender and undergone sex reassignment later in life. This has increased in the last decade. Formerly each case was judged on an individual basis by competent experts before a decision was made by the relevant sports authority. Recently the IAAF guidelines were updated by the IOC Medical Commission. More detailed information can be obtained by contacting the IOC Medical Commission.

Injuries

Women develop similar injuries as men as a result of training errors, but may be more prone to certain injuries because of anatomical differences.

Injuries to knee and ankle are common but injuries to breast are rare. There is a higher incidence of anterior cruciate ligament tears in females due to the narrow intercondylar notch of the femur and subluxaion of the patella due to genu valgum. Back pain in females may be due to gynaecological causes including ovarian cysts, endometriosis, or fibroids. Water-skiing injuries during take off, failure to rise from sitting position results in retrograde douching which may result in haematoma of the vulva or laceration of vaginal wall. Female athletes who have recurrent stress fractures should have a biomechanical assessment, a DEXA scan and hormone levels after 21st day of cycle to determine oestrogen, progesterone, prolactin, cortisol levels, and thyroid function tests. If bone density is low, other causes of bone loss must be ruled out.

Aids to performance

Ergogenic aids

Sports people have long used performance-enhancing substances (or *ergogenic aids*) in an attempt to gain advantage, and many believe that most of their competitors are taking such substances. Media influences, financial rewards, and pressure from coaches, peers, and families can encourage a competitor to attempt to cheat by using drugs or other ergogenic aids. Those using such methods tend to have genuine concerns regarding their own health, but believe that taking the substances increase their chances of being successful.

Apart from supplements and drugs, other examples of ergogenic aids might include:
- Psychology imagery.
- Custom-fitted shoe orthoses.
- Blood or gene doping.
- Some of the pharmaceutical and physiological aids are outlined below.

Performance-enhancing drugs

Anabolic steroids

These are natural or synthetically made derivatives of the hormone testosterone. Their ergogenic effects are:
- Reduced recovery time after training.
- Increased lean body mass.
- Increased aggression (seen as a benefit in some contact sports).

Anabolic steroids are used orally, as a cream, or injected.

Needle sharing carries risks of HIV, hepatitis B or C, and needle abscesses are seen from contaminated injection sites.

Despite this catalogue of adverse effects, anabolic steroid abuse is still widespread as sports people and bodybuilders risk their health in the pursuit of success. Polypharmacy and massive doses of multiple drugs is common.

Commonly abused steroids include stanozolol, nandrolone, clembuterol, and dihydrotestosterone. Tetrahydrogestrinone, a new synthetic 'designer' steroid, specifically produced to be difficult to detect in urine samples, was discovered in 2003.

Male	Female	Both sexes
Breast enlargement	Male pattern baldness	Acne
Testicular atrophy	Deepening of voice	↑ BP
↓Sperm count	Enlarged clitoris	↑LDL/total cholesterol
	↑ facial hair	↑Risk of prem. ischaemic heart disease/death
	Irregular menses	Liver abnormalities

Erythropoetin

This is a glycoprotein, produced naturally in the body by the kidneys in response to hypoxia. Erythropoetin (EPO) can be prescribed in a recombinant form and is licensed to treat or be used in renal failure, some cancers, and AIDS. It is administered by subcutaneous injection.

Effects of erythropoetin (EPO)

- EPO exerts a direct effect on bone marrow to increase red blood cell production, particularly in the presence of iron.
- Haemoglobin levels increase so improving aerobic performance by enhanced oxygen-carrying capacity of blood.

Adverse effects

Side effects are common:

- Increased haemoglobin improves cardiac output (by increasing blood volume) and anaerobic performance by better red cell (and lactic acid) buffering.

Adverse effects

Side effects of EPO include:

- Potential life-threatening thrombosis or embolism.
- Cerebrovascular accidents.
- Seizures and encephalopathy.
- Myocardial infarction.
- Iron overload causing liver or cardiac disease.

Effects similar to using EPO can be obtained by high altitude training, blood doping, and by the use of hypoxic, hypobaric chambers at ground level.

Until 2000, EPO was undetectable. Individual sporting federations, such as cycling and triathlon have instigated blood testing with upper limits of haematocrit levels being deemed as acceptable, leading to an indirect test 'failure'. At present, blood and urine tests are based upon transferrin receptor and ferritin concentrations.

Growth hormone

Growth hormone (GH) is produced from the anterior pituitary and acts to:

- Increase protein synthesis and fat breakdown.
- Increase hepatic glucose production.
- Stimulate the liver to produce insulin-like growth factor-1 (IGF-1), which helps muscle and bone growth.

GH is now available commercially as a recombinant product, but previously was made from pituitary glands extracted post mortem. This latter process carried a risk of the recipient developing human variant CJD. GH works synergistically with testosterone. Many of its effects rely on insulin, and the two drugs are often abused in combination. Recently, a seemingly reliable blood test for recombinant GH has allowed its direct measurement. Overproduction or overdosage of GH causes acromegaly, glucose intolerance, and hypertension.

Stimulants

Amphetamines

Sports people have abused amphetamines for over 70 years and several high profile deaths have been linked to their use. The main ergogenic benefits of amphetamines are:

- Increased awareness and delayed fatigue.
- Enhancement of speed, power, endurance, and concentration.

Adverse effects of amphetamines

- Amphetamines are highly addictive.
- Delirium.
- Paranoia.
- Aggression.
- Risk of cerebral haemorrhage.

Possession and supply of amphetamines in the UK is a criminal offence.

Modafinil

Recently, Modafinil, a stimulant, licensed to treat the familial condition of narcolepsy has become a drug of abuse in sport. The drug is not thought to be performance-enhancing, but there is speculation that its main use is as a masking agent for new 'designer' steroids.

Sympathomimetics

Sympathomimetics are readily available 'over-the-counter' remedies, used as treatments for the common cold. Many of these drugs are not performance-enhancing, but have been abused for years to increase energy.

Adverse effects of sympathomimetics

- Anxiety.
- Agitation.
- Headaches.
- Hypertension.
- Tremor.
- Cardiac arrhythmias and myocardial infarction.

Most of this group of drugs were removed from the WADA banned list in 2004, although ephedrine remains included. Athletes, who require a 'cold cure', should be advised to always check with a doctor before taking any such drug, even though purchased through a pharmacy. Different countries may have the same preparation on sale, but there can be variance in the constituents, which can lead to an inadvertent doping offence particularly when travelling.

Caffeine

- No longer on the WADA banned list of drugs.
- Has been shown to be ergogenic—appears to improve endurance.
- Spares glycogen and therefore delays the onset of fatigue.

- Exerts its effect by stimulating adipose tissue to release fatty acids, and also stimulates adrenaline production from the adrenal medulla, so in turn further facilitating fatty acid release.
- Caffeine has also been shown to enhance motor unit recruitment.

Beta-2 adrenoceptor agonists

- Include the drug salbutamol and related compounds.
- Potent treatments used in everyday practice to treat asthma.
- Orally, beta-2 agonists are not permitted in sport.
- No evidence that these drugs, in inhaled form, are ergogenic in the non-asthmatic athlete.
- No longer allowable in inhaled form, unless the sports person has submitted an *abbreviated therapeutic use exemption (aTUE)*.
- aTUE must be completed by the usual prescribing doctor and sent to the involved sport's governing body with laboratory evidence confirming the diagnosis of exercise-induced asthma (EIA).

Tests for exercise-induced asthma

There are two approved methods by which sports people with EIA can meet the diagnostic criteria to obtain a TUE:

1 Spirometry pre-and post-exercise challenge, showing an increase in airway obstruction, reversed by inhaled beta-2 agonist.
2 Eucapnic voluntary hyperpnoea—EVH test. This is used by WADA as the optimal laboratory challenge to confirm EIA. The subject has to hyperventilate dry air containing 5% carbon dioxide for 6 minutes. An increase in airway obstruction of greater than 10% measured by FEV_1 confirms the diagnosis.

Dietary ergogenic aids

Carbohydrates

- The primary energy source for anaerobic activity.
- Athletic diet should include 55–70% of total calories as carbohydrate, (approximately 5–10g/kg body weight).

Proteins

- Recommended daily intake varies depending on the demands of the sport in which a person participates, with the range between 1.2 and 2g/kg body weight.
- Strength and power athletes tend to require a larger intake than those who undertake endurance exercise.
- Protein supplements are useful to gain strength during conditioning and are used post-exercise to aid recovery.

Dietary supplements

- Widespread use of supplements in sport is controversial.
- Little evidence to support the use of supplements as ergogenic aids.
- Risk of contamination of supplements by banned substances is a concern.
- A recent study, found that as many as 19% of supplements produced in a selection of countries contained banned substances that were not mentioned on the product label.

Many high-profile sports stars have blamed their failed drug tests on a contamination of their supplements, taken in good faith. Athletes should be strongly advised to be extremely cautious about the use of these—any supplements taken by an athlete are at their own personal risk of liability.

Creatine monohydrate

- Physiologically active substance needed for muscle contraction.
- Present in the normal diet, particularly in meat.
- Also synthesized in the body (liver, kidneys, and pancreas).
- Increases phosphocreatine production, theoretically increasing the available energy during maximal exercise.
- Some evidence that creatine enhances performance in short bursts of stationary cycling and weight lifting.
- Causes weight gain, though this may be due to water retention rather than muscle mass gain.

Adverse effects

Include muscle cramps, GI disturbances, possibly renal and prostate disease.

Antioxidants

- Vitamins and other compounds that occur naturally in the diet.
- Act to destroy free radicals in the body.

- Free radicals are produced as a by-product of highintensity exercise and increased oxygen consumption, or as part of the normal process of inflammation and tissue healing.
- Free radicals are known to damage DNA and RNA and to destroy important enzymes, and are linked to arteriosclerosis, some cancers, and ageing as well as exercise-associated muscle damage.
- Antioxidants such as beta-carotene (vitamin A pre-cursor), vitamins C and E, selenium, and glutathione all are present in a normal healthy diet, which should contain at least five portions of fruit and vegetables daily. Such a diet is likely to give the athlete their recommended daily allowance (RDA) of vitamins.
- Most commercial multivitamins will also contain ample to satisfy the RDA. The potential benefits of taking a simple multivitamin probably outweigh any risks, but there is not enough evidence to recommend taking supplements to reduce post-exercise muscle damage.

Chromium
- Potentiates insulin action and therefore cellular glucose and amino acid uptake.
- In theory might produce muscle mass gain, but lack of evidence.
- Also has the potential to induce iron and zinc deficiency, by competition for binding sites and reduced absorption.

Magnesium
- An essential mineral and a co-factor in many enzymatic reactions.
- A typical Western diet may be deficient in magnesium, but as yet supplementation has not been proven to be performance-enhancing.

L-carnitine
- Detoxifies ammonia, a by-product of metabolism associated with fatigue.
- In theory, muscle glycogen will be spared and fatty acid oxidation increased, but studies are inconclusive.

Beta-hydroxy-beta-methylbutyrate (HMB)
- A bioactive metabolite produced from breakdown of the amino acid leucine.
- May increase fatty acid oxidation and reduce protein loss during stress by inhibiting protein catabolism.
- Used by resistance-trained athletes.

Glutamine
- A non-essential amino acid, which is synthesized in the liver, lungs, adipose tissue, and skeletal muscle.
- Stored in muscle, and is used for immunity, as a fuel for cells, protein synthesis, and to maintain acid-base balance.
- It has been hypothesized that intense exercise can increase demand for glutamine, leading to its depletion and so an increased susceptibility to infection.

- Lack of published evidence to support its use, but it is claimed that glutamine enhances immune cell function in those at risk by undertaking high intensity exercise.

Fish and seed oils

- Athletic diets have tended to be low in these oils, which contain omega-3 oils and essential fatty acids.
- Omega-3 oils are known to have a cardioprotective effect, and it may simply be good advice for general health reasons for an athlete to include oily fish in their diet.

Lactic acid

- A by-product of anaerobic glycloysis, which builds up in muscle and blood during exercise.
- Recently, has been found to also act as a fuel during sub-maximal exercise, particularly by the heart, liver and kidneys, to generate ATP.
- The liver uses any remaining lactic acid for gluconeogenesis in an attempt to restore glycogen levels and maintain glucose levels.

Sodium bicarbonate

- Neutralizes metabolic acids, including lactic acid.
- Supplementation is said to produce an alkaline reserve, to neutralize the hydrogen ions produced in anaerobic glycloysis and so reduce the onset of fatigue.

Doping and prohibited drugs

Doping has been defined on many occasions but in 1991 the UK Sports Council stated that:

'Doping is the use by or distribution to a sports man (or woman) of any substance defined by (governing body, international federation or IOC) as a banned class.'

Brief history

- 1968 drug testing first started at Grenoble Winter Olympics.
- 1974 semi-reliable tests for anabolic steroids became available.
- 1976 8 athletes tested positive for anabolic steroids. Rumours were rife of widespread use by athletes and swimmers despite the small number of positive tests.
- 1983 urine test developed to determine the ratio between testosterone and epitestosterone. These isomers usually exist in the body in a 1:1 ratio, so any exogenous testosterone taken would alter this. A ratio of 6:1 implies suspicion that an athlete has taken an anabolic steroid, although 10:1 is more likely to produce a 'guilty' verdict in a court of law. Exogenous epitestosterone has also been abused in an attempt to mask any changes in the ratio caused by taking anabolic steroids.

World Anti-Doping Agency

The banned list is no longer operated by the International Olympic Committee, and responsibility has passed to the World Anti-Doping Agency (WADA), established in 1999 after the World Conference on Doping in Sport in Lausanne recognized the need for an independent agency. The aims of WADA are to set unified standards for anti-doping work and to co-ordinate efforts against doping, seeking to foster a drug-free culture in sport.

Out-of-competition testing is conducted by independent parties and in 2003, the World Anti-Doping Code was accepted and most sports have now agreed to implement the code. UK Sport is responsible for drug testing and education in this country, and fully supports WADA and the code.

Where can the banned list be seen?

The Banned List is available online at the WADA website, along with educational pages at http://www.wada-ama.org/en/t1.asp.

Important note

It must be stressed that it is the athletes' responsibility to adhere to WADA regulations and that ignorance is not considered a defence.

Outline of the banned classes of drugs

Stimulants

- Amphetamines and related drugs.
- Epinephrine and related drugs.
- Ephedrine.
- Cocaine.

Narcotics
- Morphine and related drugs—note that codeine is not banned.

Cannabinoids
Hashish and marijuana banned in competition.

Anabolic steroids
- Testosterone derivatives and related compounds.

Peptide hormones and analogues
- Erythropoetin.
- Growth hormone.
- Insulin.
- HCG.

Beta-2 agonists
- Salbutamol and related drugs.

Anti-oestrogens (banned in males only)
- Tamoxifen.
- Clomiphene.

Masking agents
- Probenecid.
- Diuretics.
- Epitestosterone.

Glucocorticosteroids
These drugs are banned orally, rectally, intravenous, or intramuscularly, though exemptions for genuine medical illness on production of evidence may be granted. Use in topical form is subject to TUE application.

Prohibited methods
- Blood doping.
- Chemical manipulation.
- Self-catheterisation.
- Gene doping.

Prohibited in certain sports
- Alcohol.
- Beta- blockers (shooting, archery).

Advice to doctors prescribing for athletes
Doctors who prescribe for sports people who may be liable for drug testing must be aware of the banned list of substances. Most doctors will be able to access Internet resources and a valuable site is the UK Sport Drug Information Database available at www.uksport.gov.uk/did/

This site will allow almost any drug, bought anywhere in the world to be identified and classified as either permitted, restricted, or banned. The advice is also sport-specific and can be printed out for safekeeping. Although the athlete is ultimately responsible for whatever substance is found on drug testing, incorrect prescribing by a sports doctor is a potential medico-legal issue.

If in doubt do not prescribe!

Blood doping

Blood doping occurred more commonly in the 1970s and 1980s than now, and the need for this practice has been largely superseded by the abuse of erythropoetin. Blood doping was banned by the IOC. in 1986 and involved the intravenous transfusion of blood into an individual in order to increase red cell mass and therefore improved oxygen carrying capacity. In many cases autologous transfusions were used, which involved taking two units of blood from an athlete, six weeks prior to competition (often whilst training at altitude), then re-infusing the blood on the day before competition. It is reported that this process could increase an individual's haematocrit by 5–10%.

Gene doping

The future of doping seems certain to involve genetic manipulation. WADA defines gene doping as 'the non-therapeutic use of genes, genetic elements, or of the modulation of gene expressions, having the capacity to improve athletic performance'. Gene therapy is already used to treat muscular dystrophies, and experiments in mice show that genetic manipulation can increase muscle mass by 25%. The modified gene works via IGF-1 to increase muscle cell division. The gene is attached to an inert virus, causing 'infection' in muscle cells, but no disease process in the host. Scientists are currently working on tests to detect gene doping.

Drug testing

Random out-of-competition testing started in the UK in 1981. Its aims were to deter athletes from gaining an unfair advantage, to catch athletes who had taken performance enchancing substances, and to remind them of the regulations and the inadvertent use of banned substances.

Testing procedure (from UK Sport guide to drug testing procedures)

1 At an event, during training, or at an out-of-competition location, athlete is notified of selection for a drug test, using an official sample collection form. Once informed, the athlete must stay in full view of the Doping Control Officer (DCO). World-class athletes in the UK's registered testing pool are required to be available for testing anytime and anywhere and must be prepared to provide a sample when notified.

2 Athlete is required to report to doping control station as soon as possible and no later than one hour after notification. Sealed non-alcoholic drinks are available. Privacy and integrity should be maintained.

3 Athlete will be asked to select a sealed sample collection vessel. This collection vessel must be kept in sight at all times.

4 Athlete provides a sample of urine observed directly by the DCO, in order to avoid any manipulation of the sample.

5 Athlete selects a sealed urine sampling kit from a choice of such kits stored in tamper-evident packaging. The security seal should be intact.

6 Athlete divides the sample between two bottles, labelled A and B, which are then tightly sealed (by the athlete). A small residual amount of urine is left in the collection vessel to enable testing of pH and specific gravity. The athlete should then invert the sealed sampling bottles to ensure that there are no leaks.

7 If pH or specific gravity is outside the required limits, this is recorded on the sample collection form.

8 DCO records the A and B sample numbers on the sample collection form, and the athlete is asked to declare any medications, substances, or supplements taken in the past 7 days. Athlete then checks that all information on the sample collection form is correct and together with the DCO signs the form. The athlete is given a copy of this form.

Drug test result reporting

Negative result

In the UK, following analysis of the A sample, result is reported to UK Sport, and after processing this is passed to the relevant authority, who will notify the athlete.

Positive result

If a prohibited substance is found in the A sample, UK Sport is notified of the finding. After confirmation of the accuracy of supporting documentation and supporting evidence has been confirmed, the relevant authority will notify the athlete of the result. The athlete may be suspended from competition at this point and will be invited to explain the finding. The athlete may challenge the A sample finding, and is entitled to be present at the analysis of the B sample. If this second test confirms the A sample result, the athlete must attend a disciplinary panel, which may decide a suspension, or, in some cases, a lifetime ban from competition. The athlete may appeal against any decision reached.

Blood testing

Blood testing is used in some sports to check for unusual blood profiles, such as an elevated haematocrit, using much of the same procedure as outlined for urine testing, apart from the DCO taking blood by venepuncture rather than observing the passage of a urine sample.

The team physician

The medical care of a team or squad of athletes is an integral part of the role of the sports medicine specialist, and potentially one of the most rewarding aspects of sports medicine practice.

The specifics of the team physician role will depend on a variety of issues including the sport involved, the nature of the event e.g. single sport or multi-sport, and the level of competition or ability of the athletes. There are, however, a number of general principles, which are relevant to team medical support in general, and some special circumstances.

The medical kit bag

The medical kit bag has moved on from the bucket and magic sponge. The equipment that you take to an event will depend on a number of factors.

Experience of practitioner

Carry equipment that you are competent to use. If covering a sport that might require a particular piece of equipment then seek appropriate training before agreeing to cover that event. If your level of knowledge and experience is not commensurate with that required to provide a duty of care for those you are looking after, then you should not be there, no matter how attractive the opportunity.

Medical risk assessment

A vital part of team coverage is medical risk assessment. This means identifying what problems you are likely to encounter, what facilities will be at your disposal to deal with such events, and what additional equipment you need to provide or arrange to have provided. A number of issues will govern the medical risk associated with a particular event.

Sport

Different sports clearly carry different injury profiles e.g. the high risk of contact trauma associated with rugby union compared with the low risk associated with tennis. You must have an appreciation of the injury profile of the sport to be able to adequately plan. It would, for example, be indefensible if you could not adequately immobilize the cervical spine when covering a rugby match, whereas serious cervical injury would be highly unlikely on a tennis court.

Venue or event

The venue will influence the equipment that you carry. The equipment you will need, for example, to provide medical cover at a rugby international at Twickenham will be very different from that required to cover a semi-professional game at a local centre. Similarly consider the role of the medical officers for the London marathon, run over the same distance as another on the foothills of Mount Everest. The following list, although not exhaustive, covers many of the important factors:

- Will you be a single handed practitioner or part of a team of clinicians? If part of a team what is their experience, what equipment are they likely to bring?

- What medical equipment will be provided by the venue (e.g. is there a fully equipped medical room)?
- Emergency medical support (will there be a paramedic ambulance on site)?
- Where will you be situated in relation to the field of play and what access to the field of play do you have?
- Where are the nearest emergency care/hospital facilities?
- What is the transfer time to these facilities and how might that change on the day of competition?
- Environment and climate considerations.

The team you are covering

Most athletes are by definition healthy, however, they may have medical conditions e.g. diabetes, asthma, or disabilities that will influence what equipment you require. Furthermore you will almost certainly be responsible for the health of those individuals supporting the athletes e.g. performance directors, coaches, medical and paramedical staff. Support staff may have a variety of chronic illnesses and medical requirements and you should be prepared. If you are travelling with a team with whom you don't usually work it is useful to send out a questionnaire prior to departure requesting key current and past medical history, medications, and allergies.

Touchline kit bag

The key to a basic first aid kit is to only put in what you know how to use. It should be hands-free, carried on the shoulder or waist (allowing hands free) and should be clean, compact, and secure.

Suggested contents include:

- Squirty water bottle—this allows pressure to be exerted when irrigating wounds.
- Gauze swabs.
- Disposable gloves.
- Tape.
- Scissors.
- Assorted plasters, sterile wound dressings, and bandages.
- Pen and paper or copies of a suitable incident report form.
- Clinical waste bag.

Basic medical equipment

There is a basic level of equipment to which every doctor covering sport should have immediate access and, of course, be able to use. The following list is included as a guide.

- Stethoscope.
- Portable sphygmomanometer.
- Oto/opthalmoscope/spare batteries.
- Scissors.
- Tongue depressors.
- Thermometer.
- Oropharyngeal airways (e.g. Guedel sizes 2, 3, 4).
- Nasopharyngeal airways (6–8mm).
- Petroleum gel.
- Pocket mask with mouthpiece and O_2 inlet (e.g. Laerdal).
- Alcohol wipes.
- Antimicrobial soap.
- Cleaning fluid (e.g. chlorhexidine, betadine sachets).
- Semipermeable dressing (e.g. Tegaderm) various sizes.
- Low adherence dressing (e.g. Mepore) various sizes.
- Sterile gauze swabs and cotton wool.
- Tubular bandage (e.g. Tubigrip).
- Supportive bandage (e.g. crepe).
- Cohesive bandage.
- Permeable adhesive tape.
- Blister pack.
- Sterile and non-sterile gloves.
- Adhesive strips (e.g. Steri-strip).
- Tissue adhesive (e.g. 2-octyl cyanoacrylates).
- Suture kit.
- Scalpel and blades.
- Razor.
- Sharps bin.
- Assorted needles and syringes.
- Tourniquet.
- Blood and specimen bottles.
- Peak flow meter and disposable mouthpieces.
- Assorted cannulae.
- Giving set.
- 500ml bag of dextrose/saline.
- Adjustable hard collar.
- Safety pins.
- Tape measure.
- Urinalysis testing strips (e.g. clinitest).
- Glucose testing meter and test strips.
- BNF or access to BNF online.

Don't forget the obvious non-medical items e.g. pen, paper, mobile telephone, and useful contact numbers. A driving licence is often helpful.

Essential drugs and medications

If providing medical support to a large team or squad competing internationally you will need an extensive drug list to cover most medical situations. Irrespective of what drugs you have available at base there are essential drugs/medications, which you should carry with you. This list is a guide to essentials but will be influenced by the medical history of your team members.

- Epinephrine (adrenaline) (1/10,000) 1mg in 10ml pre-filled syringe.
- Epinephrine (adrenaline) (1/1000) 1mg in 1ml pre-filled syringe.
- Parentral antihistamine e.g. chlorpheniramine (10mg/ml).
- Hydrocortisone IV 100mg vial.
- Hypostop gel (3 ampoule pack).
- Frusemide (IV and oral).
- Midazolam 1mg/ml as 50ml vial (optional).
- Parenteral opiate analgesia (e.g. pethidine 25mg/1ml amp or morphine)—depends on circumstances.
- Naloxone (optional, if carrying opiate analgesia essential).
- Anaesthetic (e.g. topical (EMLA), lidocaine, bupivicaine).
- Intra-articular steroid (e.g. triamcinolone, methylprednisolone).
- Sterile water ampoules for injections.
- Antihistamine (oral and topical).
- Paracetamol.
- Compound analgesic (e.g. co-codamol).
- Parenteral analgesia (e.g. IM diclofenac).
- Non-steroidal anti-inflammatory drug (e.g. ibuprofen 400).
- Penicillin (IV and oral).
- Alternative broad spectrum antibiotics including those for penicillin sensitive individuals e.g. erythromycin, augmentin, amoxycillin.
- Aspirin 75mg.
- Nitrolingual spray.
- Antacid e.g. algicon.
- Anti-diarrhoeal agent (e.g. loperamide).
- Rehydration scahets (e.g. diarrolyte).
- Anti-emetic (e.g. prochlorperazine, buccal and IV/IM).
- Beta-2 agonist inhaler (e.g. salbutamol).
- Anaesthetic throat lozenge (e.g. merocaine).
- Oral steroid (e.g. prednisolone).
- Flamazine or equivalent.
- Topical steroid (e.g. hydrocortisone).
- Anti-fungal cream.
- Steroid drops suitable for ocular and aural use (e.g. betnesol).
- Fluorescein/amethocaine eye drops.
- Migraine treatment (e.g. sumatriptan or equivalent).

Be up to date with current doping regulations and which apply to the athletes under your care e.g. in/out competition, IOC, WADA, International Federation. Some of the medications on this list require the completion of an abbreviated or full TUE. Carry some blank forms.

Security and insurance issues

Increased security has restricted the ease with which a doctor can transport medical equipment and medication. I would encourage you to consider taking practical steps to preempt or avoid difficulty.

- Itemize in full the contents of your medical bag.
- Write to the Embassy of the country of destination detailing your travel arrangements and seek approval for the carriage of your medical equipment being sure to include your list.
- Do not take strong opiate-based analgesia e.g. morphine unless absolutely necessary, and then seek prior agreement. Many countries restrict even moderate or weak opiates not intended for personal medical use.
- Where possible source medications in the country of destination.
- Consider writing to the airline concerned detailing your medical luggage.
- Carry a copy of your itemized medical bag and a letter confirming your medical role.
- Ensure that any prohibited 'dangerous' (or potential prohibited) items are stored in the hold.
- Do not take pressurized containers e.g. oxygen, entanox.
- Ensure that you have appropriate travel insurance.
- Ensure that you have appropriate medical insurance and indemnity in order to practice in the country of destination.
- Carry separately a photocopy of your passport.

Team travel

Providing medical support to a traveling team presents the sports physician with additional challenges and adequate and timely preparation is essential. The following considerations should help you prepare for your team travel experience.

Selecting a medical team

You may be responsible for a team of medical officers. In these circumstances you should be involved in the appointment of your medical team and it is vitally important to get your team right from the start. This process should be just as any other professional appointment with a job description (including essential and desired criteria), application process with open job advert, short-listing and interview. Your interview panel should be multi-disciplinary and might include the team manager/chef de mission (or equivalent), chief physiotherapist and a medical colleague (not involved with the sport or event in question). The appointments panel should meet prior to the interview to identify key questions that will allow the interviewee to demonstrate that they possess the necessary essential and desired qualities. In particular the ability to work effectively within a multidisciplinary team should be assessed.

It may be useful to have, within a team, doctors of differing sports medicine backgrounds e.g. primary care, musculoskeletal, emergency care. In the future with specialty recognition and certified training programmes, doctors certifying in SEM will have similar backgrounds and such distinctions may no longer hold true.

Medical preparation

Adequate preparation is essential whether you are the Chief Medical Officer to the Olympic team or the medical officer to an amateur team going on a club tour. The preparation will, of course, reflect the particular circumstances but should follow good medical practice and applies irrespective of the stature of your athletes.

Team building

Get to know your team ahead of departure. In many circumstances you will already be part of a well-established team or squad. But, for major events, the headquarters staff may be from different backgrounds and you will almost certainly be working with a number of 'strangers'. For this reason most organizations arrange team building sessions, usually residential and often at weekends, which you should attend whether medical team leader or medical officer. They are invaluable opportunities to get to know other team members and facilitate preparation and planning. You should be prepared to advise your team on relevant medical issues including the ubiquitous 'what if' scenarios e.g. what do we do if one of the team brings into camp a highly contagious form of viral gastro-enteritis?

You may attend training or preparation camps. These will serve a number of purposes, not least is the opportunity to ensure effective team working and meet any athletes or support staff who are new to a squad.

If you are part of the HQ medical team it is impossible to get to know all the athletes and support staff who will form a countries delegation at a major games. Training, preparation, or holding camps may provide an opportunity to get to know some individual squads.

Pre-travel medical assessment

Providing medical support during competition can be challenging with the additional complications of being in a foreign country with all the cultural, environmental, and linguistic differences that may exist. It helps to have as much information about your destination and team members as possible.

You may have had the luxury of a pre-games visit or training camp, in which case you should perform a medical risk assessment as described previously. If not, contact non-medical colleagues who are going on a pre-games visit, other medical colleagues who may have been to your destination previously, and try and make contact with local medical services. Internet and email facilitate communication.

Your appreciation of the team's previous medical history may vary from having a detailed knowledge of a team through years of working with the same individuals, to having virtually no prior knowledge. In either case a pre-travel questionnaire is essential and should be a pre-requisite of inclusion in the team, something that you should clarify with the team manager or equivalent. The following should be included within your pre-games questionnaire:

- Demographic information (full name, date of birth, address, telephone and email contacts, GP name and contact details, NGB medical team members contact details, and the names and contact details of 2 independent adult next of kin).
- Current health and injury status.
- Previous medical and injury history.
- Vaccination history.
- Current and accurate list of medications and supplements.
- Documented confirmation of abbreviated/therapeutic use exemptions (a/TUE).
- Allergy history.
- Recent drug test record (date, event, testing body within 6 months).
- Travel history e.g. problems with jetlag, gastrointestinal upset.
- Dental and optician check. I encourage athletes to ensure they have visited their dentist and optician prior to major tournaments. Equally if a team member has a chronic medical problem I would encourage them to attend for a specialist review prior to departure.

Such questionnaires often reveal important and relevant information and being aware of this information prior to travel can be very helpful.

Most sports will have a National Governing Body (NGB) medical officer. In addition to asking athletes to complete the pre-games questionnaire, contact the NGB doctor and ensure you have his/her contact details.

Team education

Invest time in educating your team prior to competition. Hopefully you will have the opportunity to meet your team at team building sessions, preparation, or holding camps. These will usually be arranged to replicate some of the environmental challenges that may be encountered and thus provide an ideal learning opportunity for athletes and support staff. You may wish to consider a medical fact sheet, which can be sent to those on your team who you are not able to attend.

The following are some of the issues that you might wish to cover:
● Your contact details (and those on the medical team).
● Jet lag and travel sickness.
● Environmental advice (dealing with heat, humidity, cold, altitude, insects).
● Hygiene (in particular the prevention of travel related illness).
● Fluid and nutrition.
● Immunization advice.
● Locality advice e.g. details of how to access local pharmacy, opticians, hospital services, dentist with relevant names and contact information.
● Emergency advice e.g. what to do if you are involved in a car crash.
● Medical insurance cover (what cover is provided as a member of a team and what additional cover will individuals have to arrange).
● General travel advice.

Immunization and vaccination

Exact immunization requirements depend on your destination and you must ensure that you are aware of the latest advice. The 'Yellow book' available in paper and online from the department of health is a useful resource.

Assuming that the normal vaccination program against TB, measles, mumps, rubella, pertussis, Hib, meningococcus, and polio has been completed, you may up date immunization against hepatitis A and tetanus. Vaccination should take place as early as possible to allow sufficient time to get over any reaction.

Tetanus

The initial vaccination is a 3 injection course (usually given as a baby). Two booster injections are then required to a total of 5 injections (5th injection is likely to be by the age of 18). While further injections are only required at the time of injury, for those who have *not had a booster within 10 years* a booster is recommended before foreign travel.

Hepatitis A

It is strongly recommended that athletes are vaccinated against Hepatitis A. This is a very debilitating illness, which can easily be passed through food, drinks, and via hand to mouth. A single injection will provide protection for 12 months, however, I would advocate a course of 2 injections over the 6 months prior to travel, which will provide protection for 10 years.

The journey

Your role as a team doctor goes far beyond normal medical practice, you are very much a member of a team, and may be able to help with other tasks including travel logistics e.g. helping with luggage and assisting with check in .

Ensure that you have a small medical bag in your hand luggage. It may be useful to include the following:
- Letter of authority confirming your medical role and requirement to carry medical equipment (and a list of that equipment).
- Paracetamol.
- Ibuprofen.
- Prochlorperazine (buccal).
- Loperamide.
- Antihistamine.
- Merocaine throat lozenges.
- Imigran (50mg tablets).
- Epinephrine (Epipen®).
- Laerdal pocket mask.
- Stethoscope.
- Salbutamol inhaler.
- Aspirin.
- Any specific medications depending on the regular prescriptions of team members.

Jet lag

Most of us have experienced jet lag, an almost indescribable feeling of utter uselessness. It is characterized by:
- Altered sleep pattern with daytime sleepiness and nighttime insomnia.
- Poor concentration.
- Fatigue and malaise.
- Gastrointestinal disturbance.

In addition to these generic symptoms it will impair athletic performance for several days.

Jet lag is thought to be caused by disrupted circadian rhythms in those flying across 3 or more time zones (a time zone is defined by a one hour time change for every 15 degrees traveled in either direction from the Greenwich meridian. There are of course 24). Although jet lag cannot be prevented it can be modified and its impact reduced by taking fairly simple measures:
- Ensure adequate rest and sleep prior to departure. You may want to start adjusting your time zone prior to departure e.g. going to bed and getting up an hour earlier or later.
- Aim to arrive late afternoon.
- Maintain good hydration.
- Synchronize your watch to the destination time zone upon departure.
- Ensure adequate relaxation during the flight. Try to eat and sleep in concordance with your new time zone.
- Upon arrival try to remain active during any remaining daylight hours and adjust meal and bedtimes to new time zone.
- Avoid stimulants (e.g. caffeine) at times when you should be resting.
- Try to adopt a flexible routine upon arrival, a rigid routine will prolong the effects of jet lag.
- Be prepared to allow one day of recovery for each time zone crossed (e.g. if traveling from London to Sydney you should expect to modify your normal training and expect altered performance for up to 10 days).

Melatonin is a hormone secreted in the evening by the pineal gland. It has been used in experiments to modify the symptoms of jet lag. Current evidence to support its use in reducing the symptoms of jet lag is inconclusive and there is a lack of data on its longterm safety.

Arrival—getting started

Upon arrival check that your team and their medical equipment have arrived complete and undamaged. Once appropriately refreshed and rested (if time permits) establish a well organized base from which to operate from, be if the hotel room, medical room, or medical suite. You should have considered the location of your medical room prior to arrival, however, be flexible if the situation requires it. Issues to consider when planning the location of your medical room are:

- Confidentiality and privacy.
- Accessibility.
- Security.
- Space:
  - An examination couch should be accessible from all sides.
  - In an ideal world you will need a desk, 2 chairs, storage space including secure storage and a fridge.
- Proximity to colleagues e.g. physiotherapy.
- Environment e.g. air conditioning, natural light.
- Power, communication, computer and IT connections.
- Mobile telephone with appropriate network coverage.
- Access to washing and toilet facilities.
- Drug testing facility.
- Isolation room.
- Your own privacy, ideally avoid your own room becoming the medical room although all too frequently this is what happens.
- In addition the medical team should have access to a designated car.

Managing your medical service

Organization is essential for a successful medical service. Despite best made plans, medical support in a competitive environment will constantly throw up new problems, require changes in plan, flexibility, and unreasonable deadlines which have to be met. If you are organized then managing change becomes more achievable.

Medical consultations

Athletes train and compete, eat and rest, at varying times, and your accessibility should reflect this. A flexible drop-in approach to appointments suits most athletes. This usually means being available from early morning to late evening. But you also need some rest to remain fresh and enthusiastic (and don't feel guilty about it). If single-handed make everyone aware of your availability for that day, structure any down time around the likely quiet periods e.g. athletes will frequently want to see you before and after training and competition, they are less likely to need your services during their rest time. You will of course need to provide 24 hour contact details in the case of an emergency.

You will almost certainly be required to provide cover at training and competition. This is challenging in a multi-games environment. If you are part of a team then arrange a rota.

In medical consultations remember:
- Your ethical code of practice (see GMC Good Medical Practice).
- An athlete's right to confidentiality.
- Do not practice beyond your scope of practice. If you have prepared properly you will have made arrangements to seek specialist advice when appropriate.
- The ability to ask for a second opinion. Even if you are a single-handed practitioner there is always someone somewhere available to ask advice.
- You must have professional indemnity and insurance to allow you to practice medicine in the country you are working in.
- Accurate medical record keeping is essential. The development of a web-based electronic record (injury zone (IZ) in the UK) has in my opinion made an important contribution to our ability to maintain an accurate medical record for UK athletes as patients who are constantly on the move. If it isn't documented it didn't happen.
- Most consultations reflect a primary care problem e.g. URTI, gastrointestinal upset, skin rashes.
- You must have contingency plans in the event of contagious illness.
- Any prescribing must be within the IOC, WADA, Games Organising Body or International Federation out/in competition doping regulations and you must be aware of which applies. If you prescribe or use a regulated substance then you must complete and submit the relevant aTUE or TUE and ensure copies are retained by yourself, the athlete, and scanned into any electronic record.
- Good team work and communication. You are part of a medical team and all members of that team, acknowledging any limitations imposed

by respecting an athlete's confidentiality, should be included in a multidisciplinary approach to management. You are also part of a wider athletic team and in many circumstances the coach and performance director should also be kept informed although this must be with the athlete's full consent.

Medical review

Pre-competition knowledge of the athletes under your care will vary. A medical review offers a valuable opportunity to introduce yourself and seek the following:

- Accurate demographic details including local mobile telephone number and next of kin.
- Current injury status.
- Current medical status.
- Documentation of previous relevant past injury and medical history.
- Current and complete list of all medications and supplements.
- Confirmation that abbreviated TUEs and TUEs have been completed and that you and the athlete have either a copy of the submitted forms, or confirmation from the relevant authority (UK Sport, International Federation, IOC) that the aTUE or TUE has been acknowledged.
- Allergy history.

Welcome meeting

The medical component of a generic welcome meeting or team gathering with your athletes and support staff should cover:

- Introduce yourself if not known to all.
- Your contact details including emergency telephone number.
- Arranging routine medical consultation.
- Arranging emergency medical consultation.
- What to do in the event of an emergency e.g. road accident.
- Drug testing procedure.
- Medical review.
- What if scenarios e.g. what to do if a team member develops a contagious illness.
- Advice on avoiding problems e.g. hydration, sun protection, insect problems, fluid and nutrition hygiene.
- Questions. Make it clear that you will try to accommodate your teams individual needs as far as is possible.

Drug testing

Your athletes will be required to have in or out of competition drug testing. Establish a procedure in the event of a request for a drugs test. As part of this you should identify:

- Appropriate drug testing room (within limits imposed by available facilities).
- Who should be informed upon arrival of drug testing officials.
- Your role? Will you always be available as an athlete representative? If not who will stand in should the athlete request a representative?
- What to do in the event of a positive test.

Before competition has started.
- Visit the competition or athlete village medical centre. Introduce yourself to reception staff and the lead physician if possible. Find out what facilities are on site and how to organize those tests that are not immediately available e.g. MRI.
- Where possible visit the venues you are likely to be using and assess their facilities.
- Establish where the nearest bank, telephone card sales, supermarket, opticians, dentist, pharmacist are located. You'll be amazed how much athletes rely on the doctor and physiotherapist for day to day information.

Medical management

Whether you are a single-handed medical officer or the CMO of a team of medics you will have management meetings to attend. These meetings are valuable opportunities for receiving or communicating information.
- Team leader meetings, meetings with leads within your squad or team e.g. chef de mission, camp director, individual team leaders (at a games there will be leads for a number of areas e.g. transport, nutrition, competition, media, security, etc), performance director, senior coaching staff, chief physiotherapist.
- Team meetings, meetings with all members of your team.
- Medical Meetings. As CMO you should arrange to meet with the rest of your medical team on a regular basis. This should include meetings with the chief physiotherapist and physiotherapy colleagues.
- Competition medical meetings. At major competitions there will usually be an opportunity for the games/competition medical committee to meet with medical representatives from competing teams/nations. This is a valuable opportunity to receive information on host medical protocols but more importantly to feed back on areas that require attention e.g. fluid and nutrition issues, drug testing procedure, access to investigations.

The return home

The evening after competition is usually celebrated by any closing ceremonies and time with your team. This is an important opportunity for everyone to unwind but may have medical implications.

The journey home

You are still responsible for the medical care of those in your team so ensure that you have access to appropriate equipment for all stages of the journey home.

Compile a short medical report even if you are not required to do so as part of your medical officer responsibilities. It may help improve future trips and prove useful for successors.

- Your arrival at home can be quite challenging for yourself and your partner and family. There is usually a feeling of deflation when your trip comes to an end.
- You will almost certainly be physically and more importantly mentally tired in addition to any jet lag.
- You may be making the rapid transition from an exciting period of work in a new environment back to 'the day job' with all the mundane roles and responsibilities that that involves (and all too often a backlog of work that has accumulated in your absence).
- Be appreciative and balance recounting exciting moments from your travels with showing an interest in what others have been up to.
- Allow yourself adequate time to recover from jet lag before returning to work.

Professional and ethical considerations

Medical work within sport is governed by exactly the same considerations and responsibilities that govern any other form of medical work. You have a duty of care to those that you are looking after and you must execute that duty of care within the framework of the GMC's Good Medical Practice. This encompasses all aspects of your work as a team doctor but has particular relevance to respecting patient confidentiality.

In addition to the medical work you carry out while away with a team, you have to comply with requirements for appraisal, revalidation, clinical governance, and your own continuing professional development.

Chief Medical Officer (CMO) role

If you are the CMO then you will have additional responsibilities as a medical team leader.

- It is your responsibility to ensure that all in your team are medically qualified and appropriately trained. If you were not involved with the interview process then ensure you have seen proof of GMC registration and relevant qualifications of anyone not known to you.
- Code of Conduct. Establish a code of conduct for all members of the medical team. There may well be a generic team code of conduct, which the medical team code of conduct has to incorporate. Issues to consider are:
  - Medical duties. Ensure that everyone has the same team philosophy.
  - Line management. As CMO you are responsible for all aspects of medical care and you need to ensure that your colleagues report any problems to you before they get out of hand. You will probably be responsible to a non-medical colleague e.g. chef de mission, camp director and you should equally keep them informed without breaching confidentiality.
  - On-call arrangements. You have a duty to provide 24-hour emergency medical cover or make clear what alternative arrangements are in place.
  - Rest and relaxation. You should ensure that all members of your team are taking adequate down time.
  - Alcohol consumption. Squads and teams may have their own generic views on alcohol consumption and you must abide by the team code of conduct if a dry philosophy is adopted.
  - Wearing of team kit.
- Medical representation at governing body, competition, games, and delegation management meetings.
- Clinical governance issues of your team.
- Mentoring and professional development. Be mindful that you may have considerably more experience than some of your colleagues and particularly if this is their first games be supportive to ensure that their experience is a positive one.

Patient confidentiality
- Athletes deserve the same right to confidentiality as any other patient.

Medical indemnity
- Ensure that your medical insurance and indemnity covers your scope.

Organizing a major sporting event

A major sporting event is a place of employment, of entertainment, and of competition and hence entails an unusually large and diverse number of potential areas of risk. It is vital to be able to deal with these crowds in a safe and efficient manner.

Accidents at sporting events have precipitated the development of guidelines to ensure crowd safety. The sources include the Safety of Sports Grounds Act, the Taylor report and the Green Guide. Guide to safety at sports grounds:

If a ground holds a safety certificate consultation through a local authority this will give information regarding:
The limit to number of spectators.
Duration of cover.
Details of exits, entrances, means of access, crush barriers, and means of escape in case of fire.

First aid minimum requirements

- No event should have fewer than 2 first aiders.
- If seated and standing spectators there should be 1 first aider per 1000.
- If all seated, 1 first aider per 1000 up to 20000, then 1 per 2000.
- If more anticipated then consult local ambulance service.
- First aider holds standard certificate of first aid issued by voluntary aid societies. Health and safety (first aid) regulations 1981.
- Should be 16 years or older with no other duties at ground.
- At ground prior to spectators and remain until all spectators have left the ground.
- Responsibility to provide room(s) for spectators in addition to other medical facilities.
- Should compliment the facilities provided by the ambulance services.
- Consultation with ambulance, local authority, the crowd doctor and appropriate voluntary aid services.
- Non-smoking area.
- Minimum size 15 sq m, increase to 25 sq m if >15000.
- To hold a couch, area for sitting casualties, extra couch if necessary.
- Sufficient room for equipment and materials.
- Blankets, pillows, stretchers, buckets, bowls, trolleys, and screens.
- Suitable disposal facilities for sharps and waste.
- Defibrillator if >5000 expected. Provided by other agency if required.
- Appropriate design for access and egress, fittings and facilities. Should have appropriate location.

Crowd doctor

If >2000 present there should be a crowd doctor trained in immediate care with appropriate qualifications , skills, experience, and support. Knowledge of cardiopulmonary resuscitation, airway maintenance, spinal fracture immobilization, and treatment of anaphylaxis. Training in advanced life support and paediatric life support. Governing body rules will give recommendation regarding level of qualification.

- The first duty of the 'crowd doctor' is to the spectators.
- Whereabouts known to first aid, ambulance, and control point personnel and be contactable.
- Equipment levels and clinical protocols used should conform to guidelines published by the relevant sporting body.
- In position before and remain until all spectators leave the ground.
- If <2000 spectators there should be arrangements to summon a suitably trained and experienced crowd doctor.
- Aware of the location and staffing arrangements of the first aid room and ambulance cover and emergency plans for major incidents.

Ambulance provision

- One fully equipped ambulance if >5000 spectators and sourced from approved group.
- Relationship of an ambulance, if not supplied by the NHS, to access NHS facilities should be known to management.
- Access for ambulance personnel to control point.
- Ambulance present before and after spectators access and egress ground.
- With 5000–25,000 spectators, there should be 1 accident and emergency ambulance with a paramedic crew. 1 ambulance officer, paramedic holds certificate of proficiency in ambulance paramedic skills issued by IHCD and has access to equipment including drugs.
- With 25,000–45,000 spectators, 1 accident and emergency ambulance with a paramedic crew, 1 ambulance officer, 1 major incident equipment vehicle and a paramedic crew, and 1 control unit.
- 45,000 or more 2 accident and emergency ambulances with paramedic crews otherwise as above.

Major incident plan

- Plans compatible with the local emergency services major incident plan.
- Identify areas for dealing with casualties in multiple situations, may include fire, accident, crowd disturbance, bomb scare, adverse and inclement weather.
- Identify access and egress routes and rendezvous point for vehicles.
- Agreed plan of action by all interested parties.
- Briefing of all first aid and medical staff on role in the major incident plan per event. Copy kept in the first aid room.
- Risk assessments should be performed .

International governing body check lists

- Includes review of all medical arrangements.
- Includes safety measures outside stadia.
- Will define high risk event.
- Assesses size of stadium and provision of safety and medical cover.
- Reviews risks of trouble including ticket forgery.
- Fire brigade, ambulance, and security measures.
- Practical issues regarding floodlights etc.
- General rules where appropriate regarding access of medical staff and stabilization of injuries on the field of play.

- Additional cover. Temporary insurance can often be arranged with a foreign defense organization, however, there will be an application process and in my experience it can be lengthy and very expensive.

Media issues

One of the biggest challenges of a major tournament is dealing with the media. Think very carefully before discussing any issues pertaining to the health of an athlete or group of athletes. Ideally your team will be supported by a media representative who will guide you. Leave it to the experts who will release well scribed press statements that have been cleared with all concerned, most importantly the athlete. Issues to consider are:

- Beware the quiet news day. Schedules still need filling.
- Requests for interviews are made to make news not to find out what life as a doctor is like. Ideally you should say nothing in saying something.
- Recorded interviews will be edited!
- Live interviews are less likely to be mis-represented at the time (they can be edited later for recorded news) but are extremely dangerous—interviewers are trained to produce a result.
- The media will work covertly and may pretend to be an interested fan.

Index